Contemporary Melanoma Management: A Surgical Perspective

Editor

ROHIT SHARMA

SURGICAL CLINICS
OF NORTH AMERICA

www.surgical.theclinics.com

Consulting Editor
RONALD F. MARTIN

February 2020 • Volume 100 • Number 1

ELSEVIER

1600 John F. Kennedy Boulevard • Suite 1800 • Philadelphia, Pennsylvania, 19103-2899

http://www.surgical.theclinics.com

SURGICAL CLINICS OF NORTH AMERICA Volume 100, Number 1
February 2020 ISSN 0039–6109, ISBN-13: 978-0-323-67894-0

Editor: John Vassallo, j.vassallo@elsevier.com
Developmental Editor: Casey Potter

Surgical Clinics of North America (ISSN 0039–6109) is published bimonthly by Elsevier Inc., 360 Park Avenue South, New York, NY 10010-1710. Months of publication are February, April, June, August, October, and December. Business and Editorial Offices: 1600 John F. Kennedy Blvd., Suite 1800, Philadelphia, PA 19103-2899. Periodicals postage paid at New York, NY and additional mailing offices. Subscription prices are $430.00 per year for US individuals, $891.00 per year for US institutions, $100.00 per year for US & Canadian students and residents, $507.00 per year for Canadian individuals, $1130.00 per year for Canadian institutions, $536.00 for international individuals, $1130.00 per year for international institutions and $250.00 per year for foreign students/residents. To receive student/resident rate, orders must be accompanied by name of affiliated institution, date of term, and the *signature* of program/residency coordinator on institution letterhead. Orders will be billed at individual rate until proof of status is received. Foreign air speed delivery is included in all *Clinics* subscription prices. All prices are subject to change without notice. POSTMASTER: Send address changes to *Surgical Clinics*, Elsevier Health Sciences Division, Subscription Customer Service, 3251 Riverport Lane, Maryland Heights, MO 63043. **Customer Service (orders, claims, online, change of address): Telephone: 1-800-654-2452 (U.S. and Canada); 314-447-8871 (outside U.S. and Canada). Fax: 314-447-8029. E-mail: journalscustomerservice-usa@elsevier.com (for print support); journalsonlinesupport-usa@elsevier.com (for online support).**

Reprints. For copies of 100 or more, of articles in this publication, please contact the Commercial Reprints Department, Elsevier Inc., 360 Park Avenue South, New York, New York 10010-1710. Tel. 212-633-3874, Fax: 212-633-3820, E-mail: reprints@elsevier.com.

The Surgical Clinics of North America is also published in Spanish by McGraw-Hill Interamericana Editores S.A., P.O. Box 5-237 06500 Mexico D.F. Mexico; and in Portuguese by Interlivros Edicoes Ltda., Rua Comandante Coelho 1085, CEP 21250, Rio de Janeiro, Brazil; and in Greek by Paschalidis Medical Publications, Athens Greece.

The Surgical Clinics of North America is covered in *MEDLINE/PubMed (Index Medicus), EMBASE/Excerpta Medica, Current Contents/Clinical Medicine, Current Contents/Life Sciences, Science Citation Index*, and *ISI/BIOMED*.

Contributors

CONSULTING EDITOR

RONALD F. MARTIN, MD, FACS
Colonel (retired), United States Army Reserve, Department of Surgery, York Hospital, York, Maine, USA

EDITOR

ROHIT SHARMA, MD, FACS, FRCS(GLAS)
Director Surgical Resident Research, Department of Surgery, Marshfield Medical Center, Marshfield, Wisconsin, USA

AUTHORS

JAMES F. ABDO, MD
Department of Surgery, Marshfield Medical Center, Marshfield, Wisconsin, USA

SHYAM S. ALLAMANENI, MD
Surgical Oncologist, Associate Program Director, The Jewish Hospital–Mercy Health, Mercy Health–Kenwood Surgical Oncology, Cincinnati, Ohio, USA

ALEXANDRA ALLARD-COUTU, BSc, MDCM
Department of Surgery, McMaster University, Hamilton General Hospital, Hamilton, Ontario, Canada

MICHAEL J. CARR, MD
Department of Cutaneous Oncology, Moffitt Cancer Center, Tampa, Florida, USA

STEPHANIE CARR, DO
General Surgery, Marshfield Medical Center, Marshfield, Wisconsin, USA

ASMITA CHOPRA, MBBS, MS (Surgery)
Research Scholar, Department of Surgery, Division of Surgical Oncology, University of Pittsburgh, Pittsburgh, Pennsylvania, USA

KEITH A. DELMAN, MD
Division of Surgical Oncology, Emory University School of Medicine, Atlanta, Georgia, USA

LAURA M. ENOMOTO, MSc, MD
Fellow in Surgical Oncology, Department of Surgery, Wake Forest Baptist Medical Center, Winston-Salem, North Carolina, USA

VALERIE FRANCESCUTTI, MD, MSc, FACS, FRCSC
Department of Surgery, McMaster University, Hamilton General Hospital, Hamilton, Ontario, Canada

ADRIANA C. GAMBOA, MD
Division of Surgical Oncology, Emory University School of Medicine, Atlanta, Georgia, USA

ROGEH HABASHI, MD
Department of Surgery, McMaster University, Hamilton General Hospital, Hamilton, Ontario, Canada

BARBARA HELLER, MD, FRCSC
Department of Surgery, McMaster University and St. Joseph's Healthcare, Hamilton, Ontario, Canada

DANIEL JOYCE, MD
Surgical Oncology Fellow, Roswell Park Comprehensive Cancer Center, Buffalo, New York, USA

NIKHIL I. KHUSHALANI, MD
Senior Member and Vice-Chair, Department of Cutaneous Oncology, Moffitt Cancer Center, Tampa, Florida, USA

EDWARD A. LEVINE, MD
Professor, Department of Surgery, Wake Forest Baptist Medical Center, Winston-Salem, North Carolina, USA

MICHAEL LOWE, MD, MA
Division of Surgical Oncology, Emory University School of Medicine, Atlanta, Georgia, USA

SURESH NAIR, MD
Department of Hematology/Oncology, Lehigh Valley Cancer Institute, Allentown, Pennsylvania, USA

ADEDAYO A. ONITILO, MD, PhD, MSCR, FACP
Department of Hematology/Oncology, Marshfield Clinic Weston Center, Weston, Wisconsin, USA

BHUPESH PARASHAR, MD
Professor and Vice-Chair (R) of Radiation Oncology, Co-Director, Head and Neck Cancer Service, Donald and Barbara Zucker School of Medicine at Hofstra/Northwell, Northwell Health, Center for Advanced Medicine (CFAM), Lake Success, New York, USA

DAVID T. POINTER Jr, MD
Complex General Surgical Oncology Fellow, Department of Cutaneous Oncology, Moffitt Cancer Center, Tampa, Florida, USA

SIMRAN POLCE, BS
Stony Brook Medical College, Stony Brook, New York, USA

KIRITHIGA RAMALINGAM, MD
Research Fellow and Surgical Resident, Surgical Oncology, University of New Mexico School of Medicine, UNM Comprehensive Cancer Center, Albuquerque, New Mexico, USA

UMA N.M. RAO, MD (Pathology)
Professor, Department of Pathology, University of Pittsburgh School of Medicine, Director, Section of Bone/Soft Tissue, Melanoma Pathology, UPMC Presbyterian Shadyside, Pittsburgh, Pennsylvania, USA

SARO SARKISIAN, MD, MHA
Department of Hematology/Oncology, Lehigh Valley Cancer Institute, Allentown, Pennsylvania, USA

AAYUSH SHARMA
Neuroscience Major, Ohio State University, Columbus, Ohio, USA

ROHIT SHARMA, MD, FACS, FRCS(GLAS)
Director Surgical Resident Research, Department of Surgery, Marshfield Medical Center, Marshfield, Wisconsin, USA

PERRY SHEN, MD
Professor, Department of Surgery, Wake Forest Baptist Medical Center, Winston-Salem, North Carolina, USA

JOSEPH J. SKITZKI, MD, FACS
Associate Professor of Surgical Oncology, Surgery, and Immunology, Roswell Park Comprehensive Cancer Center, Buffalo, New York, USA

CHRISTY SMITH, MD
General Surgery, Marshfield Medical Center, Marshfield, Wisconsin, USA

JAMES SUN, MD
Department of Cutaneous Oncology, Moffitt Cancer Center, Tampa, Florida, USA

KONSTANTINOS I. VOTANOPOULOS, MD, PhD
Associate Professor, Department of Surgery, Wake Forest Baptist Medical Center, Winston-Salem, North Carolina, USA

JESSICA WERNBERG, MD
General Surgery, Marshfield Medical Center, Marshfield, Wisconsin, USA

A. GABRIELLA WERNICKE, MD, MSc
Weill Cornell Medical College, New York, New York, USA

JAIMIE A. WITTIG, PharmD, BCOP
Pharmacy Services, Marshfield Medical Center, Marshfield, Wisconsin, USA

MELINDA L. YUSHAK, MD, MPH
Division of Medical Oncology, Emory University School of Medicine, Atlanta, Georgia, USA

JONATHAN S. ZAGER, MD
Associate Chief Academic Officer, Chair of Graduate Medical Education, Department of Cutaneous Oncology, Moffitt Cancer Center, Tampa, Florida, USA

Contents

The incidence of melanoma continues to increase worldwide. In the United States, melanoma is the fifth most common cancer in men and the sixth most common cancer in women. The risk factors contributing to melanoma have largely remained unchanged, but there is a new focus on modifiable risk factors including sun exposure and ultraviolet light. A large public initiative supported by the Centers for Disease Control focuses on educating the public on the risks of sun exposure and indoor tanning. Early detection and resection of melanoma lesions is necessary to prevent metastasis and reduce medical costs.

Melanoma is a deadly skin cancer linked to ultraviolet radiation exposure. Heritable traits and sporadic mutations modify an individual's risk for melanoma that may be associated with phenotype. Familial/heritable melanomas are broadly used to describe families with an increased incidence of melanomas, although the underlying mutation may be unknown. Mutations associated with melanoma occur in cell cycle regulation, tumor suppression, chromosomal stability, DNA repair, pigmentation, and melanocyte differentiation genes. Genetic testing of individuals with a family history of melanoma may provide additional etiologic information and ensure patients with known markers for cancer development are closely monitored by physicians.

The melanoma expert panel devised the evidence-based eighth edition American Joint Committee on Cancer staging system by conducting vigorous analyses of stage I, II, and III patients from the International Melanoma Database and Discovery Platform. Key changes in the eighth edition are regarding subcategorization of T1, M1, pathologic stage grouping of stage I and III, and refining the definitions and terminologies used in the staging system. As the knowledge of tumor biology improves, the staging of melanoma will continue to evolve to enable betterment of care.

Melanoma is an aggressive malignancy arising from melanocytes in the skin and rarely in extracutaneous sites. The understanding of pathology of melanoma has evolved over the years, with the initial classifications based on the clinical and microscopic features to the current use of immunohistochemistry and genetic sequencing. The depth of invasion and lymph node metastasis are still the most important prognostic features of melanoma. Other important prognostic features include ulceration, lymphovascular invasion, mitosis, and tumor-infiltrating lymphocytes. This article reviews the pathology of melanoma and its precursor lesions, along with the recent advances in pathologic diagnosis of melanoma.

Primary cutaneous melanomas are potentially curative with surgical excision alone. Surgical management is based on several factors determined from the initial biopsy, including primary tumor thickness, histologic features including ulceration, and anatomic location. Cosmesis, although important, should be a secondary consideration as oncologic principles take precedence. Pathology has evolved to synoptic reporting with key variables to assist in staging and risk stratification.

This article provides a comprehensive evaluation of surgical management of the lymph node basin in melanoma, with historical, anatomic, and evidence-based recommendations for practice.

In this article we provide a critical review of the evidence available for surgical management of the nodal basin in melanoma, with an aim to ensure an understanding of risks and benefits for all lymph node surgery offered to patients, and alternatives to surgical management where appropriate.

Melanoma has a unique propensity for locoregional metastasis secondary to intralymphatic transit not seen in other cutaneous or soft tissue malignancies. Novel intralesional therapies using oncolytic immunotherapy exhibit increasing response rates with observed bystander effect. Intralesional modalities in combination with systemic immunotherapy are the subject of ongoing clinical trials. Regional therapy is used in isolated limb locoregional metastasis whereby chemotherapy is delivered to an isolated limb avoiding systemic side effects. Multimodal treatment strategy is imperative in the treatment of locoregionally advanced melanoma. One must be versed on these quickly evolving therapeutic options.

are a devastating complication of melanoma that can be traced to derangements in cell signaling pathways, and the current evidence for targeted therapy is reviewed. Finally, activating KIT mutations are rarely found to cause melanomas and may provide an actionable target for therapy. The authors review the current evidence for targeted KIT therapy and summarize the ongoing clinical trials.

The role of radiation therapy in melanoma has evolved over the last few decades. There has been a dramatic improvement in radiation delivery with the introduction of intensity-modulated radiation therapy, image-guided radiation therapy, stereotactic radiosurgery, and stereotactic body radiation therapy/stereotactic radiation therapy. More recently, with the introduction of immunotherapy in various malignancies, including melanoma, the role of radiation therapy is being reevaluated. This article describes the evolution of the role of radiation therapy from nonimmunotherapy to the era of immunotherapy.

The treatment of metastatic melanomas revolutionized during the past decade because of a better understanding of various pathways and mutations that play different roles in the pathogenesis of this disease. The incorporation of immunotherapy was the first in these efforts, followed by targeted therapies as monotherapeutic options, and then in combinations. In this article, we review the historical and landmark clinical trials that changed our treatment paradigm for advanced melanomas, also we review ongoing clinical trials that would be applicable in the near future and would expectedly improve outcomes for these patients.

SURGICAL CLINICS
OF NORTH AMERICA

SERIES OF RELATED INTEREST

Advances in Surgery
https://www.advancessurgery.com/
Surgical Oncology Clinics
https://www.surgonc.theclinics.com/
Thoracic Surgery Clinics
http://www.thoracic.theclinics.com/

THE CLINICS ARE AVAILABLE ONLINE!
Access your subscription at:
www.theclinics.com

Foreword
Melanoma

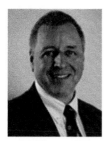

Ronald F. Martin, MD, FACS
Consulting Editor

In some respects, the goal of surgery as a discipline is in some measure to put itself out of business. I doubt that will ever happen; first, as surgeons, we are not that good at getting tasks of that magnitude done, and second, as people, we will always find a way for developing problems that surgeons will need to respond to. Still, we are in a business where the concept of preventing people from requiring some of our services is built into the profession. Despite that, we currently have a health care system that focuses more broadly on being sick as opposed to staying well. Please note, this is written with a deepest appreciation for what has been done in our field with regard to preventive care, screening, and other aspects of promoting wellness. Much has been done, and much more will need to be done.

Skin cancer and melanoma, in particular, are great examples of the need for balance of prevention and treatment. We know with a high degree of confidence the role of UV light in the cause of melanoma. We know a great deal about how to minimize our exposure to UV light by means of environmental control, protective clothing, applied sunscreens (though there may be some environmental issues caused by these), yet we will not likely reduce our photon exposure to zero. On the treatment side, we have made substantial advances in treating local disease as well as advanced disease, but still, advanced stages of melanoma carry poor prognostic outcomes.

As with many malignancies, perhaps our best outcomes have been in the area of treating early stage disease. Also, as with many other malignancies, this requires comprehensive and good-quality screening processes. Any effective screening tool needs to have a high degree of sensitivity (preferably accompanied by high specificity as well), to be utilized in an "at-risk" population, to identify a disorder that can actually be treated, and to be cost-effective. One might add that effective screening requires the people at risk to participate in the process. We have good screening tools today, and with developments in image storage and analysis capabilities, they may improve substantially.

Surg Clin N Am 100 (2020) xiii–xiv
https://doi.org/10.1016/j.suc.2019.10.002
0039-6109/20/© 2019 Published by Elsevier Inc.

Dr Sharma and his colleagues have compiled an excellent collection of articles that educate us all about melanoma from the inheritable characteristics that increase our susceptibility to the advances in immunotherapy for advanced disease. They should help us all build a solid foundation from which to deliver our own segment of care as well as speak clearly about the broader aspects of care that we may not deliver directly. We are indebted to them for their efforts on this issue.

As with so many other topics we have covered in this series, the topic of melanoma forces us to look beyond our own field of expertise and more broadly focus on how we interact with our colleagues and society in general. Melanoma is a disease of which we have a good understanding. If we can collectively put the pieces together well, we should not only improve our treatment of patients with the disease but also reduce the incidence and burden of the disease for our communities as well. As to putting ourselves out of business, I would not fear that at this time or anytime soon. Based on the current accumulated UV exposure of the world population, we likely will still have much work to do for some time to come.

Ronald F. Martin, MD, FACS
Colonel (retired), United States Army Reserve
Department of Surgery
York Hospital
16 Hospital Drive, Suite A
York, ME 03909, USA

E-mail address:
rfmcescna@gmail.com

Preface

From Melanosis to Mutations: The Present and Future of Melanoma Management

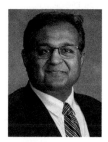

Rohit Sharma, MD, FACS, FRCS (Glas)
Editor

From the first description of an entity akin to our present understanding of Melanoma by Hippocrates of Cos in the fifth century BCE, to the coinage of the term (*melas* "dark," *oma* "tumor") by Carswell in the nineteenth century, not much changed in the understanding or the management of this disease. The next century saw the application of increasingly radical surgery in an attempt to extirpate the disease without appreciable success in the outcomes for advanced disease. From essentially useless chemotherapy in 1950 to 1980 with dacarbazine, it was not until the 1990s that first glimmer of hope was observed by the introduction of Interleukin-2 (IL-2). In 2011, an era of increasingly rapid breakthroughs in the management of advanced disease dawned with the approval of anti cytotoxic T-lymphocyte-associated protein 4 Ipilimumab and BRAF inhibitor Vemurafenib. Since the publication of the issue of *Surgical Clinics of North America* on Melanoma in 2014, the landscape for management of melanoma, in general, and advanced disease, in particular, has progressed rapidly and appreciably. PD1 inhibitors have become the preferred therapy in both the high-risk adjuvant and the metastatic setting. The variety of options available for locoregionally advanced and metastatic melanoma has expanded the therapeutic armamentarium of the physicians at the forefront of the battle. In this issue of *Surgical Clinics of North America*, world-renowned experts share their knowledge and experience.

Melanoma has one of the fastest rising frequency among all cancers in North America. The current understanding of the risk factors and epidemiology of melanoma is discussed by Dr Wernberg and colleagues.

The knowledge of the genetic basis of melanoma has improved significantly even since the last issue in 2014. Dr Abdo explores the increased understanding of role of hereditary and association with other potentially fatal visceral malignancies.

Surg Clin N Am 100 (2020) xv–xvi
https://doi.org/10.1016/j.suc.2019.10.001
0039-6109/20/© 2019 Published by Elsevier Inc.

The staging of melanoma has evolved after the publication of the American Joint Committee on Cancer, 8th manual. Dr Allamaneni discusses this change along with the potential for therapeutic implications.

Dr Chopra describes the current understanding of the histologic and molecular pathology of melanoma.

Despite the advances in the management of advanced disease, most melanomas are still cured by surgery. Dr Skitzki explains the role of surgery in the treatment of primary melanoma.

The management of lymph nodal basin at risk has changed after the publication of MSLT II and the DeCoG SLT trials. Dr Francescutti discusses the surgical and nonsurgical options for management of nodal stations.

Dr Zager describes options for locoregionally advanced melanoma, including role of oncolytic viral therapy.

Surgery still has a role in appropriately selected patients with metastatic melanoma, as described by Dr Votanopoulos.

Dr Delman discusses the implications of systemic therapy for melanoma in the surgical management.

Dr Onitilo and Khushlani introduce the principles of immunotherapy and targeted therapy for the practicing surgeons.

The role of radiation therapy in melanoma in the era of effective systemic therapy is evolving, as discussed by Dr Prashar.

Finally, Dr Sarkisian describes the ongoing clinical trials of advanced melanoma.

In the era of rapidly changing landscape of melanoma management, a multidisciplinary approach has become an essential component to optimize the care of our patients. I am thankful to all the colleagues who have taken time out of their incredibly busy schedules to provide insights about melanoma treatment and to contribute to this issue. It is my hope that the medical student and surgical community will find this issue useful for making patient care decisions. I am grateful to Dr Martin for giving me the opportunity to put this issue together, and to editorial staff at Elsevier for their assistance.

Rohit Sharma, MD, FACS, FRCS (Glas)
Department of Surgery
Marshfield Medical Center
1000 North Oak Avenue
Marshfield, WI 54449, USA

E-mail address:
sharma.rohit@marshfieldclinic.org

Epidemiology and Risk Factors of Melanoma

Stephanie Carr, DO, Christy Smith, MD, Jessica Wernberg, MD*

KEYWORDS

- Melanoma • Carcinogen • Ultraviolet radiation • Indoor tanning • Prevention

KEY POINTS

- The worldwide incidence of melanoma continues to increase.
- Ultraviolet light, especially indoor tanning, is a known carcinogen and exposure is clearly correlated with an increased incidence of melanoma.
- The average cost of diagnosis and treatment of melanoma is 10 times greater than a non-melanotic skin cancer.
- Clinicians should educate patients about risk factors for melanoma as well as the ABCDEs of melanoma to facilitate early detection and diagnosis.
- Multiple public initiatives are now underway to reduce the prevalence of indoor tanning, with 17 states now banning indoor tanning for minors.

INTRODUCTION

Melanoma is a potentially fatal skin malignancy that continues to increase in incidence worldwide . The current lifetime risk of developing melanoma is 1 in 63 in the United States, and similar ratios are noted in other Western nations.[1] Although melanoma is less common than other skin cancers, it is more lethal, accounting for nearly 73% of skin cancer–related deaths.[2] Melanoma is treatable with surgery at the localized stage and has a high 5-year relative survival rate of 98%. However, this percentage drops substantially when patients are diagnosed with advanced or metastatic melanoma (64% for regional to 23% for distant melanoma lesions) where treatment options are limited.[3]

Because of the high metastatic potential of melanoma, research is ongoing to identify the risk factors associated with melanoma and develop improved methods to diagnose and treat this aggressive skin cancer. Lifestyle and genetic risk factors are the major contributing factors to melanoma development (**Box 1**).[1] The following chapter discusses these risk factors in detail and focus on the growing health crisis involving indoor tanning.

General Surgery, Marshfield Medical Center, 1000 North Oak Avenue, Marshfield, WI 54449, USA
* Corresponding author.
E-mail address: wernberg.jessica@marshfieldclinic.org

Surg Clin N Am 100 (2020) 1–12
https://doi.org/10.1016/j.suc.2019.09.005
0039-6109/20/© 2019 Elsevier Inc. All rights reserved.

> **Box 1**
> **Risk factors of melanoma**
>
> *Modifiable Risk Factors*
>
> - Indoor tanning
> - Ultraviolet exposure
> - Medications
>
> *Nonmodifiable Risk Factors*
>
> - Genetics
> - Family history
> - Socioeconomic status
> - Nevi
> - Race
> - Age
> - Gender

EPIDEMIOLOGY
Types of Melanoma

Melanoma is a cancer that originates in the melanocytes and is broadly classified by site of presentation specifically cutaneous or noncutaneous. There are 4 major subtypes of cutaneous melanoma[4]:

- Superficial spreading melanoma (70%): the most common type of melanoma. It undergoes lateral (radial) growth before vertical (invasive) growth occurs.
- Nodular melanomas (15%–30%): rapidly enlarging elevated or polypoid lesions that are often blue or black and exhibit an early vertical growth phase.
- Lentigo maligna melanoma (4%–10%): occurs more commonly in older patients with chronically sun-exposed skin. It typically begins as a small freckle-like macule. Over time it grows, becomes darker, asymmetric, and exhibits a vertical growth phase.
- Acral lentiginous (<5%): lesions arise most commonly on palms, soles, subungual, and occasionally, mucosal surfaces.

Melanoma may also develop at any noncutaneous site where melanocytes normally occur, including ocular, gastrointestinal, genitourinary, and nasopharyngeal locations. These are much less common than cutaneous melanoma according to a review in the National Cancer Data Base, which contains records of 84,836 patients with cutaneous and noncutaneous melanoma. Cutaneous melanomas comprised 91.2% of all diagnosed melanoma. Occular melanoma represents 5.2%, with 1.3% of melanoma of mucosal primary origin, and the remaining 2.2% of cases were classified as melanoma of unknown primary site.[5] The prognosis of melanoma is based on lesion thickness with thicker lesions corresponding to a higher rate of mortality.[6] Therefore, early detection and resection of melanoma lesions is necessary to prevent metastasis.

Global Distribution

The overall incidence of melanoma has been increasing worldwide, particularly in the United States, European countries, and other countries with a predominantly Caucasian population (**Figs. 1** and **2**). Queensland, Australia, has the highest incidence of

Estimated age-standardized incidence rates (World) in 2018, melanoma of skin, both sexes, all ages

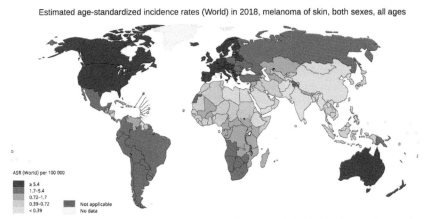

Fig. 1. Age-standardized rate of melanoma incidence worldwide for 2018. (Reproduced with permission from Ferlay J, Ervik M, Lam F, Colombet M, Mery L, Piñeros M, Znaor A, Soerjomataram I, Bray F (2018). Global Cancer Observatory: Cancer Today. Lyon, France: International Agency for Research on Cancer. Available from: https://gco.iarc.fr/today, accessed 9/13/2019; Data source: GLOBOCAN 2018. Graph production: IARC (http://gco.iarc.fr/today). World Health Organization.)

malignant melanoma in the world where melanoma is the leading malignancy and cause of cancer-related death in Australians aged 15 to 44 years.[1,7] Melanoma is the sixth most common cancer in women and the fifth most common in men in the United States.[2] Although populations with darker pigmented skin are still considered to be low risk for developing melanoma, they are not exempt from the disease and tend to develop more noncutaneous melanomas than fair-skinned individuals.[1] The

Estimated age-standardized mortality rates (World) in 2018, melanoma of skin, both sexes, all ages

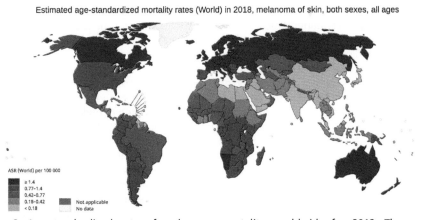

Fig. 2. Age-standardized rate of melanoma mortality worldwide for 2018. The age-standardized rate adjusts the age structure of populations to allow for comparisons that accounts for the different age structure of the populations. (Reproduced with permission from Ferlay J, Ervik M, Lam F, Colombet M, Mery L, Piñeros M, Znaor A, Soerjomataram I, Bray F (2018). Global Cancer Observatory: Cancer Today. Lyon, France: International Agency for Research on Cancer. Available from: https://gco.iarc.fr/today, accessed 9/13/2019; and Data source: GLOBOCAN 2018. Graph production: IARC (http://gco.iarc.fr/today). World Health Organization.)

incidence of melanoma has increased by 270% over the past 30 years in the United States, attributed to a variety of factors including increased exposure to ultraviolet (UV) radiation and increased surveillance.[1] Sun exposure patterns and exposure to artificial UV light can influence melanoma development.[1] A nested case-control analysis of 130 cases and 300 controls from the Nurses' Health Study cohort by Oliveria and colleagues[8] observed an increased risk of melanoma in women whose residence during the ages of 15 to 20 years was closer to the equator compared with the women living at higher latitudes during the same time periods. This risk did not continue past the age of 30 years.

Race

The incidence of melanoma varies based on race, with a lifetime risk of 2.6% for Caucasians, 0.1% for African Americans, and 0.58% for Hispanics.[9] Caucasians are at a 10-fold increased risk of developing cutaneous melanoma compared with those with dark skin pigmentation.[1] However, noncutaneous melanomas are more common in the non-Caucasian population.[1] In the United States, non-Caucasian patients have a worse outcome overall and present with a more advanced stage of melanoma compared with Caucasian patients.[10]

Age and Gender

Melanoma tends to be diagnosed in young to middle-aged adults with an average age at diagnosis of 57 years.[1] Between 25 to 50 years of age, the incidence of melanoma increases linearly; however, incidence of melanoma differs by gender as well as age. From age 25 to 40 years, women are more likely to develop melanoma than men, but after 75 years, men are 3 times more likely to develop melanoma compared with women.[1] Overall, men are 1.5 times more likely to develop melanoma.[11]

RISK FACTORS
Location

Melanoma is notorious for a wide variety of presentations depending on body site. Any melanoma at a noncutaneous location or in a location that is difficult to visualize is more likely to be diagnosed at a more advanced stage than cutaneous lesions.[1] Superficial spreading and nodular cutaneous melanomas tend to have a more classic presentation including irregular borders, asymmetry, and enlarged diameter. Lentigo maligna melanomas are more common on the face while acral lentiginous melanomas are most commonly found at the palms of the hands, soles of the feet, and nail beds.

Some patterns of melanoma distribution are related to sun exposure patterns, history of sunburns, and gender. For this reason, men are more likely to develop lesions on the back, whereas women are more likely to develop melanoma on the arms and legs.[1] Melanomas on the trunk have been associated with a history of severe sunburn, and patients with a family history of melanoma were more likely to develop lesions on the limbs, 57% versus 42%, compared with those with no family history.[7,12] Watts and colleagues[7] found that patients who self-report having "many nevi" developed truncal melanoma 41% of the time versus patients with "few" nevi who developed truncal melanoma 29% of the time.

Ultraviolet Radiation

UV radiation exposure is a clear risk factor for the development of melanoma. In 1992, solar UV radiation was classified as a carcinogen by the International Agency of Research on Cancer and in 2009 was updated to include UV radiation from indoor tanning.[13,14] In 2012, UV radiation from arc welding was also classified as carcinogenic to humans, and in 2017, this was updated to include welding fumes.[13,15] UV exposure occurs during sun exposure, indoor tanning, and welding. Sun exposure has long been associated with increased development of skin cancer. Multiple studies have demonstrated that increased exposure to ultraviolet light and many years of occupational sun exposure (>20 years) lead to increased development of melanoma.[16] Chronic sustained sun exposure is also linked to squamous and basal cell carcinomas,[17,18] whereas intermittent sun exposure and sunburns are more closely associated with melanoma.[12] A definitive link between welding and skin cancer development has not been shown; however, the full spectrum of UV radiation exposure in welding has been linked to ocular melanoma.[13,15,19,20] A French population–based case-control study showed elevated risk of ocular melanoma among welders compared with the general population (odds ratio 7.3).[19] Therefore, protection from UV radiation is paramount for preventing melanoma and nonmelanoma skin cancers.

Indoor tanning is a leisure activity with high UV exposure that is particularly popular with teenagers and young adults in affluent European and North American countries. In a 2014 survey of university students, 55% of students had tanned at least once and 43% reported having tanned in the year before the study survey.[21] Indoor tanning is a risk factor of melanoma development, and any previous indoor tanning experience is associated with a 16% to 20% increased risk of melanoma development compared with those never exposed to indoor tanning.[22]

More than 6,000 melanomas each year are thought to be caused by indoor tanning in the United States and an increased duration and earlier age at initiation of indoor tanning is associated with an even higher risk of melanoma development compared with individuals who do not engage in indoor tanning.[21,22] In women with a history of indoor tanning, melanomas were most likely to develop on the trunk, but men with the same history were more likely to develop head or neck melanomas.[23]

Exposure to UV radiation can also occur during medical treatment. Psoralen and ultraviolet A (PUVA) is used for treatment of psoriasis, eczema, and vitiligo and is associated with development of melanoma and nonmelanoma skin cancers. Patel and colleagues[24] noted that the risk of squamous cell carcinoma is increased by 100-fold in patients undergoing greater than 330 treatments, and the risk of developing malignant melanomas post-PUVA is even greater, as patients were at increased risk after 250 treatments.

Genetics

Certain skin, hair, and eye color phenotypes are associated with increased sun sensitivity and risk of skin cancer development. Freckles, light-colored eyes, red hair, fair skin, and inability to tan increase an individual's risk for melanoma by nearly 50%.[1] The red hair/fair skin phenotypes are associated with variants in melanocortin-1 receptor (MC1R), which regulates the production of pheomelanin and eumelanin.[25] Individuals with light-colored skin are more likely to develop amelanotic lesions, which often go unnoticed until the lesion becomes more advanced.[1]

In other cases, the genetic component of increased skin cancer risk is less obvious although family history of melanoma and genetic variants that alter the efficacy of UV-induced DNA repair mechanisms, cell damage–induced signaling pathways, and so forth are known to influence melanoma development. In a combined analysis from 8 case-control studies in Caucasian populations, individuals with a positive family history of melanoma have a relative risk of 2.24 for melanoma compared with individuals without a positive family history.[26] This risk was independent of age, nevus count, hair and eye color, and freckling.

The most common germline mutation identified in familial forms of melanoma is *CDKN2A*. Mutations in *CDKN2A* result in changes that alter the function of p16, which is a negative regulator of cell cycle progression.[27] A germline mutation in *CDK4* has also been identified in familial melanoma and has a similar phenotype to the *CDKN2A* mutation.[28]

Other genetic mutation syndromes that increase cancer risk overall also confer increased risk of melanoma although melanoma is not the primary tumor type. For example, whereas *BRCA1* and *BRCA2* genes are associated with increased risk of breast, ovarian, and prostate cancers, there is also an increased risk of melanoma.[29] Variants in other tumor suppressor genes such as *p53* and *RB1* are also associated with increased risk for melanoma.[30,31]

Xeroderma pigmentosum (XP) is a rare autosomal recessive disorder of DNA repair characterized by increased sensitivity to ultraviolet radiation. In a 40-year National Institutes of Health follow-up study of 106 XP patients, the risks of nonmelanoma skin cancer and melanoma were found to be 10,000-fold and 2000-fold higher, respectively, in these patients compared to the general population.[32]

Nevi

Dysplastic nevi are a relatively common occurrence in populations of Northern European descent with a frequency of about 10%.[33] The presence of dysplastic nevi is associated with a 1.5- to 10-fold increased risk of melanoma and depends on the number of dysplastic nevi present.[34] The risk for melanoma development is approximately 1.5 times higher in people with 11 to 25 nevi and seems to be doubled with every increase of 25 nevi.[11]

Personal History of Cancer

A personal history of melanoma is associated with an increased risk for a second melanoma and is greatest within the first year of index diagnosis.[35] There is also an increased risk of a second primary malignancy. Spanogle and colleagues[35] used the SEER database to analyze disease outcomes in 16,591 cutaneous melanoma survivors and found a 32% higher risk of developing any second primary malignancy, with the standardized incidence ratio being greatest for development of a second melanoma.

Smoking

A validated association between smoking and melanoma has not been established although numerous studies have reported an inverse relationship between smoking and cutaneous melanoma.[36–39] However, a direct positive correlation between current smoking and sentinel lymph node metastasis, ulceration, and increased Breslow thickness in smokers who developed melanoma was noted by Jones and colleagues.[36]

Socioeconomic Status

Lower socioeconomic status correlates with more advanced disease at diagnosis and overall worse outcomes.[40] A National Cancer Database study found that patients without insurance had a 67% greater risk of death from melanoma than those with private insurance, and Medicare and Medicaid patients had worse outcomes than those with private insurance. Furthermore, patients living in an area with a lower average income and those without a high school diploma were more likely to die of melanoma.[40] A similar study performed in California highlighted that men with a lower socioeconomic status tended to be diagnosed with more advanced melanoma including ulcerated primaries and metastases.[41]

Immunosuppression/Transplant

Patients with weakened immune systems are at increased risk for developing skin cancers. Solid organ transplant patients requiring immunosuppression have a well-known increased risk for developing skin cancers, particularly squamous cell carcinoma.[42] Patients with a history of solid organ transplant are documented to have a 2- to 4-fold increase in developing melanoma compared with the nontransplant population. Certain immunosuppressants, including cyclosporine and sirolimus, have been associated with an increased incidence of melanoma.[42,43] Individuals with human immunodeficiency virus infection are also known to have an increased risk of squamous cell carcinoma and basal cell carcinoma although multiple studies have not demonstrated an increased risk with malignant melanoma in this population.[44,45]

Similar to the general population, the incidence of melanoma is increasing in transplant recipients. Two groups of solid organ transplant patients from the years 1991 to 2000 and 2001 to 2015 were studied. The latter group had a 4 times greater risk of developing melanoma.[46] All transplant and immunosuppressed patients should undergo yearly skin examinations to ensure early identification of skin cancer.

PUBLIC AWARENESS
Early Detection

Early detection is essential to decrease mortality. Incidence of melanoma detection has increased over time due in part to increased awareness and surveillance for abnormal skin lesions. However, increased surveillance is unlikely to be the only factor for increased melanoma rate as evidenced by increased incidence in both thin and thick lesions and increase in sun bathing and sun seeking behavior over time.[2,47] Increased public awareness of self-skin assessments and recognition of the Asymmetry, irregular Borders, variation of Color, Diameter >6 mm, and Evolution (ABCDEs) of melanoma have increased the sensitivity of self-examinations to nearly 90%.[1] The ABCDE criteria for melanoma were created in 1985 to increase public awareness of the importance of early detection of skin cancer (**Fig. 3**). Any skin lesion that has one or more of these characteristics should be evaluated by a dermatologist.

Economic Impact

The medical costs associated with a diagnosis of melanoma are substantial compared with other skin cancers. The average cost per melanoma diagnosed in the United States is $32,594, whereas the average cost per nonmelanoma skin cancer is $2496. This difference is easily attributable to the more substantial cost for surgical resection and staging, imaging, and immunotherapies in advanced melanoma.[48]

Total-body skin examination (TBSE) is used to identify and diagnose melanoma at an early stage, although there are no definitive recommendations on the timing or even effectiveness of TBSE. In 2017, Matsumoto and colleagues[48] analyzed 33,647 TBSEs over a 5-year period and found a 30% biopsy rate but only a 0.46% rate of melanoma diagnosis.

Since there is a strong association between indoor tanning and melanoma development, limiting indoor tanning in minors may reduce the incidence of melanoma in teenagers and young adults. Using a cohort of 61 million individuals aged 14 years or younger, Guy and colleagues[49] estimated that 61,839 cases of melanoma and 6753 deaths attributed to melanoma could be avoided if minors were banned from indoor

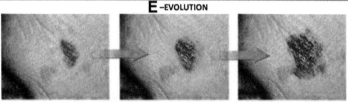

A-ASYMMETRY   **B**-BORDER   **C**-COLOR   **D**-DIAMETER

If a line is drawn down the middle of the lesion and the two sides are not identical (asymmetrical) this could be a warning sign for melanoma.

The borders of a melanoma tend to be uneven. Edges that are irregular, blurred, or notched are suspicious for melanoma.

A benign mole is a single color. Multiple colors within a skin lesion could indicate a melanoma.

Melanomas larger in diameter than 6mm can be suggestive of a melanoma.

E-EVOLUTION

A mole or skin lesion that has changed in size, shape or color is concerning for melanoma.

Fig. 3. ABCDEs of melanoma. These characteristics may be used by health care providers and patients to identify skin lesions of concerns that may necessitate a biopsy due to concerning features. ([A–D] *Courtesy of* E. Stratman, Marshfield, WI; E: From National Cancer Institute Visuals Online. Available at: https://visualsonline.cancer.gov/.)

tanning, with an estimated treatment savings of more than $340 million in the United States alone.

Prevention

Large public initiatives to decrease sun exposure, increase sunscreen utilization, and reduce indoor tanning have been present for many years. In addition, the US Surgeon General announced a Call to Action to Prevent Skin Cancer in 2014. This initiative set forth multiple goals to increase prevention of skin cancer, including increasing awareness of the effects of UV radiation, reducing indoor tanning, and promoting research in the treatment of skin cancers. Although there is no evidence to support annual skin examinations for the general population, the United States Preventative Services Task Force does recommend patient education to reduce UV radiation and indoor tanning in patients aged 10 to 24 years.[2] In the 2018 Call to Prevention Progress Report released by the Centers for Disease Control, there is a new emphasis on sun safety and sunscreen application in schools. The report also highlights the progress made to enact legislation limiting or banning indoor tanning for minors, reporting that 17 states have banned indoor tanning for minors, whereas many other states have some type of restriction for minors (**Fig. 4**). Only 6 states have no restrictions on indoor tanning for minors.[50]

Tanning Restrictions

In 2015, Guy and colleagues[51] reported that approximately 11.3 million individuals, including 1.9 million high school students, in the United States participate in indoor tanning. In a meta-analysis of multiple international databases from 2007 to 2012, Wehner and colleagues[21] determined that nearly half of university students have tanned in the previous year. Although the association between tanning and the

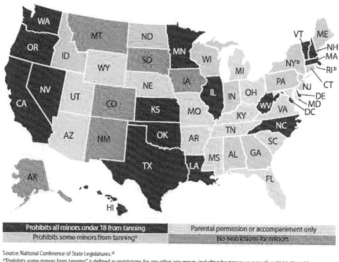

Source: National Conference of State Legislatures.[a]
[a]"Prohibits some minors from tanning" is defined as restrictions for any other age group, including for minors younger than 17, 16, 15, or 14.
[b]As of June 25, 2018, in both New York and Rhode Island, a bill prohibiting all minors under 18 from indoor tanning was awaiting the state governor's signature.

Fig. 4. Map of the United States of America demonstrating the states with restrictions on indoor tanning for minors (<18 years of age) as of June 2018. [a]"prohibits some minors from tanning" is defined as restrictions for any other age group, including for minors younger than 17,16,15,or14. [b] As of june 25,2018,in both New York and Rhode Island,a bill prohibiting all minors under 18 from indoor tanning was awating the stste governor's signature. (*From* Skin Cancer Prevention Progress Report 2018. Atlanta, GA: Centers for Disease Control and Prevention, US Dept of Health and Human Services; 2018. Available at: https://www.cdc.gov/cancer/skin/pdf/SkinCancerPreventionProgressReport-2018-508.pdf.)

increased risk of skin cancer is well known, studies have demonstrated that knowledge of this associated risk has no effect on the frequency of indoor tanning in young adults.[52] The Food and Drug Administration has proposed steps to ban indoor tanning for minors, but this legislation is not yet in place nationwide. As of June 2018, seventeen states have banned indoor tanning for minors. A 2017 study evaluating the effectiveness of state legislation found that one-third of tanning salons did not comply with their state's regulations. Tanning salons that were independently owned and those located in rural or Southern states were least likely to comply with state regulations for minors.[53]

SUMMARY

Melanoma continues to be a substantial cause of morbidity and mortality in the United States and worldwide. The increase in melanoma incidence has been attributed to increased UV radiation exposure and increased surveillance. Despite increasing public awareness of the dangers of excessive UV exposure in relation to melanoma development there has been no change in the behavior of young adults using indoor tanning beds. Current public health initiatives to reduce melanoma incidence include decreasing sun exposure, increasing sunscreen utilization, and reducing indoor tanning, especially for minors. Decreasing the morbidity and mortality associated with melanoma will require a unified effort from the public as well as health care professionals.

ACKNOWLEDGMENTS

The authors acknowledge Emily Andreae, PhD, for content editing.

DISCLOSURE STATEMENT

The authors have no conflicts of interest or financial disclosures.

REFERENCES

1. Rastrelli M, Tropea S, Rossi CR, et al. Melanoma: epidemiology, risk factors, pathogenesis, diagnosis and classification. In Vivo 2014;28(6):1005–11.
2. Gershenwald JE, Guy GP Jr. Stemming the rising incidence of melanoma: calling prevention to action. J Natl Cancer Inst 2016;108(1) [pii:djv381].
3. Survival rates for melanoma skin cancer. 2016. Available at: https://www.cancer.org/cancer/melanoma-skin-cancer/detection-diagnosis-staging/survival-rates-for-melanoma-skin-cancer-by-stage.html. Accessed December 1, 2018.
4. Schuchter L. Melanoma and non-melanoma skin cancers. In: Goldman L, Schafer AI, editors. Goldman-Cecil Medicine. 25th Edition. Philadelphia: Elsevier; 2016.
5. Chang AE, Karnell LH, Menck HR. The National Cancer Data Base report on cutaneous and noncutaneous melanoma: a summary of 84,836 cases from the past decade. The American College of Surgeons Commission on Cancer and the American Cancer Society. Cancer 1998;83(8):1664–78.
6. Shaikh WR, Dusza SW, Weinstock MA, et al. Melanoma thickness and survival trends in the United States, 1989 to 2009. J Natl Cancer Inst 2016;108(1) [pii: djv29].
7. Watts CG, Madronio C, Morton RL, et al. Clinical Features associated with individuals at higher risk of melanoma: a population-based study. JAMA Dermatol 2017; 153(1):23–9.
8. Oliveria SA, Saraiya M, Geller AC, et al. Sun exposure and risk of melanoma. Arch Dis Child 2006;91(2):131–8.
9. Key statistics for melanoma skin cancer. 2018. Available at: https://www.cancer.org/cancer/melanoma-skin-cancer/about/key-statistics.html. Accessed April 7, 2018.
10. Dawes SM, Tsai S, Gittleman H, et al. Racial disparities in melanoma survival. J Am Acad Dermatol 2016;75(5):983–91.
11. Markovic SN, Erickson LA, Rao RD, et al. Malignant melanoma in the 21st century, part 1: epidemiology, risk factors, screening, prevention, and diagnosis. Mayo Clin Proc 2007;82(3):364–80.
12. Wu S, Cho E, Li WQ, et al. History of severe sunburn and risk of skin cancer among women and men in 2 prospective cohort studies. Am J Epidemiol 2016;183(9): 824–33.
13. El Ghissassi F, Baan R, Straif K, et al. A review of human carcinogens–part D: radiation. Lancet Oncol 2009;10(8):751–2.
14. IARC monographs on the evaluation of carcinogenic risks to humans. Solar and ultraviolet radiation. IARC Monogr Eval Carcinog Risks Hum 1992;55:1–316.
15. Falcone LM, Zeidler-Erdely PC. Skin cancer and welding. Clin Exp Dermatol 2019; 44(2):130–4.
16. Nagore E, Hueso L, Botella-Estrada R, et al. Smoking, sun exposure, number of nevi and previous neoplasias are risk factors for melanoma in older patients (60 years and over). J Eur Acad Dermatol Venereol 2010;24(1):50–7.

17. Bauer A, Diepgen TL, Schmitt J. Is occupational solar ultraviolet irradiation a relevant risk factor for basal cell carcinoma? A systematic review and meta-analysis of the epidemiological literature. Br J Dermatol 2011;165(3):612–25.
18. Schmitt J, Seidler A, Diepgen TL, et al. Occupational ultraviolet light exposure increases the risk for the development of cutaneous squamous cell carcinoma: a systematic review and meta-analysis. Br J Dermatol 2011;164(2):291–307.
19. Guenel P, Laforest L, Cyr D, et al. Occupational risk factors, ultraviolet radiation, and ocular melanoma: a case-control study in France. Cancer Causes Control 2001;12(5):451–9.
20. Dixon AJ, Dixon BF. Ultraviolet radiation from welding and possible risk of skin and ocular malignancy. Med J Aust 2004;181(3):155–7.
21. Wehner MR, Chren MM, Nameth D, et al. International prevalence of indoor tanning: a systematic review and meta-analysis. JAMA Dermatol 2014;150(4): 390–400.
22. Ghiasvand R, Rueegg CS, Weiderpass E, et al. Indoor tanning and melanoma risk: long-term evidence from a prospective population-based cohort study. Am J Epidemiol 2017;185(3):147–56.
23. Lazovich D, Isaksson Vogel R, Weinstock MA, et al. Association between indoor tanning and melanoma in younger men and women. JAMA Dermatol 2016; 152(3):268–75.
24. Patel RV, Clark LN, Lebwohl M, et al. Treatments for psoriasis and the risk of malignancy. J Am Acad Dermatol 2009;60(6):1001–17.
25. Valverde P, Healy E, Jackson I, et al. Variants of the melanocyte-stimulating hormone receptor gene are associated with red hair and fair skin in humans. Nat Genet 1995;11(3):328–30.
26. Ford D, Bliss JM, Swerdlow AJ, et al. Risk of cutaneous melanoma associated with a family history of the disease. The International Melanoma Analysis Group (IMAGE). Int J Cancer 1995;62(4):377–81.
27. Goldstein AM, Chan M, Harland M, et al. Features associated with germline CDKN2A mutations: a GenoMEL study of melanoma-prone families from three continents. J Med Genet 2007;44(2):99–106.
28. Zuo L, Weger J, Yang Q, et al. Germline mutations in the p16INK4a binding domain of CDK4 in familial melanoma. Nat Genet 1996;12(1):97–9.
29. Mersch J, Jackson MA, Park M, et al. Cancers associated with BRCA1 and BRCA2 mutations other than breast and ovarian. Cancer 2015;121(2):269–75.
30. Curiel-Lewandrowski C, Speetzen LS, Cranmer L, et al. Multiple primary cutaneous melanomas in Li-Fraumeni syndrome. Arch Dermatol 2011;147(2):248–50.
31. Eng C, Li FP, Abramson DH, et al. Mortality from second tumors among long-term survivors of retinoblastoma. J Natl Cancer Inst 1993;85(14):1121–8.
32. Kraemer KH, DiGiovanna JJ. Forty years of research on xeroderma pigmentosum at the US National Institutes of Health. Photochem Photobiol 2015;91(2):452–9.
33. Goldstein AM, Tucker MA. Dysplastic nevi and melanoma. Cancer Epidemiol Biomarkers Prev 2013;22(4):528–32.
34. Gandini S, Sera F, Cattaruzza MS, et al. Meta-analysis of risk factors for cutaneous melanoma: I. Common and atypical naevi. Eur J Cancer 2005;41(1):28–44.
35. Spanogle JP, Clarke CA, Aroner S, et al. Risk of second primary malignancies following cutaneous melanoma diagnosis: a population-based study. J Am Acad Dermatol 2010;62(5):757–67.
36. Jones MS, Jones PC, Stern SL, et al. The impact of smoking on sentinel node metastasis of primary cutaneous melanoma. Ann Surg Oncol 2017;24(8):2089–94.

37. Li Z, Wang Z, Yu Y, et al. Smoking is inversely related to cutaneous malignant melanoma: results of a meta-analysis. Br J Dermatol 2015;173(6):1540–3.
38. Henderson MT, Kubo JT, Desai M, et al. Smoking behavior and association of melanoma and nonmelanoma skin cancer in the Women's Health Initiative. J Am Acad Dermatol 2015;72(1):190–1.e3.
39. Song F, Qureshi AA, Gao X, et al. Smoking and risk of skin cancer: a prospective analysis and a meta-analysis. Int J Epidemiol 2012;41(6):1694–705.
40. Sitenga JL, Aird G, Ahmed A, et al. Socioeconomic status and survival for patients with melanoma in the United States: an NCDB analysis. Int J Dermatol 2018;57(10):1149–56.
41. Clarke CA, McKinley M, Hurley S, et al. Continued increase in melanoma incidence across all socioeconomic status Groups in California, 1998-2012. J Invest Dermatol 2017;137(11):2282–90.
42. Rizvi SMH, Aagnes B, Holdaas H, et al. Long-term change in the risk of skin cancer after organ transplantation: a population-based nationwide cohort study. JAMA Dermatol 2017;153(12):1270–7.
43. Ascha M, Ascha MS, Tanenbaum J, et al. Risk factors for melanoma in renal transplant recipients. JAMA Dermatol 2017;153(11):1130–6.
44. Yanik EL, Hernandez-Ramirez RU, Qin L, et al. Brief report: cutaneous melanoma risk among people with HIV in the United States and Canada. J Acquir Immune Defic Syndr 2018;78(5):499–504.
45. Omland SH, Ahlstrom MG, Gerstoft J, et al. Risk of skin cancer in patients with HIV: a Danish nationwide cohort study. J Am Acad Dermatol 2018;79(4):689–95.
46. Fattouh K, Ducroux E, Decullier E, et al. Increasing incidence of melanoma after solid organ transplantation: a retrospective epidemiological study. Transpl Int 2017;30(11):1172–80.
47. Bataille V, Boniol M, De Vries E, et al. A multicentre epidemiological study on sunbed use and cutaneous melanoma in Europe. Eur J Cancer 2005;41(14):2141–9.
48. Matsumoto M, Secrest A, Anderson A, et al. Estimating the cost of skin cancer detection by dermatology providers in a large health care system. J Am Acad Dermatol 2018;78(4):701–709 e701.
49. Guy GP Jr, Zhang Y, Ekwueme DU, et al. The potential impact of reducing indoor tanning on melanoma prevention and treatment costs in the United States: An economic analysis. J Am Acad Dermatol 2017;76(2):226–33.
50. Skin cancer prevention progress report 2018. Centers fo Disease Control and Prevention; US Dept of Health and Human Services; 2018.
51. Guy GP Jr, Berkowitz Z, Everett Jones S, et al. Trends in indoor tanning among US high school students, 2009-2013. JAMA Dermatol 2015;151(4):448–50.
52. Nergard-Martin J, Caldwell C, Barr M, et al. Perceptions of tanning risk among melanoma patients with a history of indoor tanning. Cutis 2018;101(1):47, 50;55.
53. Williams MS, Buhalog B, Blumenthal L, et al. Tanning salon compliance rates in states with legislation to protect youth access to UV tanning. JAMA Dermatol 2018;154(1):67–72.

Role of Heredity in Melanoma Susceptibility

A Primer for the Practicing Surgeon

James F. Abdo, MD[a], Aayush Sharma[b],
Rohit Sharma, MD, FACS, FRCS (Glas)[a],*

KEYWORDS

- Melanoma • Hereditary melanoma • Familial melanoma • CDKN2A • FAMMM
- Cancer syndromes

KEY POINTS

- Heredity should be considered an independent risk factor for melanoma, that may modify environmental risk factors.
- Familial melanoma is a poorly defined term. It is most commonly understood as a syndrome based on specific phenotypic characteristics including multiple family members with melanoma, early age of onset, multiple primary melanomas, and coexistence of other primary tumors.
- Families with known germline CDKN2A mutations generally have multiple family members with melanoma, early age of onset, multiple primary melanomas in an individual, and coexistence of other primary tumors. However, germline mutations in CDKN2A are uncommon even in the presence of these phenotypic traits and family history.
- The probability of an individual with familial melanoma having an associated identifiable gene mutation will vary depending upon criteria used to define familial melanoma and geographic location.
- Genetic counseling is recommended for patients thought to be at increased risk for melanoma with either a characteristic phenotype or strong family history of melanoma to assist providers in medical decision making.

INTRODUCTION

Through clinical practice and in laboratories around the world, information accumulation in the area of melanoma genetics is being rapidly translated to actionable knowledge in the clinic. Advent of molecular and genomic evaluation techniques further our understanding of the underlying mechanisms of the complex interplay between hereditary factors and the environment. This information will help clinicians identify high risk

[a] Department of Surgery, Marshfield Medical Center, Marshfield, WI, USA; [b] Ohio State University, Columbus, OH, USA
* Corresponding author. Marshfied Clinic, Department of General Surgery, 1000 N Oak Avenue, Marshfield, WI 54449.
E-mail address: sharma.rohit@marshfieldclinic.org

Surg Clin N Am 100 (2020) 13–28
https://doi.org/10.1016/j.suc.2019.09.006
0039-6109/20/© 2019 Elsevier Inc. All rights reserved.

individuals in order to prevent, recognize and treat melanoma at an earlier stage where cure is a possibility.

In this article, we discuss hereditary as a risk factor for melanoma along with the potential indications for genetic screening. Other risk factors, such as environment, are discussed in Stephanie Carr and colleagues' article, "Epidemiology and Risk Factors of Melanoma," elsewhere in this issue.

FROM PHENOTYPE TO GENOTYPE

Melanoma is an ancient disease that has been discovered in 2400-year-old pre-Columbian mummies from Peru. It was first noted by Hippocrates in fifth century BCE[1] (**Fig. 1**). Hippocrates is credited with the name of the disease as "melas" (dark) and "oma" (tumor). The next 2000 years were the "dark" ages in our understanding of this disease. From 1600 CE, surviving European medical literature has references to "fatal black tumors" that were considered incurable and terminal.[2,3]

In 1820, Heredity was first described as a possible factor in development of melanoma along with other possible risk factors such as skin pigmentation and hair color.[1]

The first evidence based publication[4] described risk factors associated with melanoma development. The report[4] was the first to identify both environmental risk factors such as ultraviolet (UV) radiation exposure as well as genetic traits such as skin color, texture, hair color, eye color, and reaction to the sun. Further mechanistic study of this association later revealed the first identifiable gene with mutations associated with development of melanoma in the gene encoding the melanocortin receptor 1 (MC1R).[5,6]

In the following decades identification of familial clustering provided one of the first genetic insights into the heritable germline mutations that conveyed increased risk of melanoma development.[7] Approximately 5% to 12% of patients with familial clustering are estimated to be harboring a heritable genotype. Of these, only about 20% are recognized to be associated with mutation in cell cycle regulator gene cyclin dependent kinase inhibitor 2A (CDKN2A).[8,9] Typical family members have a phenotype of multiple nevi and a family history of melanoma (**Table 1**).

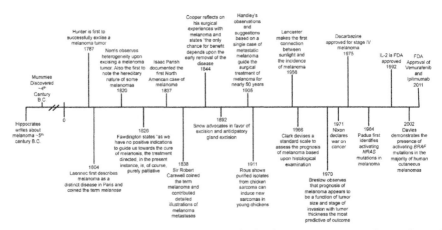

Fig. 1. Timeline of the history of melanoma with developments in our understanding of melaoma. FDA, Food and Drug Administration; IL, interleukin. (*From* Rebecca VW, Sondak VK, Smalley KS. A brief history of melanoma: From mummies to mutations. Melanoma Res 2012;22:114-122; with permission.)

Table 1
Diagnostic criteria of familial atypical multiple mole melanoma syndrome (FAMMM)

Family history	Cutaneous melanoma in ≥1 first-degree or second-degree relative
Physical examination	High total body nevi count (>50) and multiple atypical nevi in proband
Pathologic findings	Nevi with specific histologic features including asymmetry, subepidermal fibroplasia, lentiginous melanocytic hyperplasia with spindle or epithelioid melanocytes, variable dermal lymphocyte infiltration, and presence of "shouldering" phenomenon

Adapted from Soura E, Eliades PJ, Shannon K, Stratigos AJ, Tsao H. Hereditary melanoma: Update on syndromes and management: Genetics of familial atypical multiple mole melanoma syndrome. J Am Acad Dermatol 2016;74:395-407; with permission.

Recently, germline mutations in genes such as *MITF* (microphthalmia transcription factor), *TERT* (telomerase reverse transcriptase), and *BAP1* (BRCA1 associated protein) have also been associated with hereditary melanoma predisposition (**Table 2**).[10,11] Other recognized cancer syndromes caused by identifiable germline gene mutations including Li-Fraumeni (*TP53*) and Breast Ovarian Cancer syndrome (*BRCA 1&2*) also have been associated with increased relative risk of cutaneous malignant melanoma (CMM).[12]

FAMILIAL/HEREDITARY VERSUS SPORADIC MELANOMA

Sporadic melanomas are thought to arise from randomly acquired mutations in melanocytes. These mutations may be due to environment, aging, chronic sun damage (UV exposure), chance events, or other nonheritable events/factors. Differentiating familial clustering of sporadic cases from hereditary melanoma is often confounded by environmental risk factors, and traits with weak associations to melanoma, such as intense and prolonged sun exposure in susceptible skin type,[8,13,14] also influence the relative contribution of genetic factors for melanoma risk. In addition, co-inheritance of modifying genes may either inhibit or enhance the apparent penetrance of a high-risk mutation.[9,15]

Familial and Heritable Melanoma

Although generally used to refer to familial clustering of CMM cases, familial and hereditary melanoma are poorly defined terms. Not all clusters of CMM within a family have an identifiable heritable risk factor(s).[16] Some identifiable heritable mutations associated with familial melanoma are also associated with certain phenotypic traits such as high nevus count or pale skin.[5,17] However, these heritable deleterious mutations have variable penetrance.[5,17] Furthermore using these traits as markers for genetic testing has a low predictive value of finding an underlying associated deleterious germline mutations.[15,18]

Without a consensus definition of familial melanoma, collected data continue to be imprecise. Data collected with more stringent criteria in patients with suspected hereditary melanoma would produce a higher positive predictive value of genetic testing to identify mutations associated with increased risk of melanoma. Conversely, less strict criteria would be more likely to capture a larger portion of melanoma families without a recognized deleterious mutation, thus decreasing the chances of letting a life-shortening cancer syndrome go unrecognized.

Table 2
Known genes or loci with identified mutations leading to increased risk of development of cutaneous malignant melanoma (CMM)

Gene	Inheritance	Syndrome	Type of Melanoma	Phenotype	Other Cancers	Clinical Significance
CDKN2A	AD	FAMMM	Cutaneous (CMM)	>50 atypical nevi, family history of CMM	Pancreatic and nervous system	6-month annual dermatologic evaluation; consider screening for pancreatic cancer
CDK4	AD				Pancreatic and nervous system	Follow CDKN2A recommendations
POT1	AD				Glioma, CLL	No specific recommendation, may follow CDKN2A recommendations
TERT	AD				Ovarian, renal, bladder, breast, lung	No specific recommendation, may follow CDKN2A recommendations
BRCA1&2	AD	Hereditary breast and ovarian cancer	Cutaneous and uveal		Breast, ovarian	Follow NCCN recommendations[63]
BAP1	AD	BAP1 Cancer Syndrome	Cutaneous and uveal	Atypical spitz nevi	Renal and mesothelioma	Excision of atypical spitz nevi, frequent screening for high-risk ocular melanomas
MITF	AD		Cutaneous	Increased nevus count	Renal	No specific recommendation
XPC, XPD, XPA	AR	Xeroderma pigmentosum	Cutaneous	Numerous lentigines at young age, freckling, keratitis	Nonmelanoma skin cancer	Isotretinoin tumor prophylaxis
PTEN	AD	PTEN hamartoma tumor, Cowden syndrome	Cutaneous	Multiple hamartomas and trichilemmomas	Breast, colorectal, thyroid, kidney, endometrial	Specific recommendations for p53 mutations, follow NCCN guidelines[48]
TP53	AD	Li-Fraumeni	Cutaneous and uveal	Early tumors	Breast, bone, soft tissue, Colorectal, leukemia	Yearly skin examination if positive history of skin malignancy

Abbreviations: AD, autosomal dominant; AR, autosomal recessive; BAP1, BRCA1 associated protein; CDKN2A, cyclin dependent kinase inhibitor 2A; CLL, Chronic Lymphocytic Leukemia; FAMMM, familial atypical multiple mole melanoma syndrome; NCCN, National Comprehensive Cancer Network; PTEN, phosphatase and tensin homolog.

Adapted from Ransohoff KJ, Jaju PD, Tang JY, Carbone M, Leachman S, Sarin KY. Familial skin cancer syndromes: Increased melanoma risk. J Am Acad Dermatol 2016;74:423-434

Proposed Phenotypic Classification of Hereditary/Familial Melanoma Syndromes

In an attempt to standardize the classification of hereditary/familial melanoma syndromes, the following criteria are proposed: number of relatives diagnosed with CMM (1 to ≥3),[19-21] number of relatives with multiple primary CMM,[14,22] or a combination of the two. Other phenotypic traits often noted in familial clusters of CMM are early age of occurrence of CMM (**Figs. 2** and **3**) and presence of multiple typical or atypical nevi.[16] These characteristics may be phenotypically classified as 2 distinct types:

a. *Melanoma dominant:* In these disorders melanoma is the first or the most common manifestation. The most common mutations associated with this subtype occur in cyclin-dependent kinase (CDK) genes, specifically CDKN2A or *CDK4*.[8] Other recently discovered mutations have been implicated in this category, including *TERT* and *POT1* in the Shelterin complex genes.[8,11,23-29] These are generally recognized to be high-penetration genes.

b. *Melanoma subordinate*: In these disorders melanoma is not the most common, first, or predominant presentation. These included the Cowden syndrome (*PTEN*), Li-Fraumenl (*TP53*), hereditary breast and ovarian cancer (*BRCA1&2*), and BAP1 cancer syndrome (*BAP1*), among others.

MELANOMA-DOMINANT SYNDROMES

Melanoma-dominant familial melanoma are recognized *phenotypically* by (1) family history of multiple relatives with CMM, (2) relatives with multiple CMM, or (3) personal history of multiple melanomas, especially at young age. Numerous moles and nevi are often found in these families. This collection of traits has been given a variety of names because it was first described nearly in parallel as *BK mole* (named after the initials of the index patient)[30] and familial atypical multiple mole melanoma syndrome *(FAMMM) syndrome,*[7] among other eponyms (**Table 3**).

FAMMM syndrome[7] is now the name commonly used to describe the findings of families with *high total body nevi count* and a *significant family history of CMM* (see **Table 1**). Even using strict phenotypic inclusion criteria, only approximately 25% to 50% of melanoma-prone families have identifiable gene mutations,[8] and these percentages are expected to change as more knowledge accumulates. These data suggest that there are many other disease-causing mutations that are yet undiscovered.

CDK is a protein family involved in cell cycle regulation. Mutations in CDKN2A and CDK4 are associated with risk of hereditary melanoma. Deleterious mutations in the CDKN2A gene are by far most common of the identifiable mutations associated with FAMMM.[8] CDK4 is a rarer genotype associated with the FAMMM phenotype, although phenotypically these genotypes are indistinguishable.[11] The mode of inheritance seems to be autosomal dominant with high penetrance.

Table 3 Syndromes with melanoma predominance recognized by phenotype	
Syndrome Name	**Author, Year Described**
BK syndrome	Clark et al,[30] 1978
Familial atypical multiple mole melanoma syndrome	Lynch et al,[7] 1978
Dysplastic nevus syndrome	Elder,[60] 1980
Atypical mole syndrome	Newton,[64] 1993

Individuals with deleterious germline mutations in these genes not only have multiple nevi and increased likelihood of melanoma at a young age,[19] but also have a significantly increased risk for pancreatic cancer (see **Table 2**).[9] Depending on the study, the relative risk of pancreatic cancer has been estimated to range between 9.4[20] and 47.8.[21,22] Most patients with FAMMM syndrome have been reported to die of cancer. In a Dutch retrospective cohort study of FAMMM based on pedigree, presumed or proven to have CDKN2A mutations, it was estimated that excess mortality can be attributed almost entirely to cancer, specifically CMM and pancreatic cancer.[18] Individuals in this study were reported to have died from melanoma at a rate *150 times* and pancreatic cancer *67 times* greater than those without mutations.[18]

TERT promoter encodes the catalytic subunit of telomerase that is involved in telomere maintenance. TERT is often upregulated in malignancy. Germline TERT mutations can be associated with hepatocellular malignancy, bladder malignancies, thyroid cancer, and gliomas.[23,24] The combination of germline mutation of TERT promoter and a family history of melanoma has been reported to result in nearly *100% development of early CMM,*[25] and increased frequency of detection of TERT promoter genes in metastatic melanomas also have been found.[25] Based on this information, it has been suggested that TERT mutation may be an independent prognostic factor of melanoma.[26] However, the TERT promoter gene was only recently found to have an association with melanoma, so further research is required to better understand the clinical significance of TERT mutations in melanoma development.[24]

POT1 (protectin of telomeres 1), ACD (Adrenocortical Dysplasia Homolog), and TERF2IP (Telomeric Repeat-Binding Factor 2-Interacting Protein 1) are components of the telomeric shelterin complex, which functions to help protect chromosomal ends from damage degradation or inappropriate processing.[27] The association between mutations in telomerase family genes and melanoma development was discovered through genetic analysis of familial clusters of melanoma.[28] The link of POT1 to heritable melanoma was only recently discovered through whole-exome sequencing of CMM cases in melanoma-prone families without *CDKN2A* or *CDK4* mutations.[28] Mutations in *POT1, ACD,* and *TERF2IP* account for 9% of melanoma families (>3 CMM case patients) without mutations in *CDKN2A, CDK4, TERT,* and *BAP1,*[28] and *POT1* mutations appear to be highly penetrant mutations associated with risk of melanoma-predominant syndromes.[31] Studies are ongoing to elucidate the associated phenotype and prevalence of these mutations in different populations.

MELANOMA SUBORDINATE SYNDROMES

BRCA1 and *BRCA2 (Breast cancer susceptibility protein type 1 and 2)* are genes involved in DNA repair in double-strand breaks and are considered tumor suppressor genes. Mutations in *BRCA1* and *BRCA2* are associated with hereditary breast and ovarian cancer syndrome.[32] Individuals with mutations in *BRCA1* and *BRCA2* also have an increased risk of prostate, pancreatic, and other cancers in addition to melanoma in addition to melanoma.[32] However, there have been conflicting reports on the relationship between *BRCA* mutations and CMM. It is estimated that the relative risk of CMM is between 1.1 and 2.5[33] for *BRCA1* carriers and 2.6 in *BRCA2* carriers.[32]

Deleterious mutations in *BAP1 (BRCA1 associated protein)* were identified as a putative cause of inherited susceptibility by studying the genomic profiles of aggressive uveal melanomas (UMs).[34] BAP1 cancer syndrome is characterized by the development of UM, CMM, mesotheliomas, renal cell carcinoma, and other cancers.[35] Recent reports estimate 17.7% and 12.9% of *BAP1* mutant carriers develop CMM and UM, respectively.[35] Up to 67% of individuals with germline BAP1 mutation have lesions that may be characterized as a subset of atypical spitz tumors.[35] These lesions appear within the first several decades of life in germline *BAP1* mutation carriers.[35] An alternative proposed name for these lesions is Melanocytic BAP1-mutated atypical intradermal tumors (MBAITs) due to their distinct histology, genetic makeup, and their association with germline BAP1 mutations.[35] There is insufficient evidence to definitively state whether these lesions are premalignant. It has been suggested that identification of these lesions in an individual should prompt consideration for excision and evaluation in addition to genetic testing for BAP1 mutations.[29,36]

XPA (group A Xeroderma Pigmentosum [XP]), XPC (Group-C XP), DDB2 (Damage Specific DNA Binding Protein 2), ERCC1-5 (Excision Repair Cross Complementation groups 1–5), and POLH (DNA polymerase eta) are DNA damage recognition and repair factors involved in repair of UV-induced DNA damage. XP is caused by homozygous mutations in any of these DNA repair genes. Of all the melanoma-dominant syndromes, it is the only one with an *autosomal recessive* inheritance pattern.[37] XP is characterized by extreme photosensitivity and freckling starting at 1 to 2 years of age, as well as intellectual disability in up to 25% of affected individuals.[37] These individuals have a predisposition to the development of keratitis, iritis, choroidal melanoma, basal cell carcinoma, squamous cell carcinoma, and CMM at an early age. In a study of XP patients followed from 1971 to 2009, 65% of individuals were diagnosed with a skin cancer, and 31% were diagnosed with melanoma specifically.[38] Isotretinoin, a vitamin A analog, has been used as chemoprophylaxis against skin cancers, and it has been shown to be an effective chemoprophylaxis agent that reduced incidence of all skin cancers by 63% in patients with XP.[39]

PTEN (phosphatase and tensin homolog) encodes for phosphatase and tensin homolog, a tumor suppressor gene. *Cowden syndrome* is the most recognized disease entity associated with deleterious mutations in this gene.[33] This syndrome is characterized by multiple hamartomas and a high risk of breast, thyroid, and multiple other cancers.[33] Individuals with germline *PTEN* mutations were confirmed to have elevated risk for melanoma in addition to colorectal cancer and kidney cancer.[40] The estimated lifetime risk of these individuals to develop melanoma is 6%, which translates to a relative risk of 8.5.[40]

MC1R (melanocortin 1 receptor) plays a key role in pigmentation. Certain variations of *MC1R* are linked to red hair and fair skin, which are also associated with an increased risk of CMM.[4] *MC1R* not only confers independent risk of CMM, but has recently been linked to an additive increased risk of developing CMM in patients with *CDKN2A* mutations.[41] This increases the likelihood of earlier incidence of CMM, as well as incidence of multiple primary CMM.[42]

MITF is a master regulator of melanocyte development and differentiation that was previously believed to act through MC1R.[43] It has recently been identified as an independent risk factor for CMM. Individuals with mutations in this gene have fair skin, red hair, body freckling, and total nevus count varying from 40 to several hundred.[43]

TP53 (Tumor protein p53) is a master regulator of the cell cycle and tumor suppressor gene. Disruption of its function leads to unchecked progression through the cell cycle and increased genomic instability. *Li-Fraumeni syndrome* is strongly associated with germline mutations of *TP53* and individuals with Li-Fraumeni syndrome are susceptible to a variety of cancers, including early onset of soft tissue and bone sarcomas, and other cancers occurring before age 30.[44] The association of CMM and *TP53* is not clear, although there are several case reports of *TP53* patients with CMM.[45–47] However, CMM is not considered one of the typical cancers in the Li-Fraumeni syndrome. *TP53* mutations confer an increased susceptibility to UV damage, which possibly increases risk for developing CMM in germline mutation carriers.[45] Current National Comprehensive Cancer Network guidelines recommend yearly skin and organ-targeted surveillance in individuals with Li-Fraumeni syndrome and a family history of CMM.[45,48]

OTHER GENES IMPLICATED IN OUTCOME OF MELANOMA BUT NOT DIRECTLY LINKED TO HERITABILITY OF MELANOMA

Over the past 2 decades, the search for melanoma treatments has led to the study of the molecular basis of melanoma genesis. Several somatic mutations leading to uncontrolled cell growth have been identified and have been denoted "driver" mutations, as they are thought to be the underlying driving force in tumor development.[49] Driver mutations increase the risk of malignancy development and progression. Because of their essential role in melanoma development, these have become the focus of study for possible treatment. Although there may never be a "magic bullet" for melanoma cure, ongoing research has led to a better understanding of melanoma genesis, progression, and response to therapy. Some driver mutations can now be used as prognostic indicators of disease course and predict response to therapy.

BRAF encodes a serine/threonine kinase that is a member of the Raf kinase family.[2] BRAF mutations are present in approximately 50% of CMMs,[50] and BRAF mutations are generally considered to be driver mutations. These mutations are associated with melanomas occurring in younger individuals, truncal location, nonchronically sun-damaged skin, superficial spreading histology, and aggressive nature.[51] Specific BRAF mutations may be considered as a marker of worse prognosis, and BRAF (V600) mutation is also a predictor of response to BRAF inhibitor therapy inhibitor therapy.[52]

NRAS is part of the Ras superfamily of genes that are involved in various essential cell cycle functions including cell growth, differentiation, and survival. NRAS activating mutations are present in up to 15% to 20% of CMMs.[53,54] NRAS has not been found to have prognostic significance in primary melanomas. However, it has been associated with worse outcomes when present in metastatic CMM.[55] NRAS has been studied as a target for therapy, but as of today, none have made it to clinical practice.[56] NRAS and BRAF mutations are nearly mutually exclusive in sporadic melanomas, and NRAS mutations in CMM may predict a lack of response to targeted BRAF therapy.[56] Other studies have found that NRAS mutations predict treatment response to immunotherapy.[54]

GNAQ (G-protein alpha subunit) or GNA11 are genes encoding proteins involved in G-protein signaling. Mutations in this gene occur in 85% of UM and 83% of blue nevi.[57] However, UM and intradermal "blue nevi" have a distinct absence of BRAF and NRAS mutations.[58] In contrast to BRAF, GNAQ and GNA11 have not been found to be associated with worse or better outcomes,[59] and there are no currently approved GNAQ/GNA11 targeted therapies. The identification of these mutations in unknown primary metastatic tumors should prompt investigation of a primary UM.

FACTORS INFLUENCING PHENOTYPIC EXPRESSION OF DELETERIOUS MUTATION GENOTYPES

Although familial melanoma syndromes should be considered independent risk factors for development of CMM,[60] individuals are still subject to other known risk factors, such as exposure to UV light, geographic location, number of nevi and dysplastic nevi, light skin color, and propensity to sunburn.[60] Cumulative risk factors and interaction between genetic and environmental factors may influence the course of the disease and have been associated with diagnosis of CMM at an earlier age (see **Fig. 2**), increased number of CMMs in families, and increased number of primary CMMs in individuals.[11,14]

Of the heritable traits associated with increased risk of developing melanoma, *CDKN2A* mutations are by far the most common.[8] Depending upon the study, mutations in *CDKN2A* only account for 20% to 40% of familial melanomas, it is the most identifiable and most-studied gene in this high-risk population.[14] Ongoing research aims to identify the prevalence of other heritable gene mutations associated with melanoma.

Geographic Location

The likelihood of developing CMM in individuals with germline *CDKN2A* mutations varies by geography. In a meta-analysis of familial melanoma and *CDKN2A* mutations across 3 continents, the estimated penetrance rates (likelihood of developing melanoma over time) among patients 50 to 80 years of age in Australia, the United States, and Europe are 30%-91%, 50% to 76%, and 13% to 58% respectively.[11,14] Geographic location has been considered a surrogate marker for exposure to UV light,[4] therefore, UV light is considered the major factor for increasing the penetrance of *CDKN2A*-associated melanoma.[14]

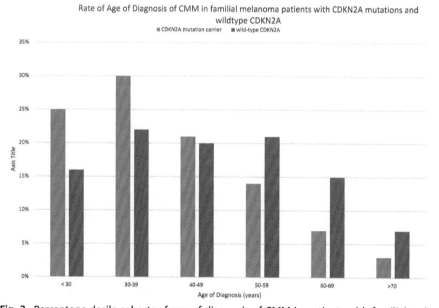

Fig. 2. Percentage decile cohorts of age of diagnosis of CMM in patients with familial melanoma with *CDKN2A* mutations and wild-type *CDKN2A*. This figure compares the rate of diagnosis of first melanoma between patients with familial melanoma with a pathogenic *CDKN2A* mutation carrier and a wild-type or nonpathogenic *CDKN2A* mutation at various age groups. This figure demonstrates that individuals with a *CDKN2A* mutation are more likely to be diagnosed with CMM at an earlier age. (*Data from* Taylor NJ, Handorf EA, Mitra N, et al. Phenotypic and histopathological tumor characteristics according to CDKN2A mutation status among affected members of melanoma families. J Invest Dermatol 2016;136:1066-1069.)

Nevi

Deleterious mutations of *CDKN2A* are associated with multiple atypical nevi. Carriers of these mutations have increased risk of developing melanoma not only associated with a patient's congenital nevi but also an increased risk for melanoma arising from non-nevus–bearing skin.[16]

ROLE OF GENETIC TESTING

The predictive value of genetic testing can be increased by strictly defining the criteria used to classify familial/hereditary melanoma. In all populations with higher incidence of CMM, such as North America, the chance of finding a germline *CDKN2A* mutation as a genetic basis of CMM in an individual diagnosed with CMM is estimated to be 2%.[61] Taking into account family history, it has been estimated that 12% of individuals from the United Kingdom with 2 or 3 family members with CMM will have an underlying *CDKN2A* mutation.[14] Enriching the population by prescreening for *CDKN2A* in addition to phenotypic criteria of familial melanoma yielded a high percentage of identifiable deleterious mutations.[14] Up to 40% of families with hereditary melanoma have germline mutations in CDK genes.[14] Families with 3 or more melanoma cases increases the likelihood of the family having a *CDKN2A* mutation associated with FAMMM to 20% in Australia, 45% in North America, and 57% in Europe.[14] A stronger family history is required to achieve the same predictive value in high-incidence populations, higher incidence have a lower likelihood of identifying an underlying deleterious *CDKN2A* mutation in melanoma families.[14] This phenomenon is likely due to increased overall incidence of "background" melanoma.[14] Lower incidence locations are associated with lower amounts of UV light, thereby decreasing an environmental risk factor for melanoma. MelaPRO is a free downloadable program included in CancerGene that uses Mendelian laws of inheritance along with best estimate penetrance to give a probability of CDKN2A mutation in a given geographic area[62] to assist provider decision making with respect to genetic testing selection.

The current American Academy of Dermatology recommendations for *CDKN2A* testing account for the degree of UV exposure and prevalence of CDKN2A mutations for a given population at a specified location (**Table 4**). Even with strict testing criteria, the identifiable germline mutation rate for patients with familial melanoma is

Table 4
Current recommendations from the American Academy of Dermatology of when to test individuals for cyclin dependent kinase inhibitor 2A (CDKN2A) mutations

Geographic Location	Number of Primary CMMs	Family History
Low melanoma incidence area (United Kingdom)	2 or more	2 first-degree or second-degree relatives with melanoma, or 1 with melanoma and 1 with pancreatic cancer
Moderate to high-incidence melanoma area (United States and Australia)	3 or more	3 melanomas or 2 melanomas and 1 pancreatic cancer or 1 melanoma and 2 pancreatic cancer

Abbreviation: CMM, cutaneous malignant melanoma.

Adapted from Leachman SA, Carucci J, Kohlmann W, et al. Selection criteria for genetic assessment of patients with familial melanoma. J Am Acad Dermatol 2009;61:677. e14; with permission.

less than 50%.[11,22] Individuals meeting the criteria outlined in **Table 4** should be considered high risk and undergo high-level skin as outlined in **Fig. 3**.[11] These individuals also should be referred to a genetic counselor and an interdisciplinary team for melanoma surveillance. A genetic counselor would discuss the likelihood of hereditary melanoma, the molecular genetics related to familial melanoma risk, testing options, costs, risks of discrimination, and possible results of genetic testing. If the individual declines genetic testing or if test results do not identify known deleterious gene mutation, the patient should still be considered high risk because of the strong family history and undergo high-level skin surveillance.[11] If any deleterious mutation is identified, then appropriate clinical management based on the known risks of development of different cancer phenotypes should be instituted (see **Table 2**).

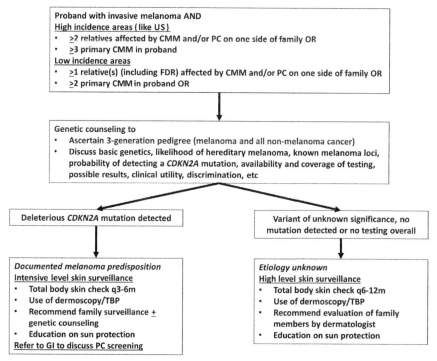

Fig. 3. Genetic counseling algorithm for patients with FAMMM. Following American Academy of Dermatology recommendations outlined by Leachman and colleagues,[22] patients would be referred to a genetic counselor for ascertainment of a 3-generation pedigree. A genetic counselor would also discuss the likelihood of hereditary melanoma, the molecular genetics related to familial melanoma risk, testing options, costs, risks of discrimination, and possible test results. If an individual undergoes testing and a deleterious CDKN2A mutation is detected, it is recommended the patient undergoes intensive skin surveillance. The individual also should be referred to a gastrointestinal (GI) specialist for discussion of pancreatic cancer screening. If an individual opts not to undergo genetic testing, or has no known deleterious mutations in CDKN2A, the patient is still considered high risk and should undergo high-level skin surveillance. FDR, first-degree relative; PC, pancreatic cancer; TBP, total body photography. (*From* Soura E, Eliades PJ, Shannon K, Stratigos AJ, Tsao H. Hereditary melanoma: Update on syndromes and management: Genetics of familial atypical multiple mole melanoma syndrome. J Am Acad Dermatol 2016;74:395-407; with permission.)

SUMMARY

- Deleterious germline mutations associated with melanoma substantially increase the risk of an individual developing melanoma.[11,15,19] Environmental risk factors may further influence the likelihood of developing melanoma for carriers of deleterious germline mutations associated with melanoma.[49]
- Family history is the strongest identifiable factor that can reliably increase the likelihood of identifying a deleterious germline mutation associated with melanoma.[11,14,16,22]
- Elevated background prevalence of melanoma may make it more difficult to identify hereditary melanoma families.[14]
- Genetic counseling and/or testing is warranted in situations in which melanoma is diagnosed at earlier than expected age, multiple relatives with melanoma, individuals with multiple primary melanomas, and other significant cancer-type history in the family.
- Multigene panel testing based on next-generation sequencing may be a more efficient method of testing rather than single gene tests for those deemed high risk based on family and personal history.
- Close appropriate clinical surveillance and modifiable risk reduction is advised for those individuals and families with identifiable deleterious mutations and increased risk of melanoma and other cancers.[11,22]
- For those individuals and families thought to be at increased risk for heritable melanoma but without identifiable deleterious germline mutation, education for melanoma risk reduction and surveillance may be considered.[11,22]

ACKNOWLEDGMENTS

The authors acknowledge Emily Andreae, PhD, for article editing.

DISCLOSURE

The authors have no personal or financial conflicts of interest to disclose.

REFERENCES

1. Urteaga BO, Pack GT. On the antiquity of melanoma. Cancer 1966;19:607–10.
2. Rebecca VW, Sondak VK, Smalley KS. A brief history of melanoma: from mummies to mutations. Melanoma Res 2012;22:114–22.
3. Mukherjee S. The emperor of all maladies: a biography of cancer. Simon and Schuster; 2010.
4. Lancaster HO. Some geographical aspects of the mortality from melanoma in Europeans. Med J Aust 1956;1:1082–7.
5. Beaumont KA, Wong SS, Ainger SA, et al. Melanocortin MC1 receptor in human genetics and model systems. Eur J Pharmacol 2011;660:103–10.
6. Valverde P, Healy E, Jackson I, et al. Variants of the melanocyte–stimulating hormone receptor gene are associated with red hair and fair skin in humans. Nat Genet 1995;11:328.
7. Lynch HT, Frichot BC 3rd, Lynch JF. Familial atypical multiple mole-melanoma syndrome. J Med Genet 1978;15:352–6.
8. Potrony M, Badenas C, Aguilera P, et al. Update in genetic susceptibility in melanoma. Ann Transl Med 2015;3(15):210.

9. Goldstein AM, Chan M, Harland M, et al. High-risk melanoma susceptibility genes and pancreatic cancer, neural system tumors, and uveal melanoma across GenoMEL. Cancer Res 2006;66:9818–28.
10. Yokoyama S, Woods SL, Boyle GM, et al. A novel recurrent mutation in MITF predisposes to familial and sporadic melanoma. Nature 2011;480:99.
11. Soura E, Eliades PJ, Shannon K, et al. Hereditary melanoma: update on syndromes and management: genetics of familial atypical multiple mole melanoma syndrome. J Am Acad Dermatol 2016;74:395–407.
12. Breast Cancer Linkage Consortium. Cancer risks in BRCA2 mutation carriers. J Natl Cancer Inst 1999;91:1310–6.
13. Goldstein AM, Tucker MA. Genetic epidemiology of cutaneous melanoma: a global perspective. Arch Dermatol 2001;137:1493–6.
14. Goldstein AM, Chan M, Harland M, et al. Features associated with germline CDKN2A mutations: a GenoMEL study of melanoma-prone families from three continents. J Med Genet 2007;44:99–106.
15. Goldstein AM, Martinez M, Tucker MA, et al. Gene-covariate interaction between dysplastic nevi and the CDKN2A gene in American melanoma-prone families. Cancer Epidemiol Biomarkers Prev 2000;9:889–94.
16. Bishop JAN, Wachsmuth RC, Harland M, et al. Genotype/phenotype and penetrance studies in melanoma families with germline CDKN2A mutations. J Invest Dermatol 2000;114:28–33.
17. Ransohoff KJ, Jaju PD, Tang JY, et al. Familial skin cancer syndromes: increased melanoma risk. J Am Acad Dermatol 2016;74:423–34.
18. Hille ET, van Duijn E, Gruis NA, et al. Excess cancer mortality in six Dutch pedigrees with the familial atypical multiple mole-melanoma syndrome from 1830 to 1994. J Invest Dermatol 1998;110:788–92.
19. Bataille V. Genetic epidemiology of melanoma. Eur J Cancer 2003;39:1341–7.
20. Moskaluk CA, Hruban RH, Schutte M, et al. Genomic sequencing of DPC4 in the analysis of familial pancreatic carcinoma. Diagn Mol Pathol 1997;6:85–90.
21. De Snoo FA, Bishop DT, Bergman W, et al. Increased risk of cancer other than melanoma in CDKN2A founder mutation (p16-leiden)-positive melanoma families. Clin Cancer Res 2008;14:7151–7.
22. Leachman SA, Carucci J, Kohlmann W, et al. Selection criteria for genetic assessment of patients with familial melanoma. J Am Acad Dermatol 2009;61:677.e14.
23. Killela PJ, Reitman ZJ, Jiao Y, et al. TERT promoter mutations occur frequently in gliomas and a subset of tumors derived from cells with low rates of self-renewal. Proc Natl Acad Sci U S A 2013;110:6021–6.
24. Huang FW, Hodis E, Xu MJ, et al. Highly recurrent TERT promoter mutations in human melanoma. Science 2013;339:957–9.
25. Horn S, Figl A, Rachakonda PS, et al. TERT promoter mutations in familial and sporadic melanoma. Science 2013;339:959–61.
26. Griewank KG, Murali R, Puig-Butille JA, et al. TERT promoter mutation status as an independent prognostic factor in cutaneous melanoma. J Natl Cancer Inst 2014;106(9) [pii:dju246].
27. Shi J, Yang XR, Ballew B, et al. Rare missense variants in POT1 predispose to familial cutaneous malignant melanoma. Nat Genet 2014;46:482.
28. Aoude LG, Pritchard AL, Robles-Espinoza CD, et al. Nonsense mutations in the shelterin complex genes ACD and TERF2IP in familial melanoma. J Natl Cancer Inst 2014;107 [pii:dju408].

29. Soura E, Eliades PJ, Shannon K, et al. Hereditary melanoma: update on syndromes and management: emerging melanoma cancer complexes and genetic counseling. J Am Acad Dermatol 2016;74:411–20.
30. Clark WH, Reimer RR, Greene M, et al. Origin of familial malignant melanomas from heritable melanocytic lesions: the BK mole syndrome. Arch Dermatol 1978;114:732–8.
31. Read J, Wadt KA, Hayward NK. Melanoma genetics. J Med Genet 2016;53:1–14.
32. Moran A, O'hara C, Khan S, et al. Risk of cancer other than breast or ovarian in individuals with BRCA1 and BRCA2 mutations. Fam Cancer 2012;11:235–42.
33. Eng C. PTEN: one gene, many syndromes. Hum Mutat 2003;22:183–98.
34. Harbour JW, Onken MD, Roberson ED, et al. Frequent mutation of BAP1 in metastasizing uveal melanomas. Science 2010;330:1410–3.
35. Carbone M, Ferris LK, Baumann F, et al. BAP1 cancer syndrome: malignant mesothelioma, uveal and cutaneous melanoma, and MBAITs. J Transl Med 2012; 10:179.
36. Stefanaki C, Stefanaki K, Chardalias L, et al. Differential diagnosis of spitzoid melanocytic neoplasms. J Eur Acad Dermatol Venereol 2016;30:1269–77.
37. DiGiovanna JJ, Kraemer KH. Shining a light on xeroderma pigmentosum. J Invest Dermatol 2012;132(3, Part 2):785–96.
38. Bradford PT, Goldstein AM, Tamura D, et al. Cancer and neurologic degeneration in xeroderma pigmentosum: long term follow-up characterises the role of DNA repair. J Med Genet 2011;48:168–76.
39. Kraemer K. Dysplastic nevi as precursors to hereditary melanoma. J Dermatol Surg Oncol 1983;9:619–22.
40. Tan M, Mester JL, Ngeow J, et al. Lifetime cancer risks in individuals with germline PTEN mutations. Clin Cancer Res 2012;18:400–7.
41. Puntervoll HE, Yang XR, Vetti HH, et al. Melanoma prone families with CDK4 germline mutation: phenotypic profile and associations with MC1R variants. J Med Genet 2013;50:264–70.
42. Goldstein AM, Landi MT, Tsang S, et al. Association of MC1R variants and risk of melanoma in melanoma-prone families with CDKN2A mutations. Cancer Epidemiol Biomarkers Prev 2005;14:2208–12.
43. Sturm RA, Fox C, McClenahan P, et al. Phenotypic characterization of nevus and tumor patterns in MITF E318K mutation carrier melanoma patients. J Invest Dermatol 2014;134:141–9.
44. Birch JM, Hartley AL, Tricker KJ, et al. Prevalence and diversity of constitutional mutations in the p53 gene among 21 Li-Fraumeni families. Cancer Res 1994;54: 1298–304.
45. Curiel-Lewandrowski C, Speetzen LS, Cranmer L, et al. Multiple primary cutaneous melanomas in Li-Fraumeni syndrome. Arch Dermatol 2011;147:248–50.
46. Pötzsch C, Voigtländer T, Lübbert M. p53 germline mutation in a patient with Li-Fraumeni syndrome and three metachronous malignancies. J Cancer Res Clin Oncol 2002;128:456–60.
47. Hartley AL, Birch JM, Marsden HB, et al. Malignant melanoma in families of children with osteosarcoma, chondrosarcoma, and adrenal cortical carcinoma. J Med Genet 1987;24:664–8.
48. National comprehensive cancer network screening recommendations for Li-Fraumeni syndrome. 2019. Available at: https://www.nccn.org/professionals/ physician_gls/pdf/genetics_screening.pdf.
49. Meyle KD, Guldberg P. Genetic risk factors for melanoma. Hum Genet 2009;126: 499–510.

50. Morris LG, Tuttle RM, Davies L. Changing trends in the incidence of thyroid cancer in the United States. JAMA Otolaryngol Head Neck Surg 2016;142:709–11.
51. Kim SY, Kim SN, Hahn HJ, et al. Metaanalysis of BRAF mutations and clinicopathologic characteristics in primary melanoma. J Am Acad Dermatol 2015;72:1046.e2.
52. Sosman JA, Kim KB, Schuchter L, et al. Survival in BRAF V600–mutant advanced melanoma treated with vemurafenib. N Engl J Med 2012;366:707–14.
53. Jovanovic B, Egyhazi S, Eskandarpour M, et al. Coexisting NRAS and BRAF mutations in primary familial melanomas with specific CDKN2A germline alterations. J Invest Dermatol 2010;130:618.
54. Muñoz-Couselo E, Adelantado EZ, Ortiz C, et al. NRAS-mutant melanoma: current challenges and future prospect. Onco Targets Ther 2017;10:3941.
55. Houben R, Becker JC, Kappel A, et al. Constitutive activation of the ras-raf signaling pathway in metastatic melanoma is associated with poor prognosis. J Carcinog 2004;3:6.
56. Ascierto PA, Schadendorf D, Berking C, et al. MEK162 for patients with advanced melanoma harbouring NRAS or Val600 BRAF mutations: a non-randomised, open-label phase 2 study. Lancet Oncol 2013;14:249–56.
57. Van Raamsdonk CD, Bezrookove V, Green G, et al. Frequent somatic mutations of GNAQ in uveal melanoma and blue naevi. Nature 2009;457:599.
58. Tsao H, Chin L, Garraway I A, et al. Melanoma: from mutations to medicine. Genes Dev 2012;26:1131–55.
59. Field MG, Harbour JW. Recent developments in prognostic and predictive testing in uveal melanoma. Curr Opin Ophthalmol 2014;25:234.
60. Elder DE, Goldman LI, Goldman SC, et al. Dysplastic nevus syndrome: a phenotypic association of sporadic cutaneous melanoma. "Cancer 1980;46(8):1787–94.
61. Thomas NE, Busam KJ, From L, et al. Tumor-infiltrating lymphocyte grade in primary melanomas is independently associated with melanoma-specific survival in the population-based genes, environment and melanoma study. J Clin Oncol 2013;31:4252–9.
62. Wang W, Niendorf KB, Patel D, et al. Estimating CDKN2A carrier probability and personalizing cancer risk assessments in hereditary melanoma using MelaPRO. Cancer Res 2010;70:552–9.
63. National comprehensive cancer network screening recommendations for BRCA-Related Breast and/or Ovarian Cancer Syndromes. 2019. Available at: https://www.nccn.org/professionals/physician_gls/pdf/genetics_screening.pdf. Accessed October 24, 2019.
64. Newton JA, Bataille V, Griffiths K, et al. How common is the atypical mole syndrome phenotype in apparently sporadic melanoma? J Am Acad Dermatol 1993;29(6):989–96.

Glossary:
Carrier A person who carries a mutated copy of a gene that can be passed onto offspring. This person may or may not manifest the phenotypes associated with this mutation.
Genome-wide association study A tool used to identify genes involved in human disease by searching for single nucleotide polymorphisms that have a higher level of incidence in people with a disease compared with people without a disease.
Genotype The genetic makeup of an organism. Governed by allelic combinations that result in various observable phenotypes.

Germline mutation (hereditary) A genetic change that is incorporated into the DNA of the organism and is therefore passed on to offspring.

Linkage analysis A biological tool used to detect the chromosomal location of disease genes. The basis of this tool is that genes that are physically close to a chromosome remain linked during meiosis.

Phenome-wide association study Used to survey which phenotypes are associated with particular genetic variations.

Phenotype The observable physical characteristics of an organism that result from the genotype of the particular organism. Some examples include height, hair and iris color, and so forth.

Proband The individual through whom a family with a genetic disorder is determined. Male individuals are referred to as propositus, and female individuals are referred to proposita.

Somatic mutation (sporadic) A genetic change that occurs within an organism after its conception. These mutations are not passed on to offspring and are often associated with various cancers.

Wild type A gene in its natural, nonmutated form.

Staging Melanoma
What's Old and New

Kirithiga Ramalingam, MD[a], Shyam S. Allamaneni, MD[b],*

KEYWORDS

- Melanoma • Cutaneous melanoma • Melanoma staging
- American Joint Committee on Cancer (AJCC)

KEY POINTS

- Mitotic count as a subcategorizing factor for T1 has been replaced with tumor thickness in the eighth edition staging system.
- Tumor thickness measurement is approximated to the nearest 0.1 mm instead of 0.01 mm.
- Elevated lactate dehydrogenase (LDH) level no longer qualifies for categorizing M to M1c. Instead, LDH is used to dichotomize all the subcategories of M1 as 0 and 1 based on the levels.
- M1d and pathologic stage IIID are the new additions to the current staging system.
- The terminologies and definitions used in staging are refined with detailed explanations.

INTRODUCTION AND IMPORTANCE OF STAGING

The incidence of cutaneous melanoma is increasing at a rate of 3% per year in the United States.[1] Although melanoma is relatively uncommon among the cutaneous malignancies, it has the highest mortality. The prognosis for early-stage cutaneous melanoma (ie, stages I and II) is favorable[2]; however, the prognosis is extremely poor for the advanced stages. Recent advances in molecular targeted therapies and immunotherapies have improved the survival of advanced stage melanoma.[3–6] Thus, it is important to stage patients appropriately so as to enable identification of those who would benefit from recent advances in therapy.

Understanding the staging of melanoma is essential for optimizing communication between treating physicians of different specialties, in assessing the prognosis, and on guiding disease management. Staging is also vital for designing clinical trials and reporting to cancer registries. In this article, the authors focus primarily on the staging of cutaneous melanoma.

[a] Department of General Surgery, Cleveland Clinic, 9500 Euclid Avenue, Cleveland, OH 44195, USA; [b] The Jewish Hospital - Mercy Health Surgical Residency Program, Department of Surgery, 4777 East Galbraith Rd, Cincinnati, OH 45236, USA
* Corresponding author.
E-mail address: drallamaneni@gmail.com

Surg Clin N Am 100 (2020) 29–41
https://doi.org/10.1016/j.suc.2019.09.007
0039-6109/20/© 2019 Elsevier Inc. All rights reserved.

surgical.theclinics.com

SUPPORTIVE DATA AND METHODS FOR THE CURRENT AMERICAN JOINT COMMITTEE ON CANCER EIGHTH EDITION STAGING OF CUTANEOUS MELANOMA

The seventh edition of the American Joint Committee on Cancer (AJCC) staging system for melanoma was published in 2010. With better understanding of the biology of melanoma over the last few years, the new eighth edition AJCC staging system for melanoma was implemented on January 1, 2018. The evidence for the formulation of the eighth edition derives from the International Melanoma Database and Discovery Platform.[7]

Unlike the seventh edition database, which included patients diagnosed as long ago as the 1960s,[8] the eighth edition includes only patients who were diagnosed since 1998. Such an inclusion criterion enabled the exclusion of patients who were diagnosed earlier than 1998, thereby omitting patients who were managed during the highly evolving era in which the investigations and treatment were not standardized.[2] To be included in the eighth edition analysis, patients were required to have sentinel lymph node biopsy (SLN) if their primary lesions were T2 or thicker. Also, only stage I, II, and III patients were included in the analysis, because the management of stage IV melanoma was rapidly evolving and the approval of new treatment agents was variable with variable prognosis during the above time period. The eighth edition includes both the anatomic "TNM" prognostic factors and the nonanatomic factors, such as lactate dehydrogenase (LDH) levels.

CHANGES FROM THE AMERICAN JOINT COMMITTEE ON CANCER SEVENTH EDITION TO THE EIGHTH EDITION
T Category

The changes between eighth and seventh editions for cutaneous melanoma are described in detail by Keung and Gershenwald[9] with tables of comparison between the 2, and explanation of the clinical implications of the current staging system. There is a clear description of Tis, T0, and Tx in the eighth edition. Tis is used for in situ melanoma with no invasive component. T0 indicates no evidence of primary tumor, for example, a patient with axillary nodal disease with no evidence of primary tumor in the draining area. Tx is assigned when the tumor thickness cannot be assessed, for example, lack of curettage specimen, or when perpendicular sections are unavailable. Tx is also applicable when the information regarding tumor thickness was unavailable because of unmaintained records of the primary melanoma that would have been resected years ago.

Mitotic rate as a dichotomous variable to subcategorize T1 is not included in the eighth edition. The current subcategorization of T1 is based on a tumor thickness threshold of 0.8 mm. The concept of using tumor thickness to subcategorize T1 melanoma was considered and evaluated by the melanoma expert panel based on the evidence seen in studies that reported poorer prognosis associated with thicker T1 melanoma compared with thin T1 melanoma.[2,10–12] The evidence for subcategorizing T1 based on tumor thickness comes from the multivariate analysis of tumor thickness, ulceration, mitotic rate, and melanoma-specific survival (MSS). Also, the likelihood of having SLN positivity for tumors of thickness less than 0.8 mm (<5%) is much less compared with the tumors of thickness of 0.8 to 1.0 mm (5%–12%).[13–16] However, mitotic rate remains an important prognostic factor across all the T stages and should be documented.

In the seventh edition, it was recommended that tumor thickness be measured to the nearest 0.01 mm. However, in the current edition, to accommodate the difficulty in measuring tumor thickness to the nearest 0.01 mm, especially for tumors greater than 1 mm in thickness, it is sufficient to approximate to the nearest 0.1 mm. For example, if the tumor thickness ranges from 0.75 to 0.84 mm, thickness would be rounded off to 0.8 mm and, accordingly, assigned to T1b.

N Category

Previously used terminology for "a" and "b" subcategories of N staging, that is, "microscopic" and "macroscopic" nodal diseases, has been replaced with the terminologies "clinically occult" and "clinically evident" nodal diseases, respectively. "Clinically occult" nodal diseases are identified by SLN, and "clinically evident" is identified by clinical and/or radiological examination.

The eighth edition melanoma staging system gives a better definition of nonnodal metastases, such as microsatellite, satellite, and in-transit lesions that are included in the N staging matrix.[7] A microsatellite is defined as any microscopic focus of metastatic tumor cells in the skin or subcutaneous tissue, adjacent to, or deep to but discontinuous from the primary lesion, that are not clinically identifiable. A satellite metastasis is defined as any foci of clinically evident cutaneous and/or subcutaneous metastasis, occurring discontinuous, but within the 2 cm of the primary tumor. An in-transit lesion is defined as a clinically evident cutaneous and/or subcutaneous metastasis, occurring beyond 2 cm from primary lesion, in the region between primary lesion and draining regional lymph nodes. In the eighth edition, a correlation of lymph node metastases, microsatellite, satellite, and in-transit lesions to MSS[2] was noted, indicating that all nonnodal regional lesions had similar survival rates compared with each other. Hence, the nonnodal lesions were grouped together in the same subcategories of N staging, that is, "c" (**Fig. 1**).

The eighth edition allows the possibility of reporting patients who undergo only SLN and not have completion lymph node dissection (CLND) even if the SLN results are positive. The evidence for such a practice is based on the results of 2 trials, namely DeCOG-SLT[17] and MSLT-II.[18] These trials showed that there is no difference in the overall survival between nodal observation group and those who had CLND following positive SLN. Patients who do not undergo CLND following a positive SLN are to be reported with a suffix "(sn)."

M Category

The melanoma expert panel concluded that it is premature to perform a broad-based analysis for M categorization because the treatment of metastatic melanoma is rapidly evolving. However, the eighth edition has included an additional subcategory of "M1d," which exclusively includes patients with central nervous system (CNS) metastases with or without metastases at other sites, because of the worst prognosis associated with CNS metastases.[19–22] This subcategorization is especially important for clinical trials with respect to the design, stratification, and analyses of results.

According to the eighth edition, site of metastases still remains the main criteria based on which M staging is subcategorized. M1a signifies nonvisceral metastasis: that is, distant cutaneous, subcutaneous, or nodal metastases. M1a patients have a better prognosis than those with distant metastases to other sites. M1b includes patients with pulmonary metastases only. These patients have an intermediate prognosis compared with those with metastases to other sites. M1c includes patients with metastases to sites other than nonvisceral, pulmonary, and CNS. M1d includes patients with CNS metastasis.

An elevated LDH level no longer qualifies for subcategorizing M staging to M1c in the eighth edition. Instead, each of the M subcategories has been dichotomized into "0" and "1" based on LDH level. Patients with normal LDH levels are labeled as

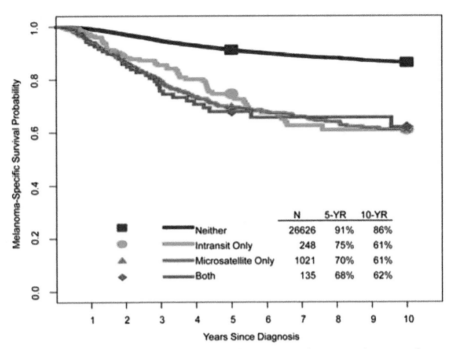

			N	5-YR	10-YR
■	Neither		26626	91%	86%
●	Intransit Only		248	75%	61%
▲	Microsatellite Only		1021	70%	61%
◆	Both		135	68%	62%

Fig. 1. Kaplan-Meier melanoma-specific survival curves according to T subcategory for patients with stage I and II melanoma from the eighth edition International Melanoma Database. (*From* Gershenwald JE, Scolyer RA, Hess KR, et al. Melanoma staging: Evidence-based changes in the American Joint Committee on Cancer eighth edition cancer staging manual. CA Cancer J Clin. 2017 Nov;67(6):472-492. https://doi.org/10.3322/caac.21409. Epub 2017 Oct 13; with permission.)

"0" and those with elevated LDH levels are labeled as "1." For example, a patient with metastasis only to the lung with elevated LDH levels would be assigned M1b 1 for M staging.

Clinical Stage Grouping

The clinical stage groups are unchanged between the seventh and eighth edition staging systems. To assess the T, N, and M for clinical stage grouping, microstaging of the excision biopsy of the primary and clinical/radiologic findings for the evidence of regional and distant metastases is performed. If chemotherapy or targeted therapy is administered in the neoadjuvant setting, the SLN pathology report is included in the N status assessment for clinical stage grouping. For example, for a patient with T1a disease on excision biopsy and 1 node positive on SLN but no evidence of distant metastasis, the clinical stage would be cT1aN1aM0, that is, stage IIIA.

Pathologic Stage I and II

MSS for stage I and II patient population of the eighth edition[2] is better than the MSS of stage I and II patients of the seventh edition.[8] The difference in survival is due to the fact that the patient population of the eighth edition was staged for nodal disease with SLN for clinical stages II and above. Performing SLN resulted in upstaging patients with clinical stage I/II disease to stage III based on a positive SLN finding.

Pathologic T1bN0M0 is grouped into pathologic stage IA instead of stage IB in the eighth edition. This change was made owing to the evidence of better prognosis of pathologic T1bN0M0 compared with clinical T1bN0M0 (because of the possibility of clinically occult nodal disease).

Pathologic Stage III

Both T and N categories are considered for stage III subgrouping in the eighth edition, unlike in the seventh edition where only tumor ulceration and N category were considered. The evidence behind this decision comes from the eighth-edition data analysis that identified the heterogeneity among stage III patients in terms of MSS based on the difference in both T and N categories. Furthermore, it is important to note that the N subcategories are different for eighth and seventh editions, resulting in a difference in the overall stage III subgrouping. The current edition stage III subgrouping has 4 subgroups, namely III A, B, C, and D, in contrast to the seventh edition, which had 3 pathologic subgroups (ie, IIIA, IIIB, and IIIC). These changes reflect a difference in the MSS between the stage III subgroups of the 2 editions with better survival seen in the eighth edition on stage-to-stage comparison. To be able to efficiently identify eighth edition stage III subgroup, stage III subgroup grids are available in several different versions[2] (**Fig. 2**).

There are no differences in pathologic stage IV groups between the seventh and eighth editions. Following neoadjuvant therapy and surgery, the pathologic stage is identified as "ypTNM." After definitive systemic or radiotherapy, the staging is represented as "ycTNM." In the eighth edition, patients who recur are represented with the staging label "rTNM." Recurrent disease is further specified as "rcTNM" when staging is based on clinical and radiological evaluation and "rpTNM" when the staging is based on pathologic findings.

IMAGING IN STAGING WORKUP
Clinical Stage I and II

For clinical stage I and II, no radiological imaging, including chest radiograph[23,24] and ultrasound,[25–27] of the draining nodes is recommended to look for distant or regional metastases. However, when the clinical examination is equivocal, or clinical assessment is inadequate because of obesity, and/or in high-risk clinical stage II melanoma (T4cN0M0), ultrasound examination of the draining nodal basin is advised.

For patients who undergo SLN, radionuclide lymphoscintigraphy is recommended, especially for primary tumors located in the head and neck region or trunk, because the drainage can vary between these subsites.[28] Lymphoscintigraphy is also helpful in identifying minor nodal basins, such as epitrochlear and popliteal nodes, and interval nodes located outside the major and minor nodal basins.[29]

Clinical Stage III and IV

For clinical stage III disease, in order to detect occult distant metastases, 2 imaging options are available: contrast-enhanced computed tomography (CT) and integrated whole-body PET/CT. The advantage of PET/CT is that it screens the entire body for metastases.[30–35] However, the CT portion of the integrated whole-body PET/CT scan does not provide the same high resolution of a contrast-enhanced CT scan to detect low-volume disease. If contrast-enhanced CT scanning is used to survey for distant metastasis, in addition to studying thorax and abdomen, CT of pelvis and neck should be included for primaries of the lower body and head and neck, respectively.[36,37] Also, brain MRI is recommended for screening of brain metastases in stage

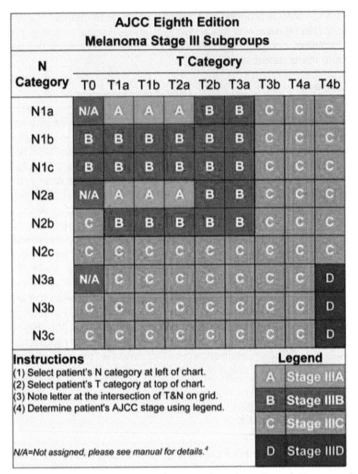

N Category	T Category								
	T0	T1a	T1b	T2a	T2b	T3a	T3b	T4a	T4b
N1a	N/A	A	A	A	B	B	C	C	C
N1b	B	B	B	B	B	B	C	C	C
N1c	B	B	B	B	B	B	C	C	C
N2a	N/A	A	A	A	B	B	C	C	C
N2b	C	B	B	B	B	B	C	C	C
N2c	C	C	C	C	C	C	C	C	C
N3a	N/A	C	C	C	C	C	C	C	D
N3b	C	C	C	C	C	C	C	C	D
N3c	C	C	C	C	C	C	C	C	D

AJCC Eighth Edition Melanoma Stage III Subgroups

Instructions
(1) Select patient's N category at left of chart.
(2) Select patient's T category at top of chart.
(3) Note letter at the intersection of T&N on grid.
(4) Determine patient's AJCC stage using legend.

N/A=Not assigned, please see manual for details.[4]

Legend

A	Stage IIIA
B	Stage IIIB
C	Stage IIIC
D	Stage IIID

Fig. 2. AJCC eighth edition stage III subgroups based on T and N categories. (*From* Gershenwald JE, Scolyer RA, Hess KR, et al. Melanoma staging: Evidence-based changes in the American Joint Committee on Cancer eighth edition cancer staging manual. CA Cancer J Clin. 2017 Nov;67(6):472-492. https://doi.org/10.3322/caac.21409. Epub 2017 Oct 13; with permission.)

III C and higher disease. To assess the location and complete extent of distant metastases in clinical stage IV disease, whole-body PET/CT scan and contrast-enhanced MRI brain are recommended.[38]

Recent Advances in Imaging for Staging Melanoma

Laser-based pump-probe microscopy to assess the nature of the primary lesion in terms of aggressiveness, metastatic potential, and thickness assessment has been studied and might help in prognostication and decision when performing SLN in the future.[39] For clinical evaluation of primary lesions, satellite lesions, and in-transit lesions, use of high-frequency ultrasound examination with 3-dimensional component and contrast modalities is primitive and needs further evaluation.[40] Single-photon emission computed tomography (SPECT)/CT is the fusion of the functional SPECT component with the anatomic CT component. Use of SPECT/CT in preoperative and intraoperative (using Freehand SPECT) SLN procedure as an adjunct to lymphoscintigraphy has several advantages. Three-dimensional visualization using SPECT/CT provides accurate information regarding the anatomic location of SLN with respect to the adjacent structures. SPECT/CT also aids in identification of SLN in challenging scenarios where lymphoscintigraphy use alone would have resulted in misinterpreted images because of skin contamination, injection site proximity (shine-through effect), or excess overlaid fat (obesity or deep-seated sentinel nodes), thereby enhancing the SLN procedure.[41,42] SPECT/CT identifies 26% more sentinel nodes than lymphoscintigraphy alone[41] and is especially useful for primary lesions located in head and neck, axilla, and groin regions.

Various modalities have been studied in an effort to enhance the sensitivity and specificity of the SLN procedure, including CT lymphotropic tracers (gold nanoparticles), magnetic lymphotropic tracers (iron oxide nanoparticles), optical lymphotropic tracers (fluorophores), and targeted SLN contrast agents (mannose-based radiolabeled contrast agents).[43] However, these methods are still in the experimental stage of development. The use of ^{18}F-5-FPN in place of ^{18}F-5-FDG in performing PET has increased the sensitivity of PET in identifying disease-positive lymph nodes; however, it requires further study to validate its use in detecting metastatic disease.[44] Whole-body MRI has been compared in several studies to PET-CT as a modality to diagnose metastatic disease, and the results are encouraging.[45]

PATHOLOGY AND LABORATORY TESTING IN STAGING WORKUP
Excision Biopsy of the Primary Tumor

Tumor thickness determination, as described by Breslow, is measured in millimeters using the ocular micrometer, starting vertically from the top of the granular layer of the epidermis to the deepest invasive cell. If the overlying epidermis is ulcerated, the thickness must be measured from the base of the ulcer to the deepest invasive cell. The thickness of the excised biopsy is used to assign the clinical T staging in melanoma. Additional parameters of the primary lesion that should be reported and which have prognostic significance include histologic subtype, Clark level of invasion, mitotic rate of the tumor per square millimeter, degree of atypia, tumor infiltrating lymphocytes, lymphovascular invasion, neurotropism, ulceration or tumor regression, microsatellitosis, and margins.

Sentinel Lymph Node Biopsy

SLN biopsy is recommended for clinical stage II and above. Also, consensus based on several published reports states that high-risk stage I tumors, such as T1b, should have SLN to stage the draining lymph node region.[38,46] The other features of SLN that are recommended for documentation because they have prognostic value include the number of tumor-involved SLN, tumor burden of SLN (ie, the single largest maximum dimension measured to the nearest 0.1 mm), the location of tumor in the SLN, that is, subcapsular versus parenchymal, and presence of extranodal extension.

Laboratory Tests

Serum LDH determination is a valuable prognostic tool for cutaneous melanoma.[47,48] Documentation of baseline LDH before starting systemic therapy for advanced melanoma is vital because it has prognostic value and aids in monitoring the response to therapy and progression-free survival.[49–51]

Table 1
Differences between the eighth and seventh editions with respect to cutaneous melanoma TNM staging are highlighted with bold type

T	Eighth Edition	Seventh Edition
T1	≤1 mm	≤1 mm
T1a	**<0.8 mm + no ulceration**	≤1 mm + no ulceration + <1 **mitosis** per mm^2
T1b	**<0.8 mm + ulceration, or 0.8–1 mm ± ulceration**	≤1 mm + (ulceration or >1 **mitosis** per mm^2)
T2	>1–2 mm	1.01–2 mm
T3	>2–4 mm	2.01–4 mm
T4	>4 mm	>4 mm
T2a, 3a, 4a	Without ulceration	Without ulceration
T2b, 3b, 4b	With ulceration	With ulceration
N terminologies	**Clinically occult** **Clinically evident**	**Micrometastasis** **Macrometastasis**
N2	2 or 3 positive lymph node (LN) or in-transit lesion (IT) or satellite lesion (SL) and/or microsatellite lesion (MSL) **+ at least 1 positive LN**	2–3 positive LN or IT or SL and/or MSL
N3	(≥4 positive LN or ITL or SL and/or MSL **+ ≥2 positive LN**) or (matted nodes)	(≥4 positive LN) or (≥4 lesions of ITL or SL or MSL with positive LN) or (matted nodes)
N1a	1 clinically occult LN	1 positive LN with micrometastasis
N1b	1 clinically evident LN	1 positive LN with macrometastatis
N2a	2 or 3 clinically occult LN	2–3 positive LNs with micrometastasis
N2b	2 or 3 clinically evident LN	2–3 positive LN with macrometastatis
N3a	≥4 clinically occult LN	—
N3b	≥4 with at least 1 clinical detected or matted nodes	—
N_c	ITL or SL or MSL	ITL or SL or MSL
N1c	**No positive LN + 1 ITL or SL or MSL**	—
N2c	**1 clinically occult or clinically detected LN** + ITL or SL or MSL with a total number of regionally lesions being 2–3	No positive LN + 2–3 ITL or SL or MSL
N3c	**≥2 clinically occult or clinically detected LN** + ITL or SL or MSL with total number of regional lesions being 4 and above	—
M1_(0)	**LDH levels are normal**	—
M1_(1)	**LDH levels are elevated**	—
M1a	Distant metastasis to skin, soft tissue, and/or nonregional LNs	Distant metastasis to skin, soft tissue, and/or nonregional LNs

(continued on next page)

Table 1 (continued)		
T	**Eighth Edition**	**Seventh Edition**
M1b	Lung metastasis ± metastasis to skin, soft tissue, and/or nonregional LNs	Lung metastasis
M1c	Distant metastasis to non-CNS visceral metastasis ± metastasis to skin, soft tissue, and/or nonregional LNs	Metastasis to sites other than skin, subcutaneous tissue, nonregional nodes, lungs, or any metastasis with **elevated LDH**
M1d	**CNS metastasis** ± metastasis in other sites	—

Abbreviations: CNS, central nervous system; ITL, in-transit lesions; LDH, lactate dehydrogenase; LN, lymph node; MSL, microsatellite lesion; SL, satellite lesion.

Data from 8th edition AJCC staging system and 7th edition AJCC staging manual; and Amin MB, Edge S, Greene F, et al. (eds.). AJCC Cancer Staging Manual, 8th edition. Springer International Publishing: American Joint Commission on Cancer; 2017 and Edge SB, Byrd DR, Compton CC, et al, (eds.) AJCC cancer staging manual, 7th edition. France: Springer; 2010.

STAGING OF MELANOMA WITH UNKNOWN PRIMARY AND NONSKIN MELANOMA

The staging criteria of melanoma with unknown primary are essentially the same as that of known primary cutaneous melanomas, because the prognosis is similar in both cases. If the patient initially presents with nodal metastases with no evidence of primary melanoma, then these nodal lesions should be considered regional and not distant. Head and neck mucosal melanoma, melanoma of the conjunctiva and uvea, and mucosal melanoma of urethra, vagina, rectum, and anus have their own staging system that is described in detail in the AJCC eighth edition and are beyond the scope of the current discussion.

SCOPE OF FURTHER IMPROVEMENT IN THE CURRENT STAGING OF MELANOMA

Inclusion of prognostic factors, such as histopathologic parameters mentioned earlier, and immune markers, based on definitive scientific evidence, would enhance the current AJCC staging system. In light of the success of BRAF, MEK, and KIT inhibitors in the management of melanoma in metastasis and adjuvant setting,[52] somatic tumor genetic profiling for BRAF and KIT has become the norm for stage III and IV melanoma. Currently, comprehensive genetic tumor sequencing is widely available for identifying the various types of melanoma, including BRAF, KIT, NRAS, GNAQ, GNA11, NF1, CDK4/6, PI3K/AKT, and NTRK/ROS1/ALK. Furthermore, genomic sequencing of melanoma can help in assigning patients to clinical trials. Chromosome aberration testing is available for assessing the prognosis of cutaneous melanoma in terms of the risk of metastasis.[53] Although genomic profiling of cutaneous melanoma is not routinely used at the present time, there is a potential for its application in staging to optimize surveillance in patients with high-risk characteristics but an early-stage disease (based on AJCC staging system).[53] Various risk-assessment statistical models have been described based on the clinical evidence for tailored approaches to individual patients. These modules should be evaluated by the precision medicine core criteria for appropriate usage.

SUMMARY

The melanoma expert panel that revised the evidence-based eighth edition AJCC staging system did so by rigorously analyzing stage I, II, and III patients included in the International Melanoma Database and Discovery Platform. Key changes in the eighth edition apply mainly to subcategorization of T1, M1, and pathologic stage grouping of stage I and III and refine the definitions and terminologies used in the staging system (**Table 1**). As the knowledge of tumor biology improves, the staging of melanoma will continue to evolve to enable betterment of care.

DISCLOSURE

Authors have nothing to disclose.

REFERENCES

1. Siegel RL, Miller KD, Jemal A. Cancer statistics, 2019. CA Cancer J Clin 2019; 69(1):7–34.
2. Gershenwald JE, Scolyer RA, Hess KR, et al. Melanoma staging: evidence-based changes in the American Joint Committee on Cancer eighth edition cancer staging manual. CA Cancer J Clin 2017;67(6):472–92.
3. Niezgoda A, Niezgoda P, Czajkowski R. Novel approaches to treatment of advanced melanoma: a review on targeted therapy and immunotherapy. Biomed Res Int 2015. https://doi.org/10.1155/2015/851387.
4. Luke JJ, Flaherty KT, Ribas A, et al. Targeted agents and immunotherapies: optimizing outcomes in melanoma. Nat Rev Clin Oncol 2017;14(8):463–82.
5. Domingues B, Lopes JM, Soares P, et al. Melanoma treatment in review. ImmunoTargets Ther 2018;7:35–49.
6. Henriques V, Martins T, Link W, et al. The emerging therapeutic landscape of advanced melanoma. Curr Pharm Des 2018;24(5):549–58.
7. AJCC cancer staging manual. 8th edition. New York: Springer; 2017. p. 563–85.
8. Balch CM, Gershenwald JE, Soong S-J, et al. Final version of 2009 AJCC melanoma staging and classification. J Clin Oncol 2009;27(36):6199–206.
9. Keung EZ, Gershenwald JE. The eighth edition American Joint Committee on Cancer (AJCC) melanoma staging system: implications for melanoma treatment and care. Expert Rev Anticancer Ther 2018;18(8):775–84.
10. Gimotty PA, Elder DE, Fraker DL, et al. Identification of high-risk patients among those diagnosed with thin cutaneous melanomas. J Clin Oncol 2007;25(9): 1129–34.
11. Green AC, Baade P, Coory M, et al. Population-based 20-year survival among people diagnosed with thin melanomas in Queensland, Australia. J Clin Oncol 2012; 30(13):1462–7.
12. Lo SN, Scolyer RA, Thompson JF. Long-term survival of patients with thin (T1) cutaneous melanomas: a Breslow thickness cut point of 0.8 mm separates higher-risk and lower-risk tumors. Ann Surg Oncol 2018;25(4):894–902.
13. Andtbacka RHI, Gershenwald JE. Role of sentinel lymph node biopsy in patients with thin melanoma. J Natl Compr Cancer Netw 2009;7(3):308–17.
14. Murali R, Haydu LE, Quinn MJ, et al. Sentinel lymph node biopsy in patients with thin primary cutaneous melanoma. Ann Surg 2012;255(1):128–33.
15. Han D, Zager JS, Shyr Y, et al. Clinicopathologic predictors of sentinel lymph node metastasis in thin melanoma. J Clin Oncol 2013;31(35):4387–93.

16. Cordeiro E, Gervais M-K, Shah PS, et al. Sentinel lymph node biopsy in thin cutaneous melanoma: a systematic review and meta-analysis. Ann Surg Oncol 2016; 23(13):4178–88.

17. Leiter U, Stadler R, Mauch C, et al. Complete lymph node dissection versus no dissection in patients with sentinel lymph node biopsy positive melanoma (De-COG-SLT): a multicentre, randomised, phase 3 trial. Lancet Oncol 2016;17(6): 757–67.

18. Faries MB, Thompson JF, Cochran AJ, et al. Completion dissection or observation for sentinel-node metastasis in melanoma. N Engl J Med 2017;376(23):2211–22.

19. Staudt M, Lasithiotakis K, Leiter U, et al. Determinants of survival in patients with brain metastases from cutaneous melanoma. Br J Cancer 2010;102(8):1213–8.

20. Davies MA, Liu P, McIntyre S, et al. Prognostic factors for survival in melanoma patients with brain metastases. Cancer 2011;117(8):1687–96.

21. Glitza IC, Heimberger AB, Sulman EP, et al. Chapter 19–prognostic factors for survival in melanoma patients with brain metastases. In: Hayat MA, editor. Brain metastases from primary tumors, vol. 3. San Diego (CA): Academic Press; 2016. p. 267–97. https://doi.org/10.1016/B978-0-12-803508-5.00019-6.

22. Frinton E, Tong D, Tan J, et al. Metastatic melanoma: prognostic factors and survival in patients with brain metastases. J Neurooncol 2017;135(3):507–12.

23. Vermeeren L, van der Ent FW, Hulsewé KW. Is there an indication for routine chest X-ray in initial staging of melanoma? J Surg Res 2011;166(1):114–9.

24. Gjørup CA, Hendel HW, Pilegaard RK, et al. Routine X-ray of the chest is not justified in staging of cutaneous melanoma patients. Dan Med J 2016;63(12) [pii: A5317].

25. Starritt EC, Uren RF, Scolyer RA, et al. Ultrasound examination of sentinel nodes in the initial assessment of patients with primary cutaneous melanoma. Ann Surg Oncol 2005;12(1):18–23.

26. Sabel MS, Wong SL. Review of evidence-based support for pretreatment imaging in melanoma. J Natl Compr Cancer Netw 2009;7(3):281–9.

27. Chai CY, Zager JS, Szabunio MM, et al. Preoperative ultrasound is not useful for identifying nodal metastasis in melanoma patients undergoing sentinel node biopsy. Ann Surg Oncol 2012;19(4):1100–6.

28. Chapman BC, Gleisner A, Kwak JJ, et al. SPECT/CT improves detection of metastatic sentinel lymph nodes in patients with head and neck melanoma. Ann Surg Oncol 2016;23(8):2652–7.

29. Zager JS, Puleo CA, Sondak VK. What is the significance of the in transit or interval sentinel node in melanoma? Ann Surg Oncol 2011;18(12):3232–4.

30. Tan JC, Chatterton BE. Is there an added clinical value of "true"whole body(18)F-FDG PET/CT imaging in patients with malignant melanoma? Hell J Nucl Med 2012;15(3):202–5.

31. Brady MS, Akhurst T, Spanknebel K, et al. Utility of preoperative [(18)]f fluorodeoxyglucose-positron emission tomography scanning in high-risk melanoma patients. Ann Surg Oncol 2006;13(4):525–32.

32. Perng P, Marcus C, Subramaniam RM. (18)F-FDG PET/CT and melanoma: staging, immune modulation and mutation-targeted therapy assessment, and prognosis. AJR Am J Roentgenol 2015;205(2):259–70.

33. Wong ANM, McArthur GA, Hofman MS, et al. The advantages and challenges of using FDG PET/CT for response assessment in melanoma in the era of targeted agents and immunotherapy. Eur J Nucl Med Mol Imaging 2017;44(Suppl 1):67–77.

34. Scheier BY, Lao CD, Kidwell KM, et al. Use of preoperative PET/CT staging in sentinel lymph node-positive melanoma. JAMA Oncol 2016;2(1):136–7.

35. Schröer-Günther MA, Wolff RF, Westwood ME, et al. F-18-fluoro-2-deoxyglucose positron emission tomography (PET) and PET/computed tomography imaging in primary staging of patients with malignant melanoma: a systematic review. Syst Rev 2012;1:62.

36. Hoffend J. Staging of cutaneous malignant melanoma by CT. Radiologe 2015; 55(2):105–10. https://doi.org/10.1007/s00117-014-2760-1, 112. [in German].

37. Ferrándiz L, Silla-Prósper M, García-de-la-Oliva A, et al. Yield of computed to-mography at baseline staging of melanoma. Actas Dermosifiliogr 2016;107(1): 55–61.

38. Wong SL, Faries MB, Kennedy EB, et al. Sentinel lymph node biopsy and manage-ment of regional lymph nodes in melanoma: American Society of Clinical Oncology and Society of Surgical Oncology clinical practice guideline update. Ann Surg On-col 2018;25(2):356–77.

39. Puza CJ, Mosca PJ. The changing landscape of dermatology practice: mela-noma and pump-probe laser microscopy. Lasers Med Sci 2017;32(8):1935–9.

40. Bard RL. High-frequency ultrasound examination in the diagnosis of skin cancer. Dermatol Clin 2017;35(4):505–11.

41. Tardelli E, Mazzarri S, Rubello D, et al. Sentinel lymph node biopsy in cutaneous melanoma: standard and new technical procedures and clinical advances. A systematic review of the literature. Clin Nucl Med 2016;41(12):e498–507.

42. Stodell M, Thompson JF, Emmett L, et al. Melanoma patient imaging in the era of effective systemic therapies. Eur J Surg Oncol 2017;43(8):1517–27.

43. Cousins A, Thompson SK, Wedding AB, et al. Clinical relevance of novel imaging technologies for sentinel lymph node identification and staging. Biotechnol Adv 2014;32(2):269–79.

44. Wang Y, Li M, Zhang Y, et al. Detection of melanoma metastases with PET-comparison of 18F-5-FPN with 18F-FDG. Nucl Med Biol 2017;50:33–8.

45. Petralia G, Padhani AR, Pricolo P, et al. Whole-body magnetic resonance imaging (WB-MRI) in oncology: recommendations and key uses. Radiol Med 2018. https://doi.org/10.1007/s11547-018-0955-7.

46. Wong SL, Faries MB, Kennedy EB, et al. Sentinel lymph node biopsy and man-agement of regional lymph nodes in melanoma: American Society of Clinical Oncology and Society of Surgical Oncology clinical practice guideline update. J Clin Oncol 2018;36(4):399–413.

47. Petrelli F, Cabiddu M, Coinu A, et al. Prognostic role of lactate dehydrogenase in solid tumors: a systematic review and meta-analysis of 76 studies. Acta Oncol 2015;54(7):961–70.

48. Gao D, Ma X. Serum lactate dehydrogenase is a predictor of poor survival in ma-lignant melanoma. Panminerva Med 2017;59(4):332–7.

49. Kelderman S, Heemskerk B, van Tinteren H, et al. Lactate dehydrogenase as a selection criterion for ipilimumab treatment in metastatic melanoma. Cancer Im-munol Immunother 2014;63(5):449–58.

50. Long GV, Grob J-J, Nathan P, et al. Factors predictive of response, disease pro-gression, and overall survival after dabrafenib and trametinib combination treat-ment: a pooled analysis of individual patient data from randomised trials. Lancet Oncol 2016;17(12):1743–54.

51. Puri S, Markowitz J. The use of baseline biomarkers to predict outcome in mel-anoma patients treated with pembrolizumab. Ann Res Hosp 2017;1(2).

Available at: http://arh.amegroups.com/article/view/3700. Accessed February 27, 2019.

52. Rothermel LD, Sarnaik AA, Khushalani NI, et al. Current immunotherapy practices in melanoma. Surg Oncol Clin N Am 2019. https://doi.org/10.1016/j.soc.2019. 02.001.

53. Funchain P, Tarhini AA. Using genomic sequencing to improve management in melanoma. Oncology (Williston Park) 2018;32(3):98–101, 104.

Pathology of Melanoma

Asmita Chopra, MBBS, MS (Surgery)[a],*, Rohit Sharma, MD, FACS, FRCS (Glas)[b],
Uma N.M. Rao, MD (Pathology)[c]

KEYWORDS

- Melanoma • Pathology • Melanocyte • Congenital nevus • Sentinel node
- Cutaneous • Extra-cutaneous

KEY POINTS

- Melanoma is a melanocytic malignant tumor. Melanocytes are pigmented cells arising from neural crest and migrating to basal epidermis, mucosal surfaces, and uvea.
- Cutaneous melanomas are classified into 4 major histologic subtypes. Variants, such as desmoplastic melanoma, although rare, have management implications.
- Immunohistochemistry aids in diagnosing melanomas, especially amelanotic and extracutaneous lesions.
- Biopsy of suspicious lesions is still the mainstay of diagnosis. Narrow margin excision biopsy is preferred.
- Pathologic characteristics, such as tumor depth and lymph node positivity, are the most important prognostic features. Other characteristics, such as ulceration, mitosis, lymphovascular invasion, and tumor-infiltrating lymphocytes, also are important in predicting outcomes.

Glossary

BRAF:	B-Raf proto-oncogene; serine-threonine kinase
NRAS:	N-Ras proto-oncogene; GTPase
HRAS:	H-Ras proto-oncogene; GTPase
BAP 1:	BRCA-1 associated protein 1
KIT:	kit proto-oncogene; tyrosine kinase
GNAQ:	G protein subunit alpha Q
GNA11:	G protein subunit alpha 11

Disclosure Statement: We disclose that we have no relationship with a commercial company that has a direct financial interest in subject matter or materials discussed in article or with a company making a competing product.
[a] Department of Surgery, Division of Surgical Oncology, University of Pittsburgh, Room A-422, Scaife Hall, 3550 Terrace Street, Pittsburgh, PA 15261, USA; [b] Department of Surgery, Marshfield Medical Center, 1000 North Oak Avenue, Marshfield, WI 54449, USA; [c] Department of Pathology, University of Pittsburgh School of Medicine, Section of Bone/Soft Tissue, Melanoma Pathology, UPMC Presbyterian Shadyside, Room WG2.9, 5230 Centre Avenue, Pittsburgh, PA 15232, USA
* Corresponding author.
E-mail address: asmita.chopra89@gmail.com

INTRODUCTION

Melanoma is the third most common skin cancer. It is responsible, however, for the highest number of deaths due to skin cancer.[1] The overall incidence of melanoma is higher in white populations compared with Asian and African populations.[2] Whites also have longest survival after diagnoses, which may be explained by lower rates of ulcerated lesions and metastasis and earlier stage at diagnosis.[3]

The prognosis and oncological outcomes are greatly influenced by the pathologic and clinical stages of melanoma.

CELL OF ORIGIN

Melanocytes originate from the neural crest cells and migrate to the basal layer of the epidermis of the skin.[4] A small proportion also migrate to the uvea, meninges, and mucosal surfaces.[5] Atypical and genetically mutated melanocytes give rise to malignant melanoma.[6]

The density of melanocytes in the skin varies based on age, number of nevi, body site, and sun exposure. There is known to be a regulatory cross-talk between melanocytes and keratinocytes. Site-specific assessment shows maximum melanocyte density in the face, neck, back, and shoulders.[7] Intermittent sun exposure is one of the important risk factors for development of melanoma.[8]

BENIGN NEVI

Nevus is defined as a visible, well-circumscribed, long-standing, benign, melanocytic lesion of the skin that can be congenital or acquired.[9]

Congenital Melanocytic Nevi

Congenital melanocytic nevi (CMN) are present at birth or infancy. They are associated with an increased risk of cutaneous melanomas as well as with neurocutaneous melanosis and primary central nervous sytem melanomas.

An analysis of the Surveillance, Epidemiology and End Results (SEER) database showed that CMN carry a 465-times increased relative risk of developing melanomas in childhood and adolescence.[10]

CMN are classified based on the maximum diameter of their projected adult size. CMN greater than 20 cm are called large CMN and those greater than 40 cm are known as giant CMN.[11] The risk of melanoma increases with the projected adult size of the CMN, with CMN greater than 20 cm carrying a lifetime risk of 5.7% to 12%.[12,13] The SEER database analysis also showed highest incidence and fatalities in patients with giant CMN.[12] In contrast, small and medium CMN have less than 1% risk of melanoma.[14,15]

Giant CMN, especially those associated with multiple smaller nevi, may be associated with leptomeningeal melanosis. This is known as neurocutaneous melanosis, or CMN syndrome.[16]

CMN commonly show *BRAF* mutations, similar to acquired nevi.[17] Giant CMN associated with neurocutaneous syndrome are associated with *NRAS* mutations in 80% of cases.[18]

Acquired Nevi

Acquired nevi are nevi seen after infancy. They can develop in both children and adults.

Those that appear before puberty show clinical features and evolution similar to small and moderate-sized CMN.[9]

Acquired nevi also are associated with an increased risk of melanoma, especially when associated with increased number, atypical features, and ultraviolet light exposure.[19]

DYSPLASTIC NEVI

Dysplastic nevi are defined based on atypical clinical and pathologic characteristics.

The International Agency for Research on Cancer defines dysplastic nevi, based on clinical characteristics, as single or multiple, slightly raised, irregularly pigmented lesions with vague borders and asymmetric shape, usually measuring greater than 0.5 mm in maximum dimension.[20]

Pathologically, cellular atypia and/or architectural abnormality can suggest dysplasia.[21] Dysplastic nevi may show melanocyte hyperplasia, occasional macronuclei, few mitotic figures, bridging of rete ridges, and lymphocytic infiltrate.[22]

Although risk factors for dysplastic nevi are not well established, they show a predilection for intermittent sun-exposed sites.[23]

Dysplastic nevi are associated with an increased risk of melanoma.[24,25] Melanoma in situ (MIS) can be seen arising in a background of dysplastic junctional nevus (**Fig. 1**). This warrants patients with dysplastic nevi to be followed-up at more frequent intervals.

SPITZOID LESIONS

Spitz nevi were originally described as juvenile melanomas with low malignant potential and good prognosis.[26] Over the years, the lesions described by Spitz were found to be benign. Spitz nevi appear as pinkish or pigmented lesions on the face and extremities, with histology depicting epithelioid and spindle-shaped melanocytes.[27] They show epidermal hyperplasia with junctional nests showing vertical orientation of cells.[28]

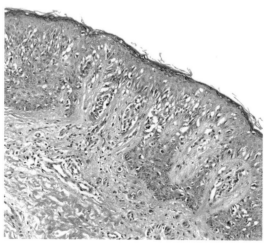

Fig. 1. MIS arising in a background of dysplastic junctional nevus. Hematoxylin-eosin, magnification original x20

Lesions with features similar to Spitz nevi but carrying a higher malignant potential also are recognized. These lesions are grouped together as spitzoid lesions.

Most investigators classify the spitzoid lesions into 3 categories—spitz nevus, atypical spitz nevus, and spitzoid melanoma.[29,30] The major challenge is to differentiate these lesions. Histologically, spitzoid melanomas show high-grade cellular atypia with pleomorphism and hyperchromasia. Mitotic figures may be seen in all types of spitzoid lesions; however, atypical mitosis and their presence in deeper portions of the lesion are indicative of spitzoid melanoma.[28,31]

Malignant lesions are uniformly positive for S-100, HMB-45, and Melan-A, unlike benign lesions that stain for p-16.[31]

Genetically, the benign lesions show *HRAS* mutations, whereas the atypical spitzoid lesions show chromosomal abnormalities, such as *BAP1* loss. Spitzoid melanomas show *NRAS* and *BRAF* mutations.[28,30]

EVOLUTION OF MELANOMA

Malignant change of a benign lesion is suggested by asymmetry, irregular borders, variable color, diameter greater than 6 mm, and evolution (ABCDE).[32] Evolution of a benign melanocytic lesion is an important clinical feature suggestive of a malignant change.

Histologically, proliferation of basal melanocytes in a lentiginous and nested pattern along the epidermis constitutes the radial growth phase. Invasion of the deeper layers constitutes the vertical growth phase and this is a temporal event.[33] Melanoma in the vertical growth phase has the potential to metastasize.[34]

MELANOMA IN SITU

MIS is defined as proliferation of large atypical melanocytes in the epidermis of the skin, without invasion to the dermis[35] (**Fig. 2**). It has been identified in all types of cutaneous melanomas except occasionally in nodular melanomas (NMs).

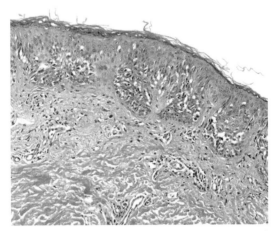

Fig. 2. MIS displaying junctional proliferation of large atypical basal melanocytes and pagetoid spread. Hematoxylin-eosin, magnification original x20.

A variant of MIS, usually confined to sun-exposed skin, is known as lentigo maligna.[36] It progresses to gives rise to lentigo maligna melanoma (LMM), with an estimated lifetime risk of 5%.[37] It is histologically seen as proliferation of atypical melanocytes in the dermoepidermal junction and along skin appendages.[38] It is important to differentiate lentigo maligna from melanocytic changes due to chronic sun exposure. Immunohistochemistry may aid in the confirmation of MIS.[39]

Presence of MIS in a lesion may help differentiate true cutaneous recurrence from in-transit and satellite lesions, in patients with melanoma.[40]

TYPES OF MELANOMA

Melanoma can be classified broadly as cutaneous and extracutaneous. The extracutaneous melanomas include ocular, mucosal, and leptomeningeal.

Cutaneous Melanomas

Cutaneous melanomas are the most common type of malignant melanomas. They are classified into 4 histologic subtypes: LMM, superficial spreading, nodular, and acral lentiginous melanomas (ALMs).[41,42]

Lentigo maligna melanoma

LMM is the second most common type of cutaneous melanoma.[37] Clinically this is a large, flat, pigmented lesion found in the chronically sun-exposed areas of the head and neck region. Classic histology shows intraepidermal proliferation of individual melanocytes, localized to the basal layer of the epidermis (dermoepidermal junction) and along skin appendages.[43] LMMs also may show features of chronic sun exposure, such as junctional melanocytic proliferation and bridging of rete ridges.[44]

Because LMM is found on visibly accessible areas, it is typically diagnosed early. It shows slowest progression among all histologic types and has a good prognosis.[45,46]

Superficial spreading melanoma

Superficial spreading melanoma (SSM) is the most common type of melanoma.[47] It is seen on intermittently sun-exposed skin, especially on the trunk and extremities.[8] Clinically, SSM sharply marginated with a raised surface and haphazard coloration. Histologically, they show an intraepidermal spread of tumor that shows pagetoid and nested growth pattern.[48] Unlike LMMs, SSMs show presence of relatively monomorphic atypical melanocytes and atypical melanocytic nests.[49] There generally is lack of maturation in deeper areas of the dermal component.

SSMs grow faster than LMMs; however, they also are associated with good prognosis.[45,46]

Nodular melanoma

NM presents as a smooth, uniform pigmented nodule with lack of surrounding flat discoloration (unlike SSM and LMM). This is predominantly a dermal tumor.[43] It has scant radial growth phase that may be difficult to find in ulcerated lesions.[41]

NMs have higher incidence of ulceration, mitosis, and thickness at the time of diagnosis. They also are reported to be more aggressive compared with other types of melanomas.[50]

Genetic analysis of the histologic subtypes has shown that *BRAF* mutations are more common in SSM, whereas *NRAS* mutation is more common in NM.[51]

Acral lentiginous melanoma

ALM is the rarest histologic type of melanoma seen in United States.[52] It is seen as a pigmented or amelanotic lesion on the soles, palms, or the nail beds (subungual). The most common site is the plantar surface.[53] Histologically, ALMs show broad lentiginous growth with invasion of the dermis and atrophy of the papillary dermis.[54] They show growth of predominantly singular cells, with poorly circumscribed nests, often located parallel to the epidermis.[55,56] ALMs have a higher rate of *NRAS* and *KIT* mutations.[56]

They have been associated with poor prognosis, which may be due to an advanced stage at presentation.[57,58] When statistically controlled for stage, the survival of patients with ALM may not be significantly different from the other histologic types.[59]

Desmoplastic Melanoma

Desmoplastic melanoma (DM) is not recognized as a separate histologic type of melanoma. It is a variant of melanoma, which shows predominance of spindle cells and fibrous stroma.[60] DMs can be mistaken for a benign spindle cell lesion. They usually present as an amelanotic, scar like, indurated lesion on sun-exposed skin.[61] Histologically, amajority have an epidermal junctional component with abundant collagenous matrix around the spindle cells in the dermis (**Fig. 3**). They show a predilection for perineural invasion. DMs are uniformly positive for S-100.[62]

Based on the density of malignant cells and stroma, they are classified as pure and mixed DMs.[63] The pure type has been shown to have higher thickness at diagnosis but shows lower rate of sentinel lymph node (SLN) positivity and ulceration along with better prognosis.[64,65] Pure DM also shows prolonged local growth with late metastasis. When compared with traditional histologic subtypes, DMs have a higher rate of local recurrence.[66] Although SLN biopsy may have a role in the mixed form, current literature shows no proved advantage in the pure DM and its role is controversial.[64,67]

Primary Mucosal Melanoma

Primary mucosal melanoma (PMMs) arise from the melanocytes found in the mucosal surface of the respiratory, gastrointestinal and genitourinary tracts. They constitute 1.4% of all melanomas.[68]

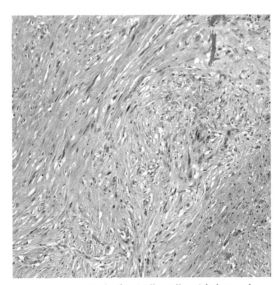

Fig. 3. DM showing tumor comprised of spindle cells with hyperchromatic nuclei. Micrograph demonstrates perineural invasion. Hematoxylin-eosin, magnification original x40.

These melanomas, unlike cutaneous melanomas, are not accessible to inspection and are identified at a later stage, when they become symptomatic.

They have no established risk factors and there is currently no defined staging system (except for head and neck mucosal melanomas by the American Joint Committee on Cancer [AJCC]).[69]

It is important to differentiate PMM from a metastatic lesion of a cutaneous primary. The presence of MIS, intact overlying epithelium, and radial growth phase may be markers of primary malignancy.[70,71]

A high rate of amelanotic lesions also pose a diagnostic challenge. Tumor markers, however, such as S-100, tyrosinase, HMB-45, and MART-1, confirm melanocytic origin.[72]

Genetically, PMMs show a higher frequency of *KIT* mutations.[73]

Ocular Melanoma

Ocular melanomas constitute 3.7% of all melanomas. They include uveal and conjunctival melanomas.[68]

Uveal melanomas

Uveal melanomas arise from melanocytes in the uvea (includes iris, ciliary body, and choroid). They have a higher incidence in patients with choroidal nevus and dysplastic nevi syndrome.[74] Diagnosis is based on clinical features, ocular ultrasound, and fundoscopy. Pathologic analysis is utilized when clinical characteristics are uncertain, such as amelanotic lesions. In such cases, fine-needle aspiration may be done.[75] Prognosis is dependent on morphology, cell type (spindle vs epithelioid type), tumor thickness, and extent of scleral and orbital involvement.

Uveal melanomas show *GNAQ/GNA11* gene mutations in up to 77% of the cases.[76] Studies have shown that certain chromosomal abnormalities can predict worse prognosis and high risk of metastasis.[77,78] Gene expression profiling for uveal melanomas, however, is a better prognostic indicator than chromosomal analysis or TNM staging.[74]

Uveal melanomas are staged and managed differently than are cutaneous melanomas.[69]

Conjunctival melanomas

Conjunctival melanomas are a rare form of ocular melanoma. They are distinct from uveal melanomas in clinical appearance and genetics. They appear as pigmented lesions of the conjunctiva.[79] Unlike uveal melanomas, their diagnosis involves an excisional biopsy. As with cutaneous melanomas, they commonly show *BRAF* mutations.[79,80]

BIOPSY OF A MELANOMA

The mainstay of diagnosis of cutaneous and mucosal melanomas is an adequate biopsy, which allows pathologists to accurately microstage and assess the depth of invasion of the melanoma. A narrow margin excision biopsy is preferred. Wide biopsy margins hamper SLN mapping and biopsy.[81] In large lesions, especially giant congenital nevi, incisional/punch biopsy may be used. Shave biopsies are discouraged, if there is high clinical suspicion of melanoma.

PATHOLOGIC STAGING OF MELANOMA

Pathologic staging is still the most important prognostic indicator in melanoma. The AJCC staging system is the most accepted system in the United States.

The National Comprehensive Cancer Network (NCCN) recommends that the pathology report of melanoma include (1) Breslow thickness (to the nearest 0.1 mm), (2) ulceration (present or absent), (3) mitotic rate, (4) margin status (deep and peripheral), (5) microsatellites (presence or absence), (6) pure desmoplasia, and (7) Clark level (for nonulcerated lesion, <1 mm, mitotic rate not determined).[81]

College of American Pathologists guidelines recommend synoptic reporting of the pathologic specimen, which includes histologic type, tumor thickness, ulceration, macroscopic satellite nodules, microsatellite lesions, margins (peripheral and deep), mitotic rate, lymphovascular invasion, neurotropism, tumor-infiltrating lymphocytes (TILs), and tumor regression.[82]

Tumor Depth or Thickness

Tumor depth or thickness is one of the most important prognostic factors in melanoma, especially for predicting SLN positivity and recurrence-free survival.[83,84] Breslow described it as thickness of melanoma measured from the top of the granular layer of epidermis, in millimeters.[85] This classification is still widely used to determine the T stage. It is also used to classify melanomas as thin (<1 mm), intermediate (1–4 mm), or thick melanomas (>4 mm) (**Figs. 4** and **5**).

Another classification was suggested by Clark and colleagues,[41] based on the layer of the reticular dermis invaded by the tumor. Although Clark thickness did show prognostic significance, its reliability is questioned because of the variability of skin thickness at different sites.

Lymph Node Status and Sentinel Lymph Node Biopsy

In patients with positive nodal status, the number of positive nodes serves as an important prognostic factor.[86] The nodal tumor burden and extranodal extension also are important prognostic factors.[87]

SLN biopsy is currently recommended for all intermediate-thickness melanomas.[81] It also be may considered in thin and thick melanomas based on presence of other clinical features.

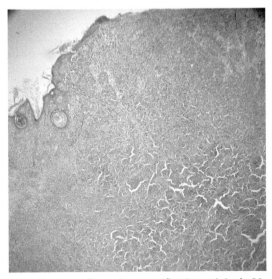

Fig. 4. Thick melanoma. Hematoxylin-eosin, magnification original x20.

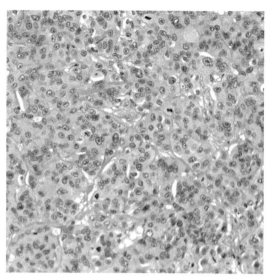

Fig. 5. Thick melanoma: high magnification of invasive component showing mitotic figures. Hematoxylin-eosin, magnification original x40.

Among the histologic types, ALM is associated with the highest rate of SLN-positive disease.[88]

Frozen section evaluation of SLN is not recommended, due to a high false-negative rate.[89] Accuracy of SLN evaluation is increased by a standardized protocol that includes serial sectioning of lymph node (LN) and additional examination of the sections with at least 2 immunohistochemical markers.[90]

There are various classification criteria for SLN that have been described. The Rotterdam criteria classify SLN based on the maximum diameter of the tumor deposit (<0.1 mm, 0.1–1 mm, and >1 mm). It has been shown that the tumor positivity rate in nonsentinel nodes increases with the size of the SLN tumor deposit.[91] The Dewar criteria is based on the microanatomic location of the tumor cells within the LN, classified as subcapsular, parenchymal, combined, multifocal, and extensive. Subcapsular location of the tumor deposit is associated with least tumor positivity in nonsentinel nodes and has best prognosis.[92]

Recent advances show that mitotic rate of SLN metastasis and immune response markers, such as follicular center count in the SLN, also have prognostic significance.[93,94]

Historically, SLN positivity was an indication for complete LN dissection (CLND). Although meta-analysis of studies comparing CLND versus observation in patients with SLN-positive disease have shown an advantage in disease control,[95,96] there are prospective trials that show no survival advantage of CLND, if the SLN micrometastasis is less than 1 mm.[97]

In-transit Lesions and Microsatellites

In-transit lesions appear as small pigmented or nonpigmented nodules and are a result of tumor cells getting trapped in the dermal lymphatics before reaching the draining nodal basin. These lesions are seen in 5% to 10% melanoma patients.[98] They are associated more commonly with intermediate and thick melanomas and with positive SLNs.

Microsatellite lesions were first described in 1981 as discrete tumor nests that are separated from the main body of the tumor by normal reticular dermal collagen or subcutaneous fat.[99] They have been associated with other poor prognostic features, such as increased primary tumor thickness, ulceration, and LN positivity, and associated with reduced disease-free survival (DFS) and overall survival (OS).[100]

Microsatellitosis along with macroscopic satellites and in-transit lesions are included in the AJCC stage III.[69]

Recent multi-institutional study suggests that stage IIIb patients with microsatellites, in the absence of other poor prognostic features, have better survival compared with the rest of the patients with the same stage.[101] Thus, SLN examination may be hold prognostic significance and may be considered in patients with microsatellitosis, even though it may not directly affect the staging of the disease.

Ulceration

Ulceration is defined as loss of continuity of the epidermis with surrounding inflammatory and reactive changes.[102] Ulceration has been associated with poor prognosis, with the extent of ulceration shown to be associated with higher nodal positivity rate.[84,103] It also predicts OS and DFS.[104] Ulceration has been shown to be associated with an improved response to interferon therapy.[105]

Mitotic Rate

Mitotic rate is identified per square millimeter, in the dermal hotspot (area with maximum mitosis) within the invasive melanoma. It has recently been excluded from the AJCC staging for melanoma.[69] It is an independent predictor, however, of SLN positivity and survival in melanoma patients.[106,107] Thus, the prognostic value of mitosis in melanoma may be considered in clinical decision making.

Lymphovascular Invasion

Lymphovascular invasion (LVI) is identified as presence of tumor cells in the dermal lymphatics and blood vessels around the primary tumor. It is a marker of poor prognosis that predicts SLN positivity and negatively influences OS and recurrence-free survival.[108] Although the detection of LVI can be the done with simple staining techniques, recent advancements in detection of lymphatic endothelial markers, such as D2-40, have improved the detection of LVI.[109,110]

Neurotropism or Perineural Invasion

Neurotropism or perineural invasion refers to tumor cells invading and spreading along perineural spaces. It does not have a significant effect on DFS.[111] It has been associated, however, with increased frequency of local recurrence.[112]

Tumor Margins

The surgical wide local excision of melanoma is aimed at achieving histologically clear margins. The peripheral and deep margins of the pathologic specimen are assessed for the presence of invasive melanoma or MIS. In cases of negative margins, distance of the tumor from the margin may be measured. Current NCCN guidelines suggest, however, that this distance should not play a role in the clinical decision making.[81]

In cases of a positive deep margin, it may be assumed that the tumor depth may be more than the reported depth.

Tumor-infiltrating Lymphocytes

Inflammatory cells invading all histologic types of melanoma have been described by Clark and colleagues.[41] TILs are lymphocytes that are in direct contact with tumor cells and/or infiltrate tumor nests.[113] They are prognostic markers that positively affect melanoma survival.[114] Identification of TILs in the tumor also helps predict positive response to immunotherapy.[113,115] TILs are now being used in adoptive immunotherapy for patients with metastatic melanoma and have produced successful regression of tumor in some patients.[116]

Tumor Regression

Tumor regression has been defined differently by various investigators. Most agree on lymphocytes with pigment-laden macrophages underlying an atrophic dermis.[117] College of American Pathologists guidelines define it as replacement of tumor cells with lymphocytic inflammation as well as attenuation of the epidermis and nonlaminated dermal fibrosis with inflammatory cells, melanophagocytosis, and telangiectasia.[82] The significance of tumor regression is not completely understood. Recent studies are challenging its prognostic role and have shown that it does not significantly affect LN metastasis or survival.[118,119]

In conclusion, pathologic evaluation of melanoma is important not only for diagnosis but also to identify important prognostic and predictive characteristics of the primary lesion and its local spread. Pathologic characteristics of the primary tumor must form the basis of the decision making for management of melanoma patients. In addition, new advancements in treatments targeting genetic alterations and TILS also cannot be undertaken without adequate pathologic analysis of the tumor.

REFERENCES

1. American Cancer Society. Cancer Facts & Figures 2018. Atlanta: American Cancer Society; 2018.
2. Tsai T, Vu C, Henson DE. Cutaneous, ocular and visceral melanoma in African Americans and Caucasians. Melanoma Res 2005;15(3):213–7.
3. Dawes SM, Tsai S, Gittleman H, et al. Racial disparities in melanoma survival. J Am Acad Dermatol 2016;75(5):983–91.
4. Dupin E, Calloni GW, Coelho-Aguiar JM, et al. The issue of the multipotency of the neural crest cells. Dev Biol 2018;444(Suppl 1):S47–59.
5. Kozovska Z, Gabrisova V, Kucerova L. Malignant melanoma: diagnosis, treatment and cancer stem cells. Neoplasma 2016;63(4):510–7.
6. Larribère L, Utikal J. Stem cell-derived models of neural crest are essential to understand melanoma progression and therapy resistance. Front Mol Neurosci 2019;12:111.
7. Whiteman DC, Parsons PG, Green AC. Determinants of melanocyte density in adult human skin. Arch Dermatol Res 1999;291(9):511–6.
8. Fears TR, Scotto J, Schneiderman MA. Mathematical models of age and ultraviolet effects on the incidence of skin cancer among whites in the United States. Am J Epidemiol 1977;105(5):420–7.
9. Schaffer JV. Update on melanocytic nevi in children. Clin Dermatol 2015;33(3):368–86.
10. Krengel S, Hauschild A, Schäfer T. Melanoma risk in congenital melanocytic naevi: a systematic review. Br J Dermatol 2006;155(1):1–8.

11. Krengel S, Scope A, Dusza SW, et al. New recommendations for the categorization of cutaneous features of congenital melanocytic nevi. J Am Acad Dermatol 2013;68(3):441–51.
12. Egan CL, Oliveria SA, Elenitsas R, et al. Cutaneous melanoma risk and phenotypic changes in large congenital nevi: a follow-up study of 46 patients. J Am Acad Dermatol 1998;39:923–32.
13. DeDavid M, Orlow SJ, Provost N, et al. A study of large congenital melanocytic nevi and associated malignant melanomas: review of cases in the New York University Registry and the world literature. J Am Acad Dermatol 1997;36(3 Pt 1): 409–16.
14. Sahin S, Levin L, Kopf AW. Risk of melanoma in medium-sized congenital melanocytic nevi: a follow-up study. J Am Acad Dermatol 1998;39(3):428–33.
15. Swerdlow AJ, English JS, Qiao Z. The risk of melanoma in patients with congenital nevi: a cohort study. J Am Acad Dermatol 1995;32:595–9.
16. Kinsler VA, O'Hare P, Bulstrode N. Melanoma in congenital melanocytic naevi. Br J Dermatol 2017;176(5):1131–43.
17. Roh MR, Eliades P, Gupta S, et al. Genetics of melanocytic nevi. Pigment Cell Melanoma Res 2015;28(6):661–72.
18. Kinsler VA, Thomas AC, Ishida M. Multiple congenital melanocytic nevi and neurocutaneous melanosis are caused by post zygotic mutations in codon 61 of NRAS. J Invest Dermatol 2013;133(9):2229–36.
19. Levy R, Lara-Corrales I. Melanocytic nevi in children: a review. Pediatr Ann 2016;45(8):e293–8.
20. Fritz A, Percy C, Jack A, et al, editors. International classification of diseases for oncology. 3rd edition. Geneva (Switzerland): World Health Organization; 2000.
21. Naeyaert JM, Brochez L. Clinical practice. Dysplastic nevi. N Engl J Med 2003; 349(23):2233–40.
22. Duffy K, Grossman D. The dysplastic nevus: from historical perspective to management in the modern era: part I. Historical, histologic, and clinical aspects. J Am Acad Dermatol 2012;67(1):1.e1-16 [quiz: 17–8].
23. Richard MA, Grob JJ, Gouvernet J, et al. Role of sun exposure on nevus. First study in age-sex phenotype-controlled populations. Arch Dermatol 1993; 129(10):1280–5.
24. Carey WP Jr, Thompson CJ, Synnestvedt M, et al. Dysplastic nevi as a melanoma risk factor in patients with familial melanoma. Cancer 1994;74(12): 3118–25.
25. Halpern AC, Guerry D 4th, Elder DE, et al. Dysplastic nevi as risk markers of sporadic (nonfamilial) melanoma. A case-control study. Arch Dermatol 1991; 127(7):995–9.
26. Spitz S. Melanomas of childhood. Am J Pathol 1948;24(3):591–609.
27. Ferrara G, Argenziano G, Soyer HP, et al. The spectrum of Spitz nevi: a clinicopathologic study of 83 cases. Arch Dermatol 2005;141:1381–7.
28. Harms KL, Lowe L, Fullen DR, et al. Atypical spitz tumors: a diagnostic challenge. Arch Pathol Lab Med 2015;139(10):1263–70.
29. Ferrara G, Gianotti R, Cavicchini S, et al. Spitz nevus, Spitz tumor, and spitzoid melanoma: a comprehensive clinicopathologic overview. Dermatol Clin 2013; 31(4):589–98, viii.
30. Tetzlaff MT, Reuben A, Billings SD, et al. Toward a molecular-genetic classification of spitzoid neoplasms. Clin Lab Med 2017;37(3):431–48.
31. Menezes FD, Mooi WJ. Spitz tumors of the skin. Surg Pathol Clin 2017;10(2): 281–98.

32. Rigel DS, Friedman RJ, Kopf AW, et al. ABCDE–an evolving concept in the early detection of melanoma. Arch Dermatol 2005;141(8):1032–4.
33. Clark WH Jr, Elder DE, Guerry D 4th, et al. A study of tumor progression: the precursor lesions of superficial spreading and nodular melanoma. Hum Pathol 1984;15(12):1147–65.
34. Elder DE. Melanoma progression. Pathology 2016;48(2):147–54.
35. Ackerman AB. Malignant melanoma in situ: the flat, curable stage of malignant melanoma. Pathology 1985;17(2):298–300.
36. Kallini JR, Jain SK, Khachemoune A. Lentigo maligna: review of salient characteristics and management. Am J Clin Dermatol 2013;14(6):473–80.
37. Cohen LM. Lentigo maligna and lentigo maligna melanoma. J Am Acad Dermatol 1995;33(6):923–36 [quiz: 937–40].
38. McKenna JK, Florell SR, Goldman GD, et al. Lentigo maligna/lentigo maligna melanoma: current state of diagnosis and treatment. Dermatol Surg 2006;32(4):493–504.
39. Mu EW, Quatrano NA, Yagerman SE, et al. Evaluation of MITF, SOX10, MART-1, and R21 immunostaining for the diagnosis of residual melanoma in situ on chronically sun-damaged skin. Dermatol Surg 2018;44(7):933–8.
40. Brown CD, Zitelli JA. The prognosis and treatment of true local cutaneous recurrent malignant melanoma. Dermatol Surg 1995;21(4):285–90.
41. Clark WH Jr, From L, Bernardino EA, et al. The histogenesis and biologic behavior of primary human malignant melanomas of the skin. Cancer Res 1969;29(3):705–27.
42. Coleman WP III, Loria PR, Reed RJ, et al. Acral lentiginous melanoma. Arch Dermatol 1980;116(7):773–6.
43. Duncan LM. The classification of cutaneous melanoma. Hematol Oncol Clin North Am 2009;23(3):501–13, ix.
44. Juhász ML, Marmur ES. Reviewing challenges in the diagnosis and treatment of lentigo maligna and lentigo-maligna melanoma. Rare Cancers Ther 2015;3:133–45.
45. Søndergaard K. Histological type and biological behavior of primary cutaneous malignant melanoma. 1. An analysis of 1916 cases. Virchows Arch A Pathol Anat Histopathol 1983;401(3):315–31.
46. Pollack LA, Li J, Berkowitz Z, et al. Melanoma survival in the United States, 1992 to 2005. J Am Acad Dermatol 2011;65(5 Suppl 1):S78–86.
47. Singh P, Kim HJ, Schwartz RA. Superficial spreading melanoma: an analysis of 97 702 cases using the SEER database. Melanoma Res 2016;26(4):395–400.
48. Scolyer RA, Long GV, Thompson JF. Evolving concepts in melanoma classification and their relevance to multidisciplinary melanoma patient care. Mol Oncol 2011;5(2):124–36.
49. Clark WH, Mihm MC. Lentigo maligna and lentigo-maligna melanoma. Am J Pathol 1969;55(1):39–67.
50. Green AC, Viros A, Hughes MCB, et al. Nodular melanoma: a histopathologic entity? Acta Derm Venereol 2018;98(4):460–2.
51. Lee JH, Choi JW, Kim YS. Frequencies of BRAF and NRAS mutations are different in histological types and sites of origin of cutaneous melanoma: a meta-analysis. Br J Dermatol 2011;164(4):776–84.
52. Bradford PT, Goldstein AM, McMaster ML, et al. Acral lentiginous melanoma: incidence and survival patterns in the United States, 1986-2005. Arch Dermatol 2009;145(4):427–34.
53. Piliang MP. Acral lentiginous melanoma. Surg Pathol Clin 2009;2(3):535–41.

54. Desai A, Ugorji R, Khachemoune A. Acral melanoma foot lesions. Part 2: clinical presentation, diagnosis, and management. Clin Exp Dermatol 2018;43(2): 117–23.
55. Fernandez-Flores A, Cassarino DS. Histopathological diagnosis of acral lentiginous melanoma in early stages. Ann Diagn Pathol 2017;26:64–9.
56. Nakamura Y, Fujisawa Y. Diagnosis and management of acral lentiginous melanoma. Curr Treat Options Oncol 2018;19(8):42.
57. Asgari MM, Shen L, Sokil MM, et al. Prognostic factors and survival in acral lentiginous melanoma. Br J Dermatol 2017;177(2):428–35.
58. Liu XK, Li J. Acral lentiginous melanoma. Lancet 2018;391(10137):e21.
59. Lino-Silva LS, Zepeda-Najar C, Salcedo-Hernández RA, et al. Acral lentiginous melanoma: survival analysis of 715 cases. J Cutan Med Surg 2019;23(1):38–43.
60. Conley J, Lattes R, Orr W. Desmoplastic malignant melanoma (a rare variant of spindle cell melanoma). Cancer 1971;28(4):914–36.
61. Chen LL, Jaimes N, Barker CA, et al. Desmoplastic melanoma: a review. J Am Acad Dermatol 2013;68(5):825–33.
62. Busam KJ. Cutaneous desmoplastic melanoma. Adv Anat Pathol 2005;12(2): 92–102.
63. Posther KE, Selim MA, Mosca PJ, et al. Histopathologic characteristics, recurrence patterns, and survival of 129 patients with desmoplastic melanoma. Ann Surg Oncol 2006;13(5):728–39.
64. Pawlik TM, Ross MI, Prieto VG, et al. Assessment of the role of sentinel lymph node biopsy for primary cutaneous desmoplastic melanoma. Cancer 2006; 106(4):900–6.
65. Scolyer RA, Thompson JF. Desmoplastic melanoma: a heterogeneous entity in which subclassification as "pure" or "mixed" may have important prognostic significance. Ann Surg Oncol 2005;12(3):197–9.
66. Busam KJ, Mujumdar U, Hummer AJ, et al. Cutaneous desmoplastic melanoma: reappraisal of morphologic heterogeneity and prognostic factors. Am J Surg Pathol 2004;28(11):1518–25.
67. Murali R, Shaw HM, Lai K, et al. Prognostic factors in cutaneous desmoplastic melanoma: a study of 252 patients. Cancer 2010;116(17):4130–8.
68. McLaughlin CC, Wu XC, Jemal A, et al. Incidence of non cutaneous melanomas in the U.S. Cancer 2005;103(5):1000–7.
69. Amin MB, Edge SB, Greene FL, et al. AJCC cancer staging manual. 8th edition. New York: Springer; 2017.
70. Billings KR, Wang MB, Sercarz JA, et al. Clinical and pathologic distinction between primary and metastatic mucosal melanoma of the head and neck. Otolaryngol Head Neck Surg 1995;112(6):700–6.
71. Sanchez AA, Wu TT, Prieto VG, et al. Comparison of primary and metastatic malignant melanoma of the esophagus: clinicopathologic review of 10 cases. Arch Pathol Lab Med 2008;132(10):1623–9.
72. Fitzgibbons PL, Chaurushiya PS, Nichols PW, et al. Primary malignant melanoma: an immunohistochemical study of 12 cases with comparison to cutaneous and metastatic melanomas. Hum Pathol 1989;20(3):269–72.
73. Mikkelsen LH, Larsen AC, von Buchwald C, et al. Mucosal malignant melanoma - a clinical, oncological, pathological and genetic survey. APMIS 2016;124(6): 475–86.
74. Chattopadhyay C, Kim DW, Gombos DS, et al. Uveal melanoma: from diagnosis to treatment and the science in between. Cancer 2016;122(15):2299–312.

75. Sellam A, Desjardins L, Barnhill R, et al. Fine needle aspiration biopsy in uveal melanoma: technique, complications, and outcomes. Am J Ophthalmol 2016; 162:28–34.e1.
76. Van Raamsdonk CD, Griewank KG, Crosby MB, et al. Mutations in GNA11 in uveal melanoma. N Engl J Med 2010;363(23):2191–9.
77. Staby KM, Gravdal K, Mørk SJ, et al. Prognostic impact of chromosomal aberrations and GNAQ, GNA11 and BAP1 mutations in uveal melanoma. Acta Ophthalmol 2018;96(1):31–8.
78. Shields CL, Say EAT, Hasanreisoglu M, et al. Personalized prognosis of uveal melanoma based on cytogenetic profile in 1059 patients over an 8-year period: the 2017 Harry S. Gradle Lecture. Ophthalmology 2017;124(10):1523–31.
79. Vora GK, Demirci H, Marr B, et al. Advances in the management of conjunctival melanoma. Surv Ophthalmol 2017;62(1):26–42.
80. Blum ES, Yang J, Komatsubara KM, et al. Clinical management of uveal and conjunctival melanoma. Oncology (Williston Park) 2016;30(1):29–32, 34-43, 48.
81. National Comprehensive Cancer Network. Cutaneous melanoma (Version 1.2019). Available at: https://www.nccn.org/professionals/physician_gls/pdf/cutaneous_melanoma.pdf. Accessed December 14, 2018.
82. Smoller BR, Gershenwald JE, Scolyer RA, et al. Protocol for the examination of specimens from patients with melanoma of the skin. Melanoma 4.0.0.0 (Posted June 2017). Based on AJCC/UICC TNM, 8th edition. 2017 College of American Pathologists (CAP). June 2017.
83. Cowart VS. Melanoma thickness correlates with prognosis. JAMA 1982;247(19):2656–7.
84. Namikawa K, Aung PP, Gershenwald JE, et al. Clinical impact of ulceration width, lymphovascular invasion, microscopic satellitosis, perineural invasion, and mitotic rate in patients undergoing sentinel lymph node biopsy for cutaneous melanoma: a retrospective observational study at a comprehensive cancer center. Cancer Med 2018;7(3):583–93.
85. Breslow A. Thickness, cross-sectional areas and depth of invasion in the prognosis of cutaneous melanoma. Ann Surg 1970;172(5):902–8.
86. Testori AA, Suciu S, van Akkooi ACJ, et al. Lymph node ratio as a prognostic factor in melanoma: results from European Organization for Research and Treatment of Cancer 18871, 18952, and 18991 studies. Melanoma Res 2018;28(3):222–9.
87. Frankel TL, Griffith KA, Lowe L, et al. Do micromorphometric features of metastatic deposits within sentinel nodes predict nonsentinel lymph node involvement in melanoma? Ann Surg Oncol 2008;15(9):2403–11.
88. Marek AJ, Ming ME, Bartlett EK, et al. Acral lentiginous histologic subtype and sentinel lymph node positivity in thin melanoma. JAMA Dermatol 2016;152(7):836–7.
89. Stojadinovic A, Allen PJ, Clary BM, et al. Value of frozen-section analysis of sentinel lymph nodes for primary cutaneous malignant melanoma. Ann Surg 2002;235(1):92–8.
90. Abrahamsen HN, Hamilton-Dutoit SJ, Larsen J, et al. Sentinel lymph nodes in malignant melanoma: extended histopathologic evaluationimproves diagnostic precision. Cancer 2004;100(8):1683–91.
91. van der Ploeg AP, van Akkooi AC, Schmitz PI, et al. EORTC Melanoma Group sentinel node protocol identifies high rate of submicrometastases according to Rotterdam Criteria. Eur J Cancer 2010;46(13):2414–21.

92. Dewar DJ, Newell B, Green MA, et al. The microanatomic location of metastatic melanoma in sentinel lymph nodes predicts nonsentinel lymph node involvement. J Clin Oncol 2004;22(16):3345–9.

93. Abbott J, Buckley M, Taylor LA, et al. Histological immune response patterns in sentinel lymph nodes involved by metastatic melanoma and prognostic significance. J Cutan Pathol 2018;45(6):377–86.

94. Baum C, Weiss C, Gebhardt C, et al. Sentinel node metastasis mitotic rate (SN-MMR) as a prognostic indicator of rapidly progressing disease in patients with sentinel node-positive melanomas. Int J Cancer 2017;140(8):1907–17.

95. Delgado AF, Delgado AF. Complete lymph node dissection in melanoma: a systematic review and meta-analysis. Anticancer Res 2017;37(12):6825–9.

96. Moreno-Ramírez D, Vidal-Sicart S, Puig S, et al. Should immediate lymphadenectomy be discontinued in patients with metastasis of a melanoma in the sentinel lymph node? Report of the results of the Multicenter Selective Lymphadenectomy Trial-II. Med Clin (Barc) 2018;150(8):323–6.

97. Leiter U, Stadler R, Mauch C, et al. Complete lymph node dissection versus no dissection in patients with sentinel lymph node biopsy positive melanoma (DeCOG-SLT): a multicentre, randomised, phase 3 trial. Lancet Oncol 2016;17(6):757–67.

98. Testori A, Ribero S, Bataille V. Diagnosis and treatment of in-transit melanoma metastasis. Eur J Surg Oncol 2017;43(3):544–60.

99. Day CL Jr, Harrist TJ, Gorstein F, et al. Malignant melanoma. Prognostic significance of "microscopic satellites" in the reticular dermis and subcutaneous fat. Ann Surg 1981;194(1):108–12.

100. Kimsey TF, Cohen T, Patel A, et al. Microscopic satellitosis in patients with primary cutaneous melanoma: implications for nodal basin staging. Ann Surg Oncol 2009;16(5):1176–83.

101. Karakousis GC, Gimotty PA, Leong SP, et al. Microsatellitosis in Patients with Melanoma. Ann Surg Oncol 2019;26(1):33–41.

102. Spatz A, Cook MG, Elder DE, et al. Interobserver reproducibility of ulceration assessment in primary cutaneous melanomas. Eur J Cancer 2003;39(13):1861–5.

103. Munsch C, Lauwers-Cances V, Lamant L, et al. Breslow thickness, clark index and ulceration are associated with sentinel lymph node metastasis in melanoma patients: a cohort analysis of 612 patients. Dermatology 2014;229(3):183–9.

104. Egger ME, Bhutiani N, Farmer RW, et al. Prognostic factors in melanoma patients with tumor-negative sentinel lymph nodes. Surgery 2016;159(5):1412–21.

105. Eggermont AM, Suciu S, Rutkowski P, et al. Long term follow up of the EORTC 18952 trial of adjuvant therapy in resected stage IIB-III cutaneous melanoma patients comparing intermediate doses of interferon-alpha-2b (IFN) with observation: ulceration of primary is key determinant for IFN-sensitivity. Eur J Cancer 2016;55:111–21.

106. Evans JL, Vidri RJ, MacGillivray DC, et al. Tumor mitotic rate is an independent predictor of survival for nonmetastatic melanoma. Surgery 2018;164(3):589–93.

107. Wheless L, Isom CA, Hooks MA, et al. Mitotic rate is associated with positive lymph nodes in patients with thin melanomas. J Am Acad Dermatol 2018;78(5):935–41.

108. Tas F, Erturk K. Histological lymphovascular invasion is associated with nodal involvement, recurrence, and survival in patients with cutaneous malignant melanoma. Int J Dermatol 2017;56(2):166–70.

109. Rose AE, Christos PJ, Lackaye D, et al. Clinical relevance of detection of lymphovascular invasion in primary melanoma using endothelial markers D2-40 and CD34. Am J Surg Pathol 2011;35(10):1441–9.
110. Feldmeyer L, Tetzlaff M, Fox P, et al. Prognostic implication of lymphovascular invasion detected by double immunostaining for D2-40 and MITF1 in primary cutaneous melanoma. Am J Dermatopathol 2016;38(7):484–91.
111. Varey AHR, Goumas C, Hong AM, et al. Neurotropic melanoma: an analysis of the clinicopathological features, management strategies and survival outcomes for 671 patients treated at a tertiary referral center. Mod Pathol 2017;30(11): 1538–50.
112. Baer SC, Schultz D, Synnestvedt M, et al. Desmoplasia and neurotropism. Prognostic variables in patients with stage I melanoma. Cancer 1995;76(11):2242–7.
113. Lee N, Zakka LR, Mihm MC Jr, et al. Tumour-infiltrating lymphocytes in melanoma prognosis and cancer immunotherapy. Pathology 2016;48(2):177–87.
114. Fortes C, Mastroeni S, Mannooranparampil TJ, et al. Tumor-infiltrating lymphocytes predict cutaneous melanoma survival. Melanoma Res 2015;25(4):306–11.
115. Zhu J, Powis de Tenbossche CG, Cané S, et al. Resistance to cancer immunotherapy mediated by apoptosis of tumor-infiltrating lymphocytes. Nat Commun 2017;8(1):1404.
116. Rosenberg SA, Restifo NP. Adoptive cell transfer as personalized immunotherapy for human cancer. Science 2015;348(6230):62–8.
117. Ribero S, Moscarella E, Ferrara G, et al. Regression in cutaneous melanoma: a comprehensive review from diagnosis to prognosis. J Eur Acad Dermatol Venereol 2016;30(12):2030–7.
118. Ribero S, Osella-Abate S, Dika E, et al. Prognostic role of histological regression in cutaneous melanoma. G Ital Dermatol Venereol 2017;152(6):638–41.
119. Tas F, Erturk K. Presence of histological regression as a prognostic factor in cutaneous melanoma patients. Melanoma Res 2016;26(5):492–6.

Surgical Management of Primary Cutaneous Melanoma

Daniel Joyce, MD, Joseph J. Skitzki, MD*

KEYWORDS

- Melanoma • Cutaneous melanoma • Wide local excision • Melanoma margins
- Melanoma biopsy • Melanoma synoptic report

KEY POINTS

- Melanocytic lesions require a biopsy to confirm melanoma with preference to biopsy techniques that define melanoma thickness and presence or absence of ulceration.
- Wide local excision is the definitive management of primary cutaneous melanomas and recommended margins of excision are evidence based.
- Closure of wide excision sites can vary by surgeon preference, but consideration for local recurrence, future therapies, and limiting morbidity is always warranted (eg, longitudinal incisions on the extremities).
- Although debated, the depth of excision for invasive melanomas should be to the level of the fascia, but does not need to include the fascia.
- Pathologic evaluations of melanoma before and after excision are standardized by synoptic reporting and aided by immunohistochemistry.

INTRODUCTION

Cancer arising from epidermal melanocytes is termed cutaneous melanoma. The term melanoma originated in the 1800s from the Greek for dark (*melas*) and tumor (*oma*); however, the disease was known from antiquity where it was described as a "fatal black tumor" as early as the time of Hippocrates.[1] Melanomas arising in the skin have been strongly linked to several risk factors including fair complexion, UV exposure, family history, prior melanomas, dysplastic nevi syndromes, and immunosuppression.[2] Currently in the United States, an estimated 96,480 cases of melanoma will be diagnosed in 2019 with a lifetime risk approaching 1 in 50 Caucasians. Fortunately, the death rate from melanoma is estimated to be much lower at 7230; however, this still equates to about 1 death per hour in the United States from melanoma.[3] The disparity between the number of diagnoses and attributable deaths from melanoma is

The authors have no disclosures to report.
Department of Surgical Oncology, Roswell Park Comprehensive Cancer Center, Buffalo, NY 14263, USA
* Corresponding author.
E-mail address: joseph.skitzki@roswellpark.org

likely a function of detection and treatment of localized disease. Public and medical professional awareness of the features of suspicious lesions has facilitated earlier detection. The ABCDEs define several features that indicate a pigmented lesion may be at higher risk for melanoma as opposed to a benign melanocytic lesion such as a nevus[4] (**Box 1**). Of these factors, evolution or change in the appearance, size, or characteristics is often the most useful. For example, if a pigmented lesion had several concerning features, but was present from birth and unchanged over decades, suspicion for melanoma would be low. On the contrary, even if a lesion lacks some of the A, B, C, and D hallmarks of a suspicious lesion, but is evolving and changing over time, this would be worrisome for a neoplastic lesion. This is particularly true for amelanotic melanoma lesions that lack pigment because melanoma may not be suspected based on clinical appearance. For any concerning cutaneous lesion suspicious for melanoma, a biopsy is absolutely required to obtain a tissue diagnosis and direct future definitive management.

TISSUE DIAGNOSIS

A biopsy is necessary to make a histologic diagnosis, but can also be leveraged to obtain information that will contribute to the staging of the primary tumor and dictate the subsequent definitive management. As a practical matter, all forms of biopsy can be done with local anesthesia consisting of 1% lidocaine solution in the clinic setting. Several methods of obtaining tissue can be used and the choice often depends on the level of suspicion, the anatomic location, the size of the lesion, and whether it is a primary tumor or a lesion concerning for metastasis or recurrence. Tumor thickness as defined by Breslow and the presence of ulceration are the 2 most important pieces of information that can be obtained by biopsy as these determine the T stage and are used to define the extent of margins on definitive wide local excision.[5] Therefore, biopsy techniques that include the full depth of the lesion to determine thickness and representative samples that may detect ulceration are necessary. Preferably, information from the initial biopsy should also include the status of the peripheral and deep margins, the mitotic index, the presence of microsatellite lesions, and whether the lesion is purely desmoplastic, which may further guide treatment decisions.[6] A punch biopsy is often ideal for these purposes, is well-tolerated, quick, and readily performed in the clinic (**Fig. 1**). If the entire skin lesion can be taken with a punch biopsy, the sampling of tumor thickness will be more accurate, and the presence of ulceration readily noted. If a lesion is too large to be encompassed by a single punch biopsy, the most

---

Box 1
The ABCDEs of cutaneous melanoma

A = Asymmetry
  Nonidentical sides if divided in half

B = Border irregularity
  Indistinct or ill-defined border

C = Color variegation
  Varied colors in same lesion

D = Diameter
  Larger than 6 mm (size of pencil eraser)

E = Evolution
  Change in size, shape, color, thickness, or bleeding over time

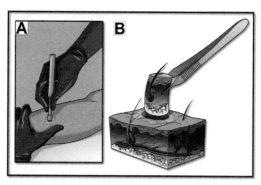

Fig. 1. A punch biopsy is performed of a suspicious lesion of the forearm (*A*) and a plug of tissue is taken down to the level of the subcutaneous fat (*B*).

suspicious areas should be sampled, especially areas that are raised (indicating vertical growth phase) or bleeding (indicating ulceration). Multiple punch biopsies can be obtained for large lesions or lesions that cover a broad area. The inclusion of normal-appearing surrounding skin may be useful in terms of orienting the sample and evaluating the potential extent and origin of the lesion that may not be evident clinically.[7] A drawback of the punch biopsy, or any other type of incisional biopsy, is the risk of underestimating the full features of the melanoma (e.g., thickness or presence of ulceration) which approximates 15% by recent reports.[8]

Alternatively, an excisional biopsy with 1- to 2-mm margins, without attempting to obtain definitive margins, can be used and has the benefit of sampling the entire lesion for accurate thickness and ulceration assessment.[9] The downside of an excisional biopsy is that it is often more involved than a simple punch biopsy and can create future issues for definitive wide local excision if not oriented correctly. An example of this would be an excisional biopsy on the extremity that is oriented transversely, especially if large. Because the resultant scar is transverse, there is more disruption of lymphatic tissue and distal drainage compared with a longitudinal scar. Compounding this issue is the need for wider margins with the definitive wide local excision and potential testing and/or removal of lymph nodes, which can all exacerbate, or at least increase, the risk for lymphedema of the extremity. When a primary tumor is large, a representative sample by punch biopsy or small incisional biopsy is preferred and attention to the likely future treatments is warranted.

A popular method of biopsy is the shave biopsy where a small blade can be used to sample the superficial layers of skin without the need for suture closure. Because the most important information to be obtained at the time of melanoma biopsy is the thickness and ulceration, there has been continued debate regarding the utility of shave biopsies because it may underestimate the total thickness of a melanoma.[10] Shave biopsies have become an acceptable practice over the last decade; studies indicate a low potential for upstaging of T stage tumor thickness and minimal impact on definitive treatment options.[11] In general shave biopsies can be slightly more cosmetic than suture closed biopsies, but this should be a secondary concern.

Fine needle aspiration (FNA) and core needle biopsies can also obtain a tissue diagnosis of melanoma, but are seldom used for suspicious primary cutaneous lesions. Rather, these techniques are useful for recurrent lesions, nodal recurrences, or concerning masses on examination or imaging. FNA is especially useful for suspected metastatic or recurrent lesions because it can be done in the clinic with immediate pathologic determination by cytology if available.[12] The advantages of FNA or core biopsy are that the diagnosis of recurrence can be made to direct additional imaging or treatment with minimal delay. Because thickness and ulceration are only necessary for classifying the primary lesion, FNA and core biopsies are adequate for the diagnosis of recurrent or metastatic disease where only the presence or absence of melanoma tumor cells is required.

Noninvasive techniques are in development to identify skin lesions that are likely to be high risk for melanoma while decreasing the need for multiple skin biopsies.[13] These technologies are not accepted practice at this time and any suspicious lesion warrants a tissue diagnosis via biopsy. Genomic testing, molecular testing, and other assays designed to provide additional prognostic or staging data regarding primary melanomas are also not accepted practice at this time and the current American Joint Committee on Cancer melanoma T staging does not include variables other than thickness and ulceration.[5] The initial biopsy dictates the subsequent definitive management and at no time should a definitive margin excision be performed without having the pathologic diagnosis, no matter how pathognomonic the lesion features may be for melanoma. The recommended definitive margins of excision completely depend on pathology evaluation and wide excision with complex closures or skin grafting in the absence of pathologic T staging data is unacceptable and often leads to greater long-term morbidity. Although sentinel node biopsy is described in Kirithiga Ramalingam and Shyam S Allamaneni's article, "Staging Melanoma: What's Old and New," in this issue and sentinel node biopsy can be performed after a wide excision, preference should always be to perform these simultaneously, especially if the nodal basin is in close proximity. In such circumstances, the background radiation at the prior excision site scar may mask the signal from the lymph node, a situation that can be avoided by doing the definitive wide local excision at the same time of sentinel node biopsy (ie, the wide excision removes the background radiation interference).

DEFINITIVE TREATMENT

The treatment for primary melanomas has evolved over time and reflects improvements in pathology and the diagnosis of early lesions. Historically, locally advanced melanomas were treated with amputation, cauterization, removal by knife or scissors, or application of caustic agents to the affected area; however, the mortality was essentially unchanged as patients died from metastatic disease that was unaffected by even amputation of the primary site.[14] The morbidity of amputation and the difficulty in treating nonextremity tumors lead to the adoption of wide excisions to treat cutaneous melanomas. The concept of margins for melanoma can be traced back to a single case report in 1907 of a young woman who died of melanoma.[15] On autopsy, several nodules were noted spreading radially from the primary site and their distance formed the basis for recommendations of excision margins. The recommended margins from this single report were approximately 5 cm and this constituted the standard margin for many decades. As anticipated, the morbidity of closure of these large wounds and total lack of impact on overall survival lead to several clinical trials regarding the optimal margin of excision. Data from these clinical trials represents some of the strongest evidence-based data in oncology and clearly demonstrated that the width of excision did not improve survival.[16–20] In fact, the concept of definitive margins is based on the thickness of the melanoma, which in turn is related to the risk of locoregional microscopic disease. It is almost certain that in widely margin negative excisions of melanoma, subsequent recurrence at the scar site is representative of local lymphatic spread and satellite or in-transit lesions that may have originally been centimeters away from the primary site.[21] The National Comprehensive Cancer Network recommended margins to be taken during wide local excision are therefore based on the melanoma thickness (**Table 1**) and are category 1 recommendations (high level of evidence, uniform consensus).[22] For simplicity, the recommended margins for melanoma in situ is 0.5 cm, invasive melanoma less than 1 mm in thickness is 1 cm, invasive melanoma between 1 and 2 mm thickness is discretionary between 1 and 2 cm, and 2 mm or greater in thickness is 2 cm. Factors that influence the decision to perform a 2-cm-wide excision in melanomas between 1 and 2 mm thickness include residual pigmentation or a positive deep margin on initial biopsy, which may indicated a thicker lesion than reported or in lesions greater than 1.5 mm in thickness with limited concern for cosmesis. As noted, the maximum margin taken for melanoma is currently 2 cm and has decreased the morbidity of resections significantly. In practice, the need for skin grafting based on the recommended margins should be less than 5%.

In lesions that have border irregularity, erythema, induration, or are depigmented at an edge, the safest place to measure from would be the abnormal appearing border with normal skin, especially because melanomas can exhibit varying degrees of regression and/or hypopigmentation. Amelanotic tumors and melanomas arising from extensive melanoma in situ lesions can be further identified with a Wood's lamp to gauge the extent and borders from which to measure margins.[23] The methods of measuring margins and converting to an ellipse of skin that can be closed primarily is demonstrated (**Fig. 2**). It needs to be emphasized that all wide excisions on the extremity need to be oriented longitudinally to limit disruption of lymphatics and facilitate re-excision and primary closure in cases of recurrence. The orientation of wide excisions of the trunk is often less critical and is best accomplished by producing the least skin tension for a primary closure. Surgeon preference often determines the type of suture closure. A single layer, interrupted deep dermal absorbable suture placed at the subcuticular layer can achieve both a strong and cosmetic closure. Spacing of sutures and performing a single layer closure limits the amount of reaction to foreign material and minimizes handling of the tissues so that healing is optimized. For closures with excessive tension, reinforcing full-thickness interrupted nonabsorbable monofilament sutures can be placed for added security and removed after 3 weeks. The epidermis can be reapproximated with strips or surgical glue based on preference. In large defects where the midportion cannot be fully approximated, a small portion of the incision can be left to heal by secondary intention with good cosmetic results. Other than local advancement flaps, complex rotational flaps, skin expansion, and skin grafting should be done only in cases where the risk of local recurrence is low and there are no concerns for margins after excision.

Table 1 Margins of excision	
Tumor Thickness	Recommended Clinical Margins (cm)
In situ	0.5–1.0
≤1.0 mm	1.0
>1.0–2.0 mm	1.0–2.0
>2.0–4.0 mm	2.0
>4.0 mm	2.0

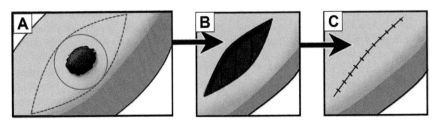

Fig. 2. A wide excision is performed by measuring the desired distance from the tumor edges (*red circle*) and converting this to an ellipse (*purple ellipse*) (*A*). The skin and underlying subcutaneous tissue is excised to the level of the fascia (*B*). The wound edges are reapproximated leaving a linear scar (*C*).

Unlike the well-described and evaluated wide excision margins, the depth of excision has been less studied.[15] There is often a lack of consensus between surgeons and limited data to drive standardized recommendations.[24] In general, for invasive melanomas requiring a wide local excision, the surrounding skin as defined by recommended margins and all the subcutaneous tissue up to the level of the fascia should be taken. This anatomic area ensures that subcutaneous lymphatic tissue and any extension of the original melanoma are removed. The fascia itself can remain intact and has not been associated with an increased risk of recurrence if not taken.[25] In lesions that are extensive, neglected, or have evidence of invasion into the fascia, the fascia and any underlying tissue may be removed as indicated; however, this would be anticipated to be the minority of wide local excisions. For melanoma in situ, a portion of subcutaneous tissue should be taken and does not require removal to the level of the fascia given the noninvasive nature of this lesion.

In acral lentiginous melanomas that arise in the fingers or toes, wide excision is often not possible without leaving exposed tendon or bone, and complex closures may offer more functional harm than benefit. The invasive nature or these acral melanomas and their often-delayed presentation and relative thickness necessitate distal amputation.[26] Standard recommended margins for wide excision are applied, but the tumor thickness may not necessarily be related to the risk of local or regional spread which is typically higher in these lesions. In rare cases of melanoma in situ, wide excisions may be possible without exposing tendons or bone, but any evidence of invasion warrants an aggressive approach. For melanomas on the palm or dorsum of the hand, heel, dorsal foot, or plantar surfaces, a wide local excision and delayed healing may be useful. Skin grafting can be considered once definitive margins are taken and healthy granulation tissue forms at the base. Immediate skin grafting is often at risk to fail from poorly vascularized tissue beds, shear forces, and the potential for a positive margin that would require re-excision. Healing by secondary intention without skin grafting should be strongly considered as the wound heals to conform to lines of tension, the skin is full thickness, and there is no need for immobility or restrictions. Contrary to skin grafting, the patient is often encouraged to maintain full range of motion and activity with no sacrifice of long-term cosmetic results (**Fig. 3**). This technique has proven to be a useful option in patients willing to put effort into wound care in the short term because the long-term results are quite favorable.

PATHOLOGY EVALUATION

The wide excision specimen can be fixed in formalin for paraffin embedding. Fresh tissue is not necessary unless specific tissue procurement or research protocols are

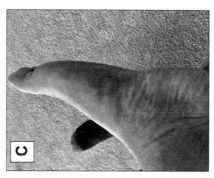
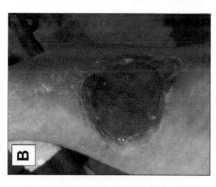
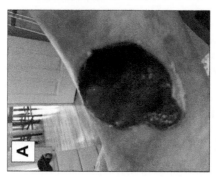

Fig. 3. Healing by secondary intention of a wide excision site on the medial plantar surface of the left foot at 1 month after excision (A), 2 months after excision (B), and 8 months after excision (C).

being used. To facilitate a proper evaluation of the margins of excision, a marking stitch is used to orient the specimen before it leaves the surgical field. A single stitch is usually adequate to denote proximal or superior as the epidermis clearly defines the superficial surface. Pathology evaluation includes the radial and deep margins which may be facilitated by immunohistochemistry. Common immunohistochemistry markers for melanoma include Melan-A, S100, HMB-45, tyrosinase, and microphthalmia-associated transcription factor (MITF).[27] The final pathology report includes the margin status, the final thickness of the melanoma, and any other histologic features, as well as the presence or absence of satellite lesions for staging.[6] In general, the distance from the tumor to the margin as reported in the final pathology specimen should not be confused with the recommended surgical margins that were measured and taken clinically. Shrinkage of the specimen occurs when it is freed from the surrounding skin and less so from formalin fixation,[28] so these measures are often not related to the clinical measures.[29] Re-excision is only recommended if clear margins are not achieved or if the melanoma has a greater thickness than anticipated from the initial biopsy that may increase the recommended margin (eg, from 1 cm to 2 cm margins).

FUTURE OF SURGICAL MANAGEMENT

The curative treatment of primary cutaneous melanomas has been the exclusive domain of surgery for the previous century. The methods of surgery are evolving and techniques such as Moh's surgery has been extended to melanoma lesions. The benefit of taking the least possible margin with Moh's surgery may be useful in melanoma in situ lesions or lentigo maligna of the face or head.[30] The concern with this approach is that ,unlike basal cell carcinomas where Moh's surgery is clearly indicated, the ability to discern melanoma cells at the margin has been limiting. With improvement in immunohistochemistry techniques, the ability of Moh's to clear melanoma in situ lesions has become increasingly accepted; however, the potential for an invasive component and the need for wide margins defined by years of clinical trials remains a concern. For these reasons, any invasive melanoma should not be addressed by Moh's surgery, because the key concept for wide excision margins is to include any tumor deposits in proximity to the primary site. There is ongoing debate as to the appropriate application of Moh's surgery for melanoma, but current guidelines do not endorse this technique.[22]

The landscape of melanoma treatment has evolved quickly in the last 5 years with the introduction of effective immunotherapies, small molecule inhibitors, and local injectables. These therapies are used in the metastatic and adjuvant settings, and are actively being investigated in the neoadjuvant setting. For primary cutaneous melanoma, wide local excision remains the fastest, cheapest, and most curative treatment to date; however, in large, neglected, or high-risk tumors, there may be a role for these agents in the near future. Last, there will be the rare patient encountered who cannot undergo a wide excision without significant morbidity. In such circumstances, radiation therapy (and several other modalities of topical and injectable therapies) have been applied. Although this strategy is not optimal for a cure, it can sometimes address symptomatic lesions in patients with limited life expectancy or limiting comorbidities.[31] These situations are rare and a wide local excision under local anesthesia can be tolerated by almost any patient.

REFERENCES

1. Gorantla VC, Kirkwood JM. State of melanoma: an historic overview of a field in transition. Hematol Oncol Clin North Am 2014;28(3):415–35.

2. Rastrelli M, Tropea S, Rossi CR, et al. Melanoma: epidemiology, risk factors, pathogenesis, diagnosis and classification. In Vivo 2014;28(6):1005–11.
3. Hurlbert M. Estimated rates of melanoma increasing in 2019, vol. 2019. Washington, DC: Melanoma Research Alliance; 2019.
4. Thomas L, Tranchand P, Berard F, et al. Semiological value of ABCDE criteria in the diagnosis of cutaneous pigmented tumors. Dermatology 1998;197(1):11–7.
5. Gershenwald JE, Scolyer RA, Hess KR, et al. Melanoma staging: evidence-based changes in the American Joint Committee on Cancer eighth edition cancer staging manual. CA Cancer J Clin 2017;67(6):472–92.
6. Maley A, Patrawala S, Stoff B. Compliance with the College of American Pathologists Protocol for Melanoma in Synoptic and Non-Synoptic reports: a cross-sectional study. J Am Acad Dermatol 2016;74(1):179–81.
7. Levitt J, Bernardo S, Whang T. Videos in clinical medicine. How to perform a punch biopsy of the skin. N Engl J Med 2013;369(11):e13.
8. Doolan BJ, Robinson AJ, Wolfe R, et al. Accuracy of partial biopsies in the management of cutaneous melanoma. Australas J Dermatol 2019;60(3):209–13.
9. Hieken TJ, Hernandez-Irizarry R, Boll JM, et al. Accuracy of diagnostic biopsy for cutaneous melanoma: implications for surgical oncologists. Int J Surg Oncol 2013;2013:196493.
10. de Menezes SL, Kelly JW, Wolfe R, et al. The increasing use of shave biopsy for diagnosing invasive melanoma in Australia. Med J Aust 2019;211(5):213–8.
11. Zager JS, Hochwald SN, Marzban SS, et al. Shave biopsy is a safe and accurate method for the initial evaluation of melanoma. J Am Coll Surg 2011;212(4):454–60 [discussion: 460–2].
12. Lindsey KG, Ingram C, Bergeron J, et al. Cytological diagnosis of metastatic malignant melanoma by fine-needle aspiration biopsy. Semin Diagn Pathol 2016;33(4):198–203.
13. Fink C, Haenssle HA. Non-invasive tools for the diagnosis of cutaneous melanoma. Skin Res Technol 2017;23(3):261–71.
14. Rebecca VW, Sondak VK, Smalley KS. A brief history of melanoma: from mummies to mutations. Melanoma Res 2012;22(2):114–22.
15. DeFazio JL, Marghoob AA, Pan Y, et al. Variation in the depth of excision of melanoma: a survey of US physicians. Arch Dermatol 2010;146(9):995–9.
16. Khayat D, Rixe O, Martin G, et al. Surgical margins in cutaneous melanoma (2 cm versus 5 cm for lesions measuring less than 2.1-mm thick). Cancer 2003;97(8):1941–6.
17. Cohn-Cedermark G, Rutqvist LE, Andersson R, et al. Long term results of a randomized study by the Swedish Melanoma Study Group on 2-cm versus 5-cm resection margins for patients with cutaneous melanoma with a tumor thickness of 0.8-2.0 mm. Cancer 2000;89(7):1495–501.
18. Veronesi U, Cascinelli N. Narrow excision (1-cm margin). A safe procedure for thin cutaneous melanoma. Arch Surg 1991;126(4):438–41.
19. Balch CM, Urist MM, Karakousis CP, et al. Efficacy of 2-cm surgical margins for intermediate-thickness melanomas (1 to 4 mm). Results of a multi-institutional randomized surgical trial. Ann Surg 1993;218(3):262–7 [discussion: 267–9].
20. Thomas JM, Newton-Bishop J, A'Hern R, et al. Excision margins in high-risk malignant melanoma. N Engl J Med 2004;350(8):757–66.
21. Wysong A, Higgins S, Blalock TW, et al. Defining skin cancer local recurrence. J Am Acad Dermatol 2019;81(2):581–99.

22. Coit DG, Thompson JA, Albertini MR, et al. Cutaneous melanoma, version 2.2019, NCCN clinical practice guidelines in oncology. J Natl Compr Canc Netw 2019; 17(4):367–402.

23. Sharma S, Sharma A. Robert Williams Wood: pioneer of invisible light. Photodermatol Photoimmunol Photomed 2016;32(2):60–5.

24. Grotz TE, Markovic SN, Erickson LA, et al. Mayo Clinic consensus recommendations for the depth of excision in primary cutaneous melanoma. Mayo Clin Proc 2011;86(6):522–8.

25. Hunger RE, Seyed Jafari SM, Angermeier S, et al. Excision of fascia in melanoma thicker than 2 mm: no evidence for improved clinical outcome. Br J Dermatol 2014;171(6):1391–6.

26. Goydos JS, Shoen SL. Acral lentiginous melanoma. Cancer Treat Res 2016;167: 321–9.

27. Ohsie SJ, Sarantopoulos GP, Cochran AJ, et al. Immunohistochemical characteristics of melanoma. J Cutan Pathol 2008;35(5):433–44.

28. Dauendorffer JN, Bastuji-Garin S, Guero S, et al. Shrinkage of skin excision specimens: formalin fixation is not the culprit. Br J Dermatol 2009;160(4):810–4.

29. Friedman EB, Dodds TJ, Lo S, et al. Correlation between surgical and histologic margins in melanoma wide excision specimens. Ann Surg Oncol 2019;26(1): 25–32.

30. Nosrati A, Berliner JG, Goel S, et al. Outcomes of melanoma in situ treated with Mohs micrographic surgery compared with wide local excision. JAMA Dermatol 2017;153(5):436–41.

31. Barker CA. Radiation therapy for cutaneous melanoma: clonogenic assays to clinical trials. Oncology (Williston Park) 2015;29(10):752, 754.

Surgical Management of Lymph Nodes in Melanoma

Alexandra Allard-Coutu, BSc, MDCM, Barbara Heller, MD, FRCSC,
Valerie Francescutti, MD, MSc, FRCSC*

KEYWORDS

- Melanoma • Sentinel lymph node (SLN) • SLN Biopsy (SLNBx)
- Completion lymph node dissection (CLND) • Regional node management
- locoregional control

KEY POINTS

- Sentinel lymph node biopsy in patients with melanoma provides important prognostic information.
- Completion lymphadenectomy is not associated with a survival benefit.
- Early nodal intervention remains controversial, without clear survival benefit.
- Clinically positive nodes are managed surgically to maintain locoregional control. Increasingly, adjuvant treatment or enrollment in clinical trials is offered.
- Either completion lymph node dissection or nodal surveillance may be offered to patients with low-risk micrometastatic nodal disease.

INTRODUCTION

The ability of melanoma to spread to lymph nodes has been well described, and regional nodal basins have long been recognized as a critical factor in clinical decision making in melanoma. Although the mainstay of treatment of melanoma continues to be resection of the primary tumor with wide local excision (WLE), the management of regional lymph nodes has evolved considerably over the past 20 years.

There remains significant controversy with regards to patient selection and clinical decision making for both sentinel lymph node (SLN) biopsy and completion lymph node dissection (CLND).[1–3] Moreover, with advances in targeted and immune adjuvant therapies, regional lymph node status for accurate prognostication has become increasingly clinically relevant.[2,4] This article reviews the literature on the importance of regional lymph node management in melanoma, focusing on patient selection for

Disclosure Statement: The authors have nothing to disclose.
Department of Surgery, McMaster University, Hamilton General Hospital, 237 Barton Street East, 6 North, Hamilton, Ontario L8L 2X2, Canada
* Corresponding author.
E-mail address: francev@mcmaster.ca

Surg Clin N Am 100 (2020) 71–90
https://doi.org/10.1016/j.suc.2019.09.002
0039-6109/20/© 2019 Elsevier Inc. All rights reserved.

surgical.theclinics.com

SLN biopsy and CLND, technical considerations, and management of patients with clinically positive nodes.

MANAGEMENT OF CLINICALLY NEGATIVE NODAL BASINS

Most primary cutaneous melanomas spread through intradermal lymphatics to the regional nodes prior to affecting to distant sites.[5-9] Early research in lymph node mapping revealed that each area of skin is connected to specific lymph nodes in the regional draining basin.[5-7] This led to the discovery of SLNs, defined as the first nodes in the drainage pathway of a cutaneous lesion, thus the first nodes to receive tumor cells from the primary site.[5-10]

Three decades of cumulative data reveal routine CLND removes detectable metastasis in only 20% of specimens, implying that 80% of patients undergoing CLND do not experience a clinical benefit from the procedure.[8-11] In addition, randomized control trials have failed to demonstrate improved overall survival for patients undergoing routine elective CLND, although there may be some survival benefit in certain subgroups.[8,9,12]

Initially described in 1992, the SLN biopsy was pioneered by Morton as a minimally invasive way to identify patients with occult nodal metastases who might benefit from early CLND.[6-11] The SLN biopsy has since become a safe and well established procedure, proved effective for prognostication and patient selection for treatment planning.[6-11,13-16] In addition, lymphatic mapping identifies lymph node basins draining from primary sites associated with unclear or multiple nodal basins.[5-7] Such sites include the trunk, head and neck, and distal extremities, where dynamic lymphatic flow studies reveal ambiguous and multidirectional drainage pathways.[5-7,17-19]

In 2009, the American Joint Committee on Cancer staging system formally recognized the prognostic value of micrometastasis to regional lymph nodes.[20-24] With increasing availability of immunohistochemical staining, nodal metastases at a microscopic level consisting of aggregates of only a few cells are readily and routinely detectable.[20-24] These micrometastases have been shown to be clinical relevant, whereby 5-year survival rates range from 70% in patients with a single SLN with micrometastases compared with 39% for patients with 4 or more involved nodes.[20,21] Taken together, these findings have shifted treatment paradigms favoring SLN biopsy in a large subset of patients.

Table 1 Predicting sentinel lymph node positivity	
Increased risk of SLN positivity[1,9,14]	• 0.8-mm thick or <0.8 mm thick + ulceration • Extracapsular extension • Concomitant microsatellitosis of primary • 3 involved nodes • 2 involved nodal basins • Immunosuppression
Variable increased risk of SLN positivity[9,14]	• Young age • Thickness of primary lesion • Infiltrating lymphocytes • LI
Increased risk of false negative[9,14]	• >60 y of age • Increased primary lesion thickness • Prior flap reconstruction or WLE • Ulcerated lesions

Sentinel Lymph Node Biopsy for Regional Nodal Staging

Coupled with lymphoscintigraphy to identify the location of tumor-draining nodal basins, the SLN biopsy is a sensitive and specific evaluation of regional nodes without the surgical morbidity of an elective lymph node dissection (**Tables 1** and **2**).[5–11,13] Literature review and meta-analysis involving the most recent large multicenter trials reveals SLN are identified in 97% to 98% of patients with melanoma, of which 20% have a positive SLN.[8–10,13–15]

The Multicenter Selective Lymphadenectomy Trial (MSLT)-I is the largest trial designed to study the accuracy of nodal staging based on SLN biopsy as well as to assess the role of lymphatic mapping with SLN biopsy in determining prognosis and the impact of SLN biopsy on survival.[8–10] A total of 1269 patients with 1.2-mm to 3.5-mm thick melanomas were randomized to either wide excision plus SLN biopsy, with immediate CLND if the nodes were positive, versus WLE followed by observation, with CLND only if there was clinical evidence of nodal recurrence.[8]

The incidence of nodal metastasis was shown to vary by primary melanoma thickness.[8–10,12,14,20,27–31] Specifically, among patients with intermediate-thickness melanoma (1.2–3.5 mm), the incidence for nodal metastasis was 19.8% in the SLN biopsy group and 42% in the thicker melanoma group (>3.5 mm).[12,30,31] Moreover, MSLT-I data confirm that regional lymph nodes are noted to be clinically detectable

Table 2 Technical considerations—sentinel node	
Accuracy	• Peritumor intradermal injection of blue dye (methylene blue, isosulfan blue) and/or radioactive tracer identifies SLNs.[5–8,11] • Preoperative lymphoscintigraphy and/or intraoperative gamma probe localization increases diagnostic accuracy.[6–9,15–17] • Blue dye identifies SLN in 82% of cases.[5–8] • Using both radiolabeled colloid and blue dye increases the identification of at least 1 SLN to more than 96%.[11,17,25,26]
Identifying SLN	• In 99% of basins, the SLN is the hottest or second-hottest node present.[25,26] • These findings led to the 10% rule, whereby nodes with a radioactive count ≥10% of the ex vivo count of the hottest node are considered SLNs. • All blue or grossly abnormal nodes also should be removed.[25]
False negatives	• Handheld gamma probes are associated with operator-dependent sensitivity. • SLNs can be missed due to unexpected topographic positions, increased body habitus, or signal error related to proximity to the injection site.[17,25,26] • The field of detection of the probe may miss smaller, mobile nodes.[25,26] • Other contributing factors include inadequate pathologic examination, poor tracer injection technique, insufficient imaging of nodal basins, failure to detect in-transit nodes, and complete neoplastic replacement of the node.[6–11,16,47,48]
Nonmapping	• If dual SLN localization technique with both blue dye/radiolabeled tracer fails, in the absence of palpable or grossly abnormal nodes, consider reinjection with tracer.[6–11] • The procedure can also be aborted to allow further discussion with the patient or a multidisciplinary tumor board. • In some circumstances, the nodal basin can be observed with serial physical examinations and ultrasound.[5–8,11] • Alternatively, if appropriate, an ELND can be considered.[8,11,27–31,38,39]

at 15 mm to 20 mm in diameter, whereby 0.05-mm micrometastases are detected in an SLN biopsy.[1,2,6–11]

These trials convincingly demonstrated the prognostic significance of the sentinel node. The presence of microscopic involvement of the SLN was found to be a significant predictor of subsequent relapse in patients with intermediate or thick primary melanomas.[8–10,12,20,27–31] For patients with intermediate-thickness melanoma, the melanoma-specific survival rate at 10 years was significantly decreased when the biopsied SLN was positive (62% vs 85%; hazard ratio [HR] 3.09; 95% CI, 2.12–4.49).[1,2,12,29–31] Similarly, in patients with thick melanoma, the melanoma-specific survival rate at 10 years was 48.0% in patients with a positive SLN versus 64.6% in patients with a negative SLN biopsy (HR 1.75; 95% CI, 1.07–2.87).[1,2,8–10,20]

Risks and Benefits

The decision to pursue SLN biopsy is based on an individualized discussion of risks and benefits for each patient as well as the predicted risk of SLN positivity (see **Table 1**). In general, the risks associated with SLN biopsy are low, including seroma, wound infection, and, rarely, lymphedema.[6–10,21–24] MSLT-I and the Sunbelt Melanoma Trial study support the claim that SLN biopsy is associated with significantly fewer complications than regional lymphadenectomy (**Table 3**).[1,2,8,34]

At a median follow-up of 16 months, the overall complication rate was significantly lower for SLN biopsy as compared to CLND (5% vs 23%), with reduced wound infection (1% vs 7%), lymphedema (0.7% vs 11.7%), hematoma/seroma (2% vs 6%), and sensory nerve injury (0.2% vs 1.8%).[6–10,34] The difference was dramatic in groin procedures, with a total complications rate of 8% with an SLN biopsy versus 51% after CLND, and the incidence of lymphedema after SLN biopsy was reduced to 2% from 32% after CLND.[10,21–24,34]

The threshold at which the risk of the SLN biopsy is justified varies by institution and by surgeon, taking into consideration patient characteristics and preferences. A predicted SLN biopsy positivity rate of greater than or equal to 10% is a reasonable threshold, below which the procedure is not recommended.[22–24,35,36]

PATIENT SELECTION AND RECOMMENDATIONS FOR SENTINEL LYMPH NODE BIOPSY
Thin Melanoma (≤1-mm Breslow Thickness)

Thin lesions represent 70% of newly diagnosed melanoma.[27–29] There is thus a substantial absolute number of patients in this subgroup predicted to have positive

Table 3
Comparative morbidity of sentinel lymph node biopsy versus completion lymph node dissection in melanoma

	Wound Infection (%)	Lymphedema (%)	Hematoma/ Seroma (%)	Sensory Nerve Injury (%)	Overall (%)
Sentinel lymph node biopsy[9,21,32]	1–3	0.7–1	0.5–2	0–0.2	3–8
CLND[9,21,32,]	8–31	12–25	6–20	3–18	23–51
Axilla[9,21,32]	3–15	12	2–17	4–45	12–45
Groin[33]	20–30	20–45	20–32	15–34	15–72

SLNs.[27] The overall risk of SLN positivity in this group is cited as approximately 5%, and thus the selection for SLN biopsy becomes controversial.[1,2,10,27–29]

At this time, routine SLN biopsy is not recommended for patients with T1a melanomas (nonulcerated, <0.8 mm).[22–24,35,36] It is reasonable, however, to offer SLN biopsy in the presence of multiple additive risk factors, such as a young patient with a thin, nonulcerated melanoma with evidence of lymphovascular invasion (LVI) and a high mitotic rate, because the predicted risk of a positive SLN increases, approaching 10%.[1,2,13–16,24,35–37] In the setting of T1b lesions (0.8–1 mm ± ulceration, <0.8 mm with ulceration), SLN biopsy should be discussed and considered.[13–16,22–24,35,36]

Intermediate-thickness melanoma (>1-mm to 4-mm Breslow Thickness)

There are strong data supporting the use of SLN biopsy in this population in the MSLT-I trial, where the estimated risk of SLN positivity is approximately 15%.[8–12,30,31] As such, based on the prognostic significance, and a potential therapeutic benefit, SLN biopsy has been widely adopted in intermediate thickness, including patients with T2 or T3 melanomas.[22–24,35,36]

The risk of SLN positivity in intermediate-thickness melanoma is based on a variety of clinicopathologic risk factors and has been shown highly variable. Multivariate analysis demonstrates that age, thickness (1.00–1.49 mm vs 1.50–4.00 mm), tumor-infiltrating lymphocytes, LVI, and microsatellites all are statistically significant predictors of sentinel node positivity in this subgroup (see **Table 1**).[8–12,30,31]

Thick Melanoma (>4-mm Breslow Thickness)

Although the risk of SLN positivity in thick melanoma approaches 30% to 40%,[9,10] there is debate with regard to routine SLN biopsy given that this subgroup also is at increased risk of distant disease at the time of diagnosis.[1,2,14–16,20] MSLT-I data on long-term outcomes of high-risk patients with thick melanomas (>3.5 mm) revealed SLN biopsy was highly prognostic of survival in this cohort (65% 10-year survival if SLN negative vs 48% if SLN positive; $P = .003$).[8–10]

This data are further corroborated by several retrospective studies demonstrating significant prognostic value of the SLN even in the setting of thick melanoma.[1,2,9,10,14–16,20] Contrary to patients with intermediate-thickness melanoma, however, there is no associated survival benefit, which is not surprising given the likelihood of distant spread at the time of initial therapy.[8–10,20] Despite this, SLN biopsy is recommended in this group of patients, for prognostication and treatment planning.[20,22–24,35,36]

Sentinel Lymph Node Biopsy for Local Recurrence

SLN biopsy is reasonable in the setting of isolated local recurrence if a positive node will inform a decision for adjuvant therapy or eligibility for clinical trials. A positive SLN biopsy in this subgroup is associated with poor outcomes, including decreased disease-specific survival and increased locoregional recurrence.[38,39] The rate of positive SLN biopsy in this population has been described as high as 40%, and the rate of non–sentinel node positivity as high as 30% to 40%.[25,38,39]

Whether CLND adds prognostic or therapeutic benefit in this setting remains unclear. Moreover, although prior WLE theoretically disrupts lymphatic drainage, multiple retrospective studies offer subgroup analysis for SLN biopsy post-WLE, and the data suggest it remains highly prognostic (**Table 4**).[32,45–47]

| Table 4 |
| Special considerations—sentinel |
Positive deep biopsy margins	• Up to 40% of skin biopsies in patients with clinically localized melanoma are found to have a positive deep margin.[40,41] • This is particularly relevant in thin melanomas, because a tenth of a millimetre may affect the decision to perform an SLN biopsy.[21,23,24,40] • Positive deep margins, however, do not confer added risk of SLN positivity in thin melanomas.[40,41] • Careful consideration of a patient's clinicopathologic risk factors is warranted for thin melanomas with positive deep margins.
Prior WLE	• Prior WLE theoretically disrupts lymphatic drainage and could limit the accuracy of the SLN biopsy. • Despite the hypothetical damage to lymphatics, multiple retrospective studies offer subgroup analysis for SLN biopsy post-WLE, and the data suggest it remains highly prognostic.[42–44] • Significant flap reconstruction is, however, associated with an increased SLN biopsy false-negative rate.[42] • To limit false negatives, SLN biopsies should be performed at the time of the definitive resection.[1,2,22–24,35,36,42]
Lesions on the trunk	• Preoperative imaging should include axillary and inguinal basins due to variable lymphatic drainage, and SLNs in multiple basins is common.[1,2,6–10,17,18] • Careful evaluation for in-transit nodes in warranted.[17,18,39,43]
Isolated local recurrence	• SLN biopsy is recommended for isolated locally recurrent melanoma as well as limited in-transit disease if a positive node informs a decision for adjuvant therapy or eligibility clinical trials. • Clinical data are limited by low event rates, and there are no available data on long-term outcomes.[42–44] • Nevertheless, a positive SLN biopsy in this subgroup is associated with poor outcomes including decreased disease-specific survival and increased locoregional recurrence.[43,44] • The rate of positive SLN biopsy in this population has been described as high as 40% and the rate of nonsentinel node positivity as high as 30%–40%.[42] • Whether CLND adds prognostic or therapeutic benefit in this setting remains unclear.

Clinically Apparent Residual Lesion

A clinically apparent residual lesion in addition to an incongruous biopsy warrants special consideration. Certain lesions are associated with higher rates of underestimated thickness, including subungual and acral melanomas.[48,49] Clinical suspicion of underestimated thickness or extent of disease should guide rebiopsy, or treatment can be planned assuming a higher T stage, if appropriate.[1,2,48,49] Some studies further suggest acral melanomas may represent an independent risk factor for SLN positivity and overall survival.[49]

Microsatellites

Microsatellites are defined as discontinuous nests of melanoma cells at least 0.3 mm in diameter, which are separated from the primary lesion by greater than 0.05 mm of normal tissue.[43,45] Representing stage III disease, they are associated with increased risk of distant metastasis at the time of diagnosis.[45] Microsatellites are an independent predictor of nodal metastasis as well as a generally poor prognosis.[43,45]

Studies dedicated to risk stratification and prognostication have found a surprising heterogeneity in survival among patients with microsatellitosis, which correlates with aggressive features of the primary tumor.[1,45] In the absence of independent negative prognostic features, such as ulceration or multiple metastatic nodes, there is a subset of patients with a considerably improved prognosis who would benefit from SLN biopsy.[45] As such, SLN biopsy may be a consideration regardless of thinness of the primary tumor if it will guide further treatment.

Pregnancy

There are no absolute contraindications to melanoma excisions during pregnancy.[22–24,35,36] Radioactive colloid tracers are considered safe in pregnancy and the standard dose can be lowered without compromising accuracy.[1,2,50] Isosulfan blue is avoided due to the rare risk of severe allergic reactions,[6,50] and methylene blue is contraindicated because it is associated with developmental malformations.[50] Although limiting exposure to radiation, staging can be safely performed.[23,35,36,50] Treatment decisions in pregnancy should be made in collaboration with a multidisciplinary medical team.

MANAGEMENT OF A POSITIVE SENTINEL LYMPH NODE BIOPSY

In the era before effective systemic therapy for melanoma, approximately 30% of patients with resected clinically palpable lymph nodes experienced long-term survival.[1,2,8–11,13,34,37,46] Thus, the removal of positive regional nodes has been shown curative in a substantial subset of patients. A subgroup analysis of patients with positive SLNs who underwent elective lymph node dissection revealed resection of occult nodal disease was associated with increased overall survival (48% at 5 years) compared with those who were observed and developed nodal recurrence (27% at 5 years).[8–11,13,46] Similar to the 20% survival benefit seen in MSLT-I, patients with a positive SLN had a 5 year melanoma-specific survival of 72% compared with 52% in the observation arm who subsequently developed nodal recurrence.[8–11,13,46]

In MSLT-I, patients with positive SLN were randomized to early CLND versus observation with delayed CLND for clinical regional recurrence.[8–11,13,22] The median interval before development of palpable nodal disease was shown to vary by primary melanoma thickness. The median interval before development of palpable nodal disease in patients randomized to nodal observation was 19 months in the intermediate-thickness group versus 9.6 months for thicker lesions.[8–11,13,22]

In addition, this trial confirmed that nodal observation increased the number of positive nodes at the time of clinical detection. This implies that microscopic nodal metastases, if left alone, in time will become clinically apparent and spread within the nodal basin.[1,22] The risk of recurrence without CLND is estimated to be 26% at 5 years.[8,9,46] This argues in favor of SLN biopsy with early CLND for patients with positive nodes. Moreover, it also has been reported that a finding of multiple tumor-positive nonsentinel nodes is associated with a significantly worse prognosis.[1,2,15,46,47]

Limitations of Completion Lymph Node Dissection

Despite the understanding of the potential for disease progression with positive SLNs, the value of CLND remains controversial in patients with an SLN metastasis. In an early proof-of-concept study, CLND post–positive SLN biopsy to verify the accuracy of intraoperative lymphatic mapping was performed in 223 patients, and of the 3079 total nonsentinel nodes examined, only 2 (0.06%) were found to contain tumor deposits.[8–10] As such, most patients have all their nodal metastasis removed with the initial SLN biopsy, and thus do not derive any therapeutic benefit from CLND.

Moreover, several retrospective studies and multivariate analysis have confirmed that even microscopic nonsentinel node metastases are independent predictors of poor prognosis, similar to that of patients with bulky, palpable, or clinically diagnosed metastases.[1,8–16,20,28–31] These patients have been shown to be unlikely to benefit from early dissection.[1,2,8–11,13–16] CLND is associated with higher morbidity than SLN biopsy alone.[10,20–24] Delayed CLND further increases the incidence of lymphedema (see **Table 3**).[10,16,20–24,31]

Neither MSLT-I nor preceding trials evaluating long-term outcomes of elective lymph node dissection have demonstrated a survival advantage with complete regional lymphadenectomy compared with nodal basin observation (**Table 5**).[8–10,22–24,46] The recent publication of 2 large randomized clinical trials has altered the recommended management of positive SLN biopsies.[10,11,13,34,36,51] Prior to these landmark trials, performing CLND after a positive SLN biopsy was the standard of care.[10,16]

The German Dermatologic Cooperative Oncology Group (DeCOG) and the MSTL-II trials were designed to determine if there is any benefit in CLND in the context of a positive SLN biopsy.[1,2,8–11,13–16,24,46] DeCOG included 483 patients randomized to CLND or observation with nodal basin ultrasound every 3 months. The study demonstrated no difference in distant metastasis-free survival, overall survival, or recurrence-free survival at 3 years.[46] Due to poor rate of accrual, however, the trial ended early, and was statistically underpowered.

MSLT-II included 1934 patients in their analysis.[8–10,24] At 3 years, there was no difference in melanoma-specific survival (86% in each arm) between patients who underwent CLND versus nodal observation.[8,9] Their data identify a modest difference in disease-free survival (68% in the CLND group vs 63% in the observation group) that was driven by an increased rate of nodal recurrence in the observation group.[8–10,24] Nodal recurrence-free survival in the CLND group was 92% versus 77% in the observation group.[8–10] The increased rate of nodal recurrence in the observation group closely correlates with the expected 20% occurrence of positive nonsentinel nodes on CLND documented in multiple retrospective studies.[1,2,8–10,12,34,37,46,47] Higher recurrence rate in the lymph node basin with observation is thus expected. In MSTL-II, lymphedema was more common in the CLND group (24.1% vs 6.3%).[8–10,24]

Nodal observation in patients with a positive SLN would spare patients from the morbidity of completion dissection. It remains unclear, however, to what extent nodal recurrences are salvageable with lymphadenectomy at the time of recurrence. Based on limited retrospective data, true loss of regional control in patients opting for nodal observation is rare.[16,37] Taken together, the findings of both studies offer compelling evidence that immediate nodal intervention does not confer survival advantage over selective nodal intervention in patients with nodal recurrence. Currently, national guidelines support both CLND and nodal surveillance.[22–24,35,36]

An Era of Nodal Observation

There may be a subset of patients with microscopic nodal disease who would benefit from CLND before the disease progression to clinically or radiographically detectable disease. Conceptually, for immediate lymphadenectomy to be therapeutic, metastatic cells in the lymph node must have the potential to metastasize systemically.[1,2,6–8] Furthermore, only patients with the lowest risk of synchronous systemic disease would benefit from early CLND because the lymph nodes would be the only source of future metastases. Moreover, only those with nodotrophic biology would

Table 5
Summarizing the evidence for regional node management in melanoma

	Multicenter Selective Lymphadenectomy Trial I — Morton et al,[24] 2014	Multicenter Selective Lymphadenectomy Trial II — Faries et al,[2] 2017	German Dermatologic Cooperative Oncology Group Selective Lymphadenectomy — Leiter et al,[46] 2016
Intervention	WLE + SLNB and immediate LND for positive nodes vs WLE + nodal observation with LND for nodal recurrence	CLND vs OBS with nodal ultrasonography + LND for dectectable nodal disease	CLND vs OBS in SLNB positive patients (majority with micrometastasis)
No. of patients	Thick melanoma (3.5 mm) SLNB: 185 OBS: 126 Intermediate-thickness melanoma (1.2–3.5 mm) SLNB: 805 OBS: 522	ITT analysis 1934 Per protocol analysis 1755 CLND: 824 OBS: 931	484 total CLND: 242 OBS: 241
Primary endpoint	Melanoma-specific survival	Melanoma-specific survival	Distant metastasis-free survival

MSS	Thin melanoma
	 10-y MSS
	   Biopsy: 58.9 +/- 4.0%
	   OBS: 64.4 +/- 4.6% (HR 1.12; P = .56)
	   OS: not reported
	 Intermediate melanoma
	 10-y MSS:
	   Biopsy: 81.4 +/- 1.5%
	   OBS: 78.3 +/- 2.0% (HR 0.84; P = .18)
	   OS: not reported
		OBS vs CLND
		 Melanoma-specific survival
		   HR 1.08 (95% CI, 0.38–1.34; P = .42)
		 Distant metastasis-free survival
		   Adjusted HR 1.10 (55% CI, 0.92–1.31; P = .31)
			OBS vs CLND
			 Overall survival
			   HR 1.02 (90% CI, 0.68–1.52; P = .95)
			 Recurrence-free survival
			   HR 0.959 (90% CI, 0.70–1.31; P = .83)
			 Distant metastasis-free survival
			   HR 1.19 (90% CI, 0.83–1.69; P = .43)

(continued on next page)

Table 5
(continued)

	Multicenter Selective Lymphadenectomy Trial I Morton et al,[24] 2014	Multicenter Selective Lymphadenectomy Trial II Faries et al,[2] 2017	German Dermatologic Cooperative Oncology Group Selective Lymphadenectomy Leiter et al,[46] 2016
DFS	Intermediate-thickness melanoma 10-y MSS: 10-y DFS*: SLNB: 50.7 +/- 4.0% OBS: 40.5 +/- 4.7% (HR 0.70; P = .03) Intermediate-thickness melanoma SLNB: 71.3 +/- 1.8% OBS: 64.7 +/- 2.3% (HR 0.76; P = .01)	CLND: 68 6 1.7% vs OBS: 63 6 1.7%; log-rank P = .05	—
Median follow-up	10 y	43 mo	35 mo
Median thickness	SLNB: 1.8 OBS:1.9 (p = 0.3927)	CLND: 2.10 (range: 0.23–28.0) OBS: 2.10 (range: 0.35–30.0)	CLND: 2.4 (1.6–4.0) OBS: 2.4 (1.5–3.85)
Positive non-SLN	—	11.50%	24%
SLN micrometastasis	—	66%	66%
Regional recurrence	—	92% vs 77% at 3 y; P<.001	8% vs 15% regional recurrence
Lymphedema (CLND vs OBS)	—	24.1% vs 6.3%	8% CLND

Abbreviations: DFS, disease-free survival; LND, lymph node dissection; MSS, melanoma-specific survival; OBS, observation group; OS, overall survival; SLNB, sentinel lymph node biopsy.

theoretically benefit from nodal removal. This favorable biology might also confine tumor cells to lymph nodes, contributing to comparable long-term outcomes in early versus delayed nodal intervention.[1,2,8–10,14–16,24]

Albeit interesting, the debate regarding early nodal intervention has limited impact on the clinical management of patients. Assuming early nodal intervention is therapeutic, it only benefits the 3% to 4% of patients with intermediate-thickness melanoma (20% survival advantage in the 15%–20% of patients with a positive SLN) and the 2% to 3% of patients with a thin melanoma (35% survival advantage in the 5%–10% of patients with a positive SLN).[1,2,24,31] Unfortunately, these differences remain too small to detect via randomized trial.

Considerations for Surveillance of Regional Nodes

Another key principle of nodal observation recommended by DeCOG and MSLT-II is the assumption that regular surveillance by high-quality ultrasound will identify recurrence earlier compared with clinical evaluation of palpable nodes.[3,9–11,13,14,51] If close nodal observation is not feasible, or there are patient factors that could mask recurrence, such as morbid obesity or concomitant unrelated lymphadenopathy, CLND may be considered.[17,35,37]

MANAGEMENT OF CLINICALLY POSITIVE NODES

Surgical lymphadenectomy is recommended for clinically palpable nodal metastasis as well as for pathologically proved regional nodal involvement in patients with melanoma (**Table 6**).[1,2,8–10,15,16,22–24,35,36] Patients with advanced disease have at least stage IIIb melanoma, with greater than 23% risk of death from melanoma at 10 years.[22–24,35,36] The high risk of additional nodal metastases within the basin

Table 6 Management of clinically positive nodes	
Palpable lymphadenopathy with unknown primary	• Represents up to 3%–5% of patients with melanoma and 10%–20% of patients presenting with regional nodal disease[15,43–45] • Once treated as metastatic disease with a poor prognosis, retrospective studies have surprisingly demonstrated that, stage for stage, long-term outcomes often are equivalent, if not better, compared with patients with a known primary.[1,3,43–45] • Recommended treatment at this time consists of regional lymphadenectomy and consideration for adjuvant therapy.[22–24,35,36,45]
Bulky nodal disease	• Therapeutic lymph node dissection is recommended for all patients presenting with bulky nodal disease.[22–24,35,36] • These patients should first be staged to rule out synchronous metastatic disease.[38]
Unresectable stage III disease	• At this time, most patients in this cohort are recommended adjuvant immune or targeted therapies.[1,2,4] Enrollment into clinical trials should be considered.[4,22–24,35,36] • When considering neoadjuvant treatment, discussion with the patient must include consideration of the risk of disease progression and/or metastasis weighed against the potential benefit of early systemic treatment of downstaging bulky disease, and the morbidity associated with CLND.

and/or extranodal spread with clinically positive nodes warrants complete regional dissection in order to prevent morbidity caused by locoregional disease, such as mass effect or skin breakdown.[15,16,36]

The morbidity of CLND varies by anatomic location and includes both short-term and long-term complications (see **Table 3**). In the axilla, common short-term complications include wound infection and breakdown, seroma formation, and shoulder dysfunction.[8–10,21,24,32] Long-term complications include lymphedema and paresthesias.[21,32] In contrast, complications are more common after groin dissection, especially lymphedema.[10,21,32,33,52,53]

TECHNICAL CONSIDERATIONS
Axillary Lymphadenectomy

The axillary space is defined by the axillary vein superiorly, the pectoralis muscles anteriorly, latissimus dorsi posterolaterally, and both teres major and subscapularis posteriorly (**Fig. 1**). Level I nodes are inferior and lateral to the pectoralis minor, level II nodes are posterior to the pectoralis minor and below the axillary vein, and level III nodes are medial to the pectoralis minor and against the chest wall, including infraclavicular nodes (**Box 1**). The angular vein, a tributary of the subscapular vein, has been described as an inferior border for the axillary space, but there is no consensus on the extent of inferior dissection.[1,54,55]

Complications

The incidence of wound infection varies from 3% to 15%, and the incidence of postoperative hematoma from 2% to 10% (see **Table 3**).[1,8–10,51,54–57] Although drains decrease seroma formation as well as the volume and frequency of postoperative seroma aspirations, they do not reduce the incidence of wound infections.[51,54–57]

Lymphedema is a serious irreversible complication of axillary dissection. Axillary radiation is associated with higher rates of lymphedema (relative risk [RR] 2.97; 95% CI, 2.06–4.28).[54,56,57] Patients with positive axillary lymph nodes also have increased rates of lymphedema (RR 1.54; 95% CI, 1.32–1.80).[56,57]

As many as 42% of patients experience shoulder stiffness, numbness, or paresthesias of the upper arm after axillary dissection.[54,56,57] The risk of significant motor nerve injury is less than 1%.[56,57] Injury to the long thoracic nerve results in a winged scapula. Injury to the thoracodorsal nerve weakens shoulder abduction and internal rotation. Injury to the medial pectoral nerve results in atrophy of the lateral aspect of the pectoralis major muscle, potentially having an impact on cosmesis. Transection of the intercostobrachial nerves causes numbness of the inner upper arm.

Groin Lymphadenectomy

Two anatomic regions harbor lymph nodes in the groin: the superficial region containing nodes in the femoral triangle and the deeper pelvic region containing nodes along the external iliac artery and obturator region (**Fig. 2**). The optimal extent of dissection remains controversial. Current guidelines advocate for inguinal dissection to optimize regional control, especially in patients with low suspicion of pelvic nodal metastasis (**Boxes 2** and **3**).[1,2,33,52]

Treatment decisions also must take into consideration tumor and patient characteristics. Moreover, some surgeons biopsy Cloquet node for additional diagnostic information.[33,52] This node lies just within the pelvis, slightly posterior and medial to the external iliac vein and has been demonstrated to be a predictor of positive pelvic nodes.[33,52]

Axillary Lymphadenectomy

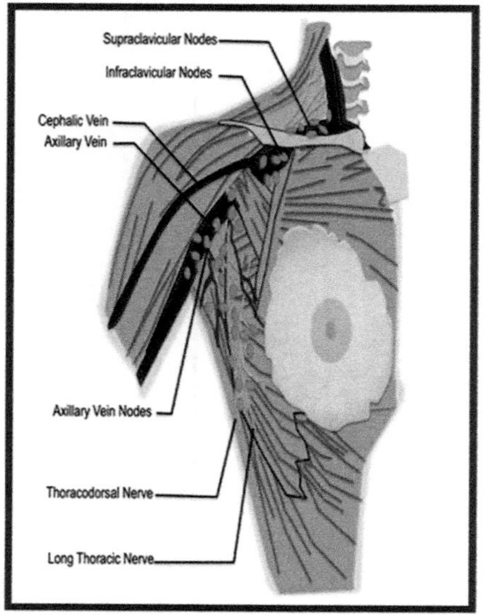

Fig. 1. Axillary Dissection.

Anatomy	• Anatomic space defined by the axillary vein superiorly, pectoralis muscles anteriorly, latissimus dorsi posterolaterally and both teres major and subscapularis posteriorly. • The angular vein, a tributary of the subscapular vein, has been described as an inferior border for the axillary space, but there is no consensus on the extent of inferior dissection.[1,49,50]
Nodes	• Level I nodes are inferior and lateral to the pectoralis minor • Level II nodes are posterior to pectoralis minor and below the axillary vein • Level III nodes are medial to pectoralis minor and against the chest wall, and include the infraclavicular nodes. • Complete dissection includes Levels I, II, and III for evaluation of at least 20 nodes. For AJCC staging, 10-12 lymph nodes are required.[27-31]
Technical Considerations	• The arm is extended with ≤90 degrees abduction from the chest wall to protect the brachial plexus • If sensory intercostobrachial nerves along the latissimus dorsi cannot be spared, ligation should be performed sharply. • Do not open the axillary sheath or skeletonize the axillary vein unless extensive nodal disease is noted. • The axillary vein often bi- or trifurcates, and venous structures high in the axilla should not be ligated. • The facial layer of serratus anterior should not be breached.

> **Box 1**
> **Axillary dissection essential steps**
>
> 1. Skin crease incision is made below the axillary hairline along the edge of pectoralis major.
> 2. Raise flaps; extend dissection superiorly to the tendinous portion of pectoralis major and inferiorly to the junction of the latissimus and serratus muscles.
> 3. Retract the lateral edge of pectoralis major exposing pectoralis minor and Rotter nodes.
> 4. Divide the clavipectoral fascia at the inferior axillary sheath, exposing underlying lymphatic tissue.
> 5. Continue dissection superiorly to the inferior border of the axillary vein, preserving the axillary artery and brachial plexus.
> 6. Dissection along latissimus dorsi is extended inferiorly toward the chest wall and superiorly to the tendon of insertion, preserving neurovascular structures.
> 7. Blunt dissection below the medial aspect of the axillary vein lateral to the chest wall reveals the long thoracic nerve.
> 8. The thoracodorsal neurovascular bundle can be identified by dissecting inferior to the axillary vein.
> 9. The specimen is dissected away from both nerve bundles, off the chest wall and inferior surface of the axillary vein.
> 10. The pectoralis minor is then elevated or divided, exposing the medial aspect of the axillary vein and level III nodes.
> 11. The remaining tissue is freed up to Halsted ligament.
> 12. Remove the specimen, confirm hemostasis, and leave a closed suction drain in the surgical bed.
> 13. The clavipectoral fascia is closed, and the wound is reapproximated in layers.

Complications

Up to 72% of groin dissections are associated with complications; 20% to 32% develop seromas, 20% to 45% experience lymphedema, 20% to 30% develop infections, and 52% have skin flap complications (see **Table 3**).[1,8–11,24,33,52] Surgical techniques, including the creation of vascularized flaps and minimally invasive

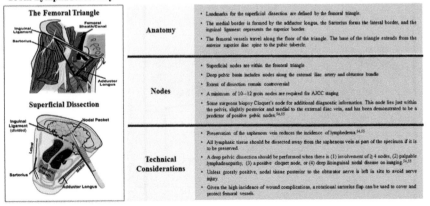

Fig. 2. Groin Dissection.

Box 2
Superficial groin dissection essential steps

1. A longitudinal, lazy-S incision is made, starting superior and medial to the anterior superior iliac spine, running parallel within the groin crease, and extending vertically to the apex of the femoral triangle.

2. Lymphatic tissue overlying the external oblique aponeurosis is swept from 5 cm above the inguinal ligament into the femoral triangle.

3. Tissue overlying the lateral border of the sartorius is mobilized, including fascia.

4. Medially, the dissection extends along the adductor longus, excluding fascia.

5. The anterior surface of the femoral artery and vein are skeletonized by dissecting the specimen off the vessels superiorly to the level of the saphenofemoral junction.

6. The saphenous vein is identified as it crosses the adductor longus and can be ligated as needed.

7. All lymphatic tissue should be dissected away from the saphenous vein as part of the specimen.

8. Lymphatics over the medial aspect of the femoral vein are ligated at the level of the femoral canal, and the specimen is detached.

9. At this point, the lacunar ligament can be divided, creating a femoral hernia through which Cloquet node can be biopsied for frozen section.

---

approaches, aim to reduce complications and improve cosmesis.[33,52] Further studies to assess feasibility of implementation and long-term outcomes are needed.

Other Anatomic Locations for Lymphadenectomy

Lymphadenectomy of epitrochlear, popliteal, and cervical lymph node basins have been described (**Figs. 3–5**).

Box 3
Deep pelvic dissection essential steps

1. The incision is extended superiorly over the abdominal wall.

2. Underlying muscles are divided.

3. The peritoneum is mobilized and retracted medially, exposing the retroperitoneum.

4. The ureter is protected and inferior epigastric vessels retracted or ligated.

5. External iliac vessels are skeletonized to the bifurcation of the common iliac vessels.

6. Grossly positive nodal disease proximal to the bifurcation can be removed but indicate stage IV disease and a poor prognosis.

7. The obturator neurovascular bundle is identified, and obturator nodes bluntly dissected.

8. Unless grossly positive, nodal tissue posterior to the obturator nerve is left in situ to avoid nerve injury.

9. Nodes are sent separately to pathology for analysis.

10. The femoral canal is closed.

11. Given the high incidence of wound complications, a rotational sartorius flap is used to cover and protect femoral vessels.

12. Hemostasis is confirmed, and a drain is placed in the superficial groin. The wound is closed in layers.

Popliteal Dissection

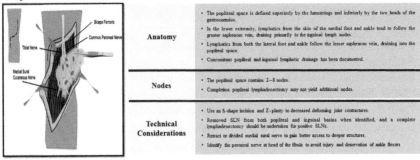

Anatomy	• The popliteal space is defined superiorly by the hamstrings and inferiorly by the two heads of the gastrocnemius. • In the lower extremity, lymphatics from the skin of the medial foot and ankle tend to follow the greater saphenous vein, draining primarily to the inguinal lymph nodes. • Lymphatics from both the lateral foot and ankle follow the lesser saphenous vein, draining into the popliteal space. • Concomitant popliteal and inguinal lymphatic drainage has been documented.
Nodes	• The popliteal space contains 2–8 nodes. • Completion popliteal lymphadenectomy may not yield additional nodes.
Technical Considerations	• Use an S-shape incision and Z-plasty to decreased deforming joint contractures. • Removed SLN from both popliteal and inguinal basins when identified, and a complete lymphadenectomy should be undertaken for positive SLNs. • Retract or divided medial sural nerve to gain better access to deeper structures. • Identify the peroneal nerve at head of the fibula to avoid injury and denervation of ankle flexors

Fig. 3. Popliteal Dissection.

Cervical Dissection

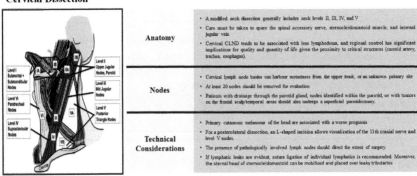

Anatomy	• A modified neck dissection generally includes neck levels II, III, IV, and V • Care must be taken to spare the spinal accessory nerve, sternocleidomastoid muscle, and internal jugular vein. • Cervical CLND tends to be associated with less lymphedema, and regional control has significant implications for quality and quantity of life given the proximity to critical structures (carotid artery, trachea, esophagus).
Nodes	• Cervical lymph node basins can harbour metastases from the upper trunk, or an unknown primary site • At least 20 nodes should be removed for evaluation • Patients with drainage through the parotid gland, nodes identified within the parotid, or with tumors on the frontal scalp/temporal areas should also undergo a superficial parotidectomy.
Technical Considerations	• Primary cutaneous melanoma of the head are associated with a worse prognosis • For a posterolateral dissection, an L-shaped incision allows visualization of the 11th cranial nerve and level V nodes. • The presence of pathologically involved lymph nodes should direct the extent of surgery. • If lymphatic leaks are evident, suture ligation of individual lymphatics is recommended. Moreover, the sternal head of sternocleidomastoid can be mobilized and placed over leaky tributaries

Fig. 4. Cervical Dissection.

Epitrochlear Dissection

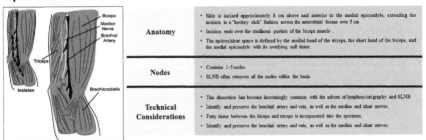

Anatomy	• Skin is incised approximately 8 cm above and anterior to the medial epicondyle, extending the incision in a "hockey stick" fashion across the antecubital fossae over 5 cm • Incision ends over the tendinous portion of the biceps muscle . • The epitrochlear space is defined by the medial head of the triceps, the short head of the biceps, and the medial epicondyle with its overlying soft tissue.
Nodes	• Contains 1-5 nodes • SLNB often removes all the nodes within the basin
Technical Considerations	• This dissection has become increasingly common with the advent of lymphoscintigraphy and SLNB • Identify and preserve the brachial artery and vein, as well as the median and ulnar nerves. • Fatty tissue between the biceps and triceps is incorporated into the specimen. • Identify and preserve the brachial artery and vein, as well as the median and ulnar nerves.

Fig. 5. Epitrochlear Dissection.

SUMMARY

Recent data from large, multicenter randomized trials have shifted paradigms in the management of regional nodes in melanoma. The SLN biopsy has been established as an effective and safe procedure yielding critical prognostic information to guide clinical decision making. Moreover, there is convincing evidence that CLND does not confer survival benefit. Clinically positive nodes continue to be managed surgically in order to maintain locoregional disease control, but adjuvant therapy is increasingly considered in this setting. Ongoing advances in targeted immunotherapies, combined with a better understanding of tumor biology, will likely continue to expand treatment options.

REFERENCES

1. Bartlett EK. Current management of regional lymph nodes in patients with melanoma. J Surg Oncol 2019;119(2):200–7.
2. Faries MB, Thompson JF, Cochran AJ, et al. Completion dissection or observation for sentinel-node metastasis in melanoma. N Engl J Med 2017;376(23):2211–22.
3. SEER cancer stat facts. Available at: https://seer.cancer.gov/statfacts/html/melan.html. Accessed Februrary 2019.
4. Kwak M, Farrow NE, Salama AK, et al. Updates in adjuvant systemic therapy for melanoma. J Surg Oncol 2019;119(2):222–31.
5. Norman J, Cruse CW, Espinosa C, et al. Redefinition of cutaneous lymphatic drainage with the use of lymphoscintigraphy for malignant melanoma. Am J Surg 1991;162(5):432–7.
6. Morton DL, Wen DR, Wong JH, et al. Technical details of intraoperative lymphatic mapping for early stage melanoma. Arch Surg 1992;(127–4):392–9.
7. Morton DL, Hoon DS, Cochran AJ, et al. Lymphatic mapping and sentinel lymphadenectomy for early-stage melanoma: therapeutic utility and implications of nodal microanatomy and molecular staging for improving the accuracy of detection of nodal micrometastases. Ann Surg 2003;238(4):538–49 [discussion: 549–50].
8. Morton DL, Cochran AJ, Thompson JF, et al. Sentinel node biopsy for early-stage melanoma: accuracy and morbidity in MSLT-I, an international multicenter trial. Ann Surg 2005;242(3):302–11 [discussion: 311–3].
9. Morton DL. Overview and update of the phase III Multicenter Selective Lymphadenectomy Trials (MSLT-I and MSLT-II) in melanoma. Clin Exp Metastatis 2002; 29(7):699–706.
10. Morton DL, Thompson JF, Cochran AJ, et al. Sentinel-node biopsy or nodal observation in melanoma. N Engl J Med 2006;355:1307.
11. Valsecchi ME, Silbermins D, de Rosa N, et al. Lymphatic mapping and sentinel lymph node biopsy in patients with melanoma: a meta-analysis. J Clin Oncol 2011;29(11):1479–87.
12. Balch CM, Soong S, Ross MI, et al. Long-term results of a multi-institutional randomized trial comparing prognostic factors and surgical results for intermediate thickness melanomas (1.0 to 4.0 mm). Intergroup Melanoma Surgical Trial. Ann Surg Oncol 2000;7(2):87–97.
13. Balch CM, Thompson JF, Gershenwald JE, et al. Age as a predictor of sentinel node metastasis among patients with localized melanoma: an inverse correlation of melanoma mortality and incidence of sentinel node metastasis among young and old patients. Ann Surg Oncol 2014;21(4):1075–81.

14. Han D, Zager JS, Shyr Y, et al. Clinicopathologic predictors of sentinel lymph node metastasis in thin melanoma. J Clin Oncol 2013;31(35):4387–93.

15. Wiener M, Acland KM, Shaw HM, et al. Sentinel node positive melanoma patients: prediction and prognostic significance of nonsentinel node metastases and development of a survival tree model. Ann Surg Oncol 2010;17(8):1995–2005.

16. Wong SL, Morton DL, Thompson JF, et al. Melanoma patients with positive sentinel nodes who did not undergo completion lymphadenectomy: a multi-institutional study. Ann Surg Oncol 2006;13(6):809–16.

17. Sinnamon AJ, Neuwirth MG, Bartlett EK, et al. Predictors of false negative sentinel lymph node biopsy in trunk and extremity melanoma. J Surg Oncol 2017;116(7): 848–55.

18. Cascinelli N, Morabito A, Santinami M, et al. Immediate or delayed dissection of regional nodes in patients with melanoma of the trunk: a randomised trial. WHO melanoma programme. Lancet 1998;351(9105):793–6.

19. de Rosa N, Lyman GH, Silbermins D, et al. Sentinel node biopsy for head and neck melanoma: a systematic review. Otolaryngol Head Neck Surg 2011; 145:375.

20. Ribero S, Osella-Abate S, Sanlorenzo M, et al. Sentinel lymph node biopsy in thick melanoma patients (N = 350): what is its prognostic role? Ann Surg Oncol 2015;22(6):1967–73.

21. Wrightson WR, Wong SL, Edwards MJ, et al. Complications associated with sentinel lymph node biopsy for melanoma. Ann Surg Oncol 2003;10:676.

22. Balch CM, Gershenwald JE, Soong SJ, et al. Update on the melanoma staging system: the importance of sentinel node staging and primary tumor mitotic rate. J Surg Oncol 2011;104(4):379–85.

23. Gershenwald JE, Scolyer RA, Hess KR, et al. Melanoma staging: Evidence-based changes in the American Joint Committee on Cancer eighth edition cancer staging manual. CA Cancer J Clin 2017;67(6):472–92.

24. Morton DL, Thompson JF, Cochran AJ, et al. Final trial report of sentinel-node biopsy versus nodal observation in melanoma. N Engl J Med 2014;370(7):599–609.

25. Murphy AD, Britten A, Powell B. Hot or not? The 10% rule in sentinel lymph node biopsy for malignant melanoma revisited. J Plast Reconstr Aesthet Surg 2014; 67(3):316–9.

26. Lee DY, Huynh KT, Teng A, et al. Predictors and survival impact of false-negative sentinel nodes in melanoma. Ann Surg Oncol 2016;23(3):1012–8.

27. Whiteman DC, Baade PD, Olsen CM. More people die from thin melanomas (1 mm) than from thick melanomas (>4 mm) in Queensland, Australia. J Invest Dermatol 2015;135(4):1190–3.

28. Bartlett EK, Gimotty PA, Sinnamon AJ, et al. Clark level risk stratifies patients with mitogenic thin melanomas for sentinel lymph node biopsy. Ann Surg Oncol 2014; 21(2):643–9.

29. Cordeiro E, Gervais MK, Shah PS, et al. Sentinel lymph node biopsy in thin cutaneous melanoma: A systematic review and meta-analysis. Ann Surg Oncol 2016;(23):4178–88.

30. Chang JM, Kosiorek HE, Dueck AC, et al. Stratifying SLN incidence in intermediate thickness melanoma patients. Am J Surg 2018;215(4):699–706.

31. Bartlett EK, Peters MG, Blair A, et al. Identification of patients with intermediate thickness melanoma at low risk for sentinel lymph node positivity. Ann Surg Oncol 2016;23(1):250–6.

32. Shaw JH, Rumball EM. Complications and local recurrence following lymphadenectomy. Br J Surg 1990;77:760.

33. Badgwell B, Xing Y, Gershenwald JE, et al. Pelvic lymph node dissection is beneficial in subsets of patients with node-positive melanoma. Ann Surg Oncol 2007; 14(10):2867–75.

34. van der Ploeg AP, Haydu LE, Spillane AJ, et al. Outcome following sentinel node biopsy plus wide local excision versus wide local excision only for primary cutaneous melanoma: analysis of 5840 patients treated at a single institution. Ann Surg 2015;260(1):149–57.

35. Coit DG, Thompson JA, Albertini MR, et al. Cutaneous melanoma, version 2.2019, NCCN clinical practice guidelines in oncology. J Natl Compr Canc Netw 2019; 17(4):367–402.

36. Wong SL, Faries MB, Kennedy EB, et al. Sentinel lymph node biopsy and management of regional lymph nodes in melanoma: American Society of Clinical Oncology and Society of Surgical Oncology clinical practice guideline update. J Clin Oncol 2018;36(4):399–413.

37. Bamboat ZM, Konstantinidis IT, Kuk D, et al. Observation after a positive sentinel lymph node biopsy in patients with melanoma. Ann Surg Oncol 2014;21(9): 3117–23.

38. Sanki A, Uren RF, Moncrieff M, et al. Targeted high-resolution ultrasound is not an effective substitute for sentinel lymph node biopsy in patients with primary cutaneous melanoma. J Clin Oncol 2009;27(33):5614–9.

39. Gonzalez AB, Jakub JW, Harmsen WS, et al. Status of the regional nodal basin remains highly prognostic in melanoma patients with in-transit disease. J Am Coll Surg 2016;223(1):77–85.e1.

40. Egnatios GL, Dueck AC, Macdonald JB, et al. The impact of biopsy technique on upstaging, residual disease, and outcome in cutaneous melanoma. Am J Surg 2011;202(6):771–7 [discussion: 777–8].

41. Herbert G, Karakousis GC, Bartlett EK, et al. Transected thin melanoma: implications for sentinel lymph node staging. J Surg Oncol 2018;117(4):567–71.

42. Ariyan S, Ali-Salaam P, Cheng DW, et al. Reliability of lymphatic mapping after wide local excision of cutaneous melanoma. Ann Surg Oncol 2007;14(8): 2377–83.

43. Yao KA, Hsueh EC, Essner R, et al. Is sentinel lymph node mapping indicated for isolated local and intransit recurrent melanoma? Ann Surg 2003;238(5):743–7.

44. Beasley GM, Hu Y, Youngwirth L, et al. Sentinel lymph node biopsy for recurrent melanoma: a multicenter study. Ann Surg Oncol 2017;24(9):2728–33.

45. Bartlett EK, Gupta M, Datta J, et al. Prognosis of patients with melanoma and microsatellitosis undergoing sentinel lymph node biopsy. Ann Surg Oncol 2014; 21(3):1016–23.

46. Leiter U, Stadler R, Mauch C, et al. Complete lymph node dissection versus no dissection in patients with sentinel lymph node biopsy positive melanoma (DeCOG-SLT): a multicentre, randomised, phase 3 trial. Lancet Oncol 2016;17(6): 757–67.

47. Ghaferi AA, Wong SL, Johnson TM, et al. Prognostic significance of a positive nonsentinel lymph node in cutaneous melanoma. Ann Surg Oncol 2009;16(11): 2978–84.

48. Cohen T, Busam KJ, Patel A, et al. Subungual melanoma: management considerations. Am J Surg 2008;195(2):244–8.

49. Marek AJ, Ming ME, Bartlett EK, et al. Acral lentiginous histologic subtype and sentinel lymph node positivity in thin melanoma. JAMA Dermatol 2016;152(7): 836–7.

50. Driscoll MS, Martires K, Bieber AK, et al. Pregnancy and melanoma. J Am Acad Dermatol 2016;75(4):669–78.
51. He XD, Guo ZH, Tian JH, et al. Whether drainage should be used after surgery for breast cancer? A systematic review of randomized controlled trials. Med Oncol 2011;28(Suppl 1):S22–30.
52. Hyde GA, Jung NL, Valle AA, et al. Robotic inguinal lymph node dissection for melanoma: a novel approach to a complicated problem. J Robot Surg 2018; 12(4):745–8.
53. Wagner T, Meyer N, Zerdoud S, et al. Fluorodeoxyglucose positron emission tomography fails to detect distant metastases at initial staging of melanoma patients with metastatic involvement of sentinel lymph node. Br J Dermatol 2011; 164(6):1235–40.
54. Kretschmer L, Preusser K. Standardized axillary lymphadenectomy improves local control but not survival in patients with palpable lymph node metastases of cutaneous malignant melanoma. Langenbecks Arch Surg 2001;386:418–25.
55. Chan CY, Tan M. Spatial relations of the angular vein, an important landmark in axillary node dissection. Br J Surg 2003;90:948–9.
56. Chang DW, Suami H, Skoracki R. A prospective analysis of 100 consecutive lymphovenous bypass cases for treatment of extremity lymphedema. Plast Reconstr Surg 2013;132:1305.
57. Ivens D, Hoe AL, Podd TJ, et al. Assessment of morbidity from complete axillary dissection. Br J Cancer 1992;66(1):136–8.

Nonsurgical Management of Lymph Node Basins in Melanoma

Rogeh Habashi, MD, Valerie Francescutti, MD, MSc, FRCSC*

KEYWORDS

- Melanoma • Sentinel lymph node biopsy • Completion lymph node dissection
- Locoregional control • Surveillance

KEY POINTS

- Offering sentinel lymph node biopsy (SLNB) to patients with thin melanomas should take into account histologic features that may increase risk of positivity, countered with comorbidities, and the implications of a positive result with respect to candidacy for adjuvant therapies.
- A preoperative workup including cross-sectional imaging is recommended in patients with thick melanomas, before offering SLNB, because of the high risk of distant metastatic disease. Preoperative discussion with patients regarding the risk a thick melanoma portends, distant metastatic risk, and what benefit the results of an SLNB may offer is suggested.
- In patients with bulky nodal metastatic melanoma, neoadjuvant systemic therapy may be an alternative, in particular when radical resection may result in significant morbidity, or the risk of distant metastatic disease is felt to be high. This treatment is recommended in the setting of a clinical trial if the nodal disease is borderline resectable.
- The use of SLNB in the setting of locally recurrent or in-transit melanoma has been shown in retrospective studies to afford prognostic information, despite the already high risk of distant metastatic disease in this group. As some of these patients will be offered adjuvant systemic therapies, the value of an SLNB in this setting should be considered.

BACKGROUND

Melanoma incidence has increased rapidly over the past 50 years, faster than many other types of cancer.[1,2] Although melanoma constitutes only 5% of all skin cancers, it accounts for the most deaths, highlighting the potential aggressiveness of the disease.[3] However, the clinical behavior of melanoma can be vastly different, ranging from localized early-stage disease to micrometastases in sentinel lymph nodes (SLNs), to bulky nodal disease or widely metastatic melanoma; this behavior can directly impact survival and other outcomes.[4]

Department of Surgery, McMaster University, Hamilton General Hospital, 237 Barton Street East, 6 North, Hamilton, Ontario L8L 2X2, Canada
* Corresponding author.
E-mail address: francev@mcmaster.ca

Surg Clin N Am 100 (2020) 91–107
https://doi.org/10.1016/j.suc.2019.09.008
surgical.theclinics.com

A great deal of attention has been paid to lymph node evaluation and dissection in melanoma. Although positive lymph nodes generally carry a worse prognosis, in some patients, lymph node dissection can be therapeutic. As such, the prognostic argument behind SLN biopsy (SLNB) centers around 2 hypotheses championed by Donald Morton: the "Incubator Hypothesis" versus the "Marker Hypothesis." The Incubator Hypothesis posits the primary melanoma metastasizes via lymphatics to the SLN, which is "suppressed" by factors released from the primary melanoma tumor site, remaining latent and incubating before spreading to other sites. In this situation, removing the SLN gives information regarding the ability of the melanoma to spread outside of the skin, and removal of the SLN before spread past lymph nodes should be preventive in further spread of melanoma. The Marker Hypothesis differs in that parallel and simultaneous spread of melanoma via lymphatic and hematogenous routes occur. In this situation, a positive SLNB is a marker of metastatic ability, but would not affect growth of distant metastatic disease and would not be considered therapeutic.[5]

This review focuses on the cases in which lymph node evaluation or treatment in melanoma may not be necessary, either forgoing the lymph node evaluation or treatment altogether, replacing the pathologic lymph node evaluation with an alternative strategy, or offering the patient a nonsurgical treatment option.

SENTINEL LYMPH NODE BIOPSY: APPLICATION AND ALTERNATIVES

Initial management of the regional lymph node basin in patients with cutaneous melanoma has remained a controversial topic of discussion for many decades. As nodal basins were considered the most common initial route of melanoma spread, lymph node dissection has been recognized as a possible option. Although routine elective complete lymphadenectomy of the nodal basin in all patients at diagnosis was recommended in the distant past, subsequent randomized trials indicated select patients with melanoma may benefit from elective lymphadenectomy.[6–10] The rationale in such a situation was that further spread could be curtailed before metastatic spread to the body by removing the potentially involved lymph nodes. Despite some small single-center series of patients undergoing elective lymph node dissection immediately along with wide excision of the primary melanoma site showing survival improvements, the high risk of lymphedema, surgical site infections, and other complications raised concerns about this routine practice.[11–13]

Since 1977, nodal lymphoscintigraphic studies have revealed that early-stage melanoma metastases usually target the most 1 to 2 proximal lymph nodes within the drainage basin.[14,15] Thus, sentinel lymph node biopsy (SLNB) was developed as a more minimally invasive option with lower complication rates, identifying the first node(s) within a basin as representative of the drainage pattern and tumor status of other nodes within that nodal basin.[16,17]

The Multicenter Selective Lymphadenectomy Trial (MSLT-I) was designed to determine if occult lymph node micrometastases could be identified in this manner, to reduce morbidity but preserve the potential prognostic value of lymph node involvement. This trial specifically addressed the intermediate-thickness group (per the trial defined as 1.2–3.5 mm Breslow depth) and also the thick primary melanoma group (>3.5 mm Breslow depth).[18] Patients were randomized to wide local excision alone with clinical observation of the nodal basin with subsequent lymphadenectomy for those developing clinical nodal recurrence versus wide excision with SLNB followed by immediate completion lymph node dissection for patients with micrometastases on SLNB. This study of 1327 patients showed the prognostic value of the SLNB procedure, with 5-year overall survival (OS) of 90% in the SLNB-negative group, and 72% in the SLNB-positive group. There was, however, no difference in melanoma-specific survival rates in the 2 groups (87% for the SLNB group vs 86.6% in the observation groups).

Since the MSLT-I trial, SLNB has become the standard of care for assessing occult metastases and staging lymph node basins of primary cutaneous melanoma (Breslow thickness ≥1 mm with Clark level ≥III or any thickness with Clark level ≥IV). SLNB primarily offers prognostic value in both intermediate and thick melanoma groups. With respect to patient selection for SLNB aside from Breslow depth, the decision is based on patient characteristics including comorbidities along with the estimated risk from the procedure, which in most series has been cited at 5%, including surgical site infection, seroma formation, and lymphedema risk.[19]

In addition, although an SLNB may be negative, patients should be always informed that there is a 1.7% to 6.0% (59/944; 18) chance of nodal basin recurrence in the dissected (81%) or other drainage basins (19%[20]) after adjustment for risk factors. With 88% of the nodal basin recurrences in context of negative SLNB being local or in-transit recurrence, it remains unclear if the nodal recurrence is secondary to local microscopic disease or missed micrometastases.[18] Further complicating the picture is surgical failure of identifying the true SLN and sample error related to limited assessment by pathology as less than 2% of sentinel node (SN) volume is actually sectioned and only 8 to 20 sections are assessed for metastases.[5]

Thin Melanomas

The group that has generated the most discussion is the thin melanoma (<1 mm thick) population, which in fact represents most newly diagnosed patients.[21] Overall, the risk of SLN positivity in patients with thin melanoma remains very low, at approximately 5%.[22–24] Risk factors for SLNB positivity identified based on retrospective cohorts of patients with thin melanomas undergoing the procedure include male gender, higher Clark level, presence of ulceration, lymphovascular invasion, increasing mitotic index, and increasing Breslow thickness.[25–27] Current guidelines recommend patients with melanomas smaller than 0.8 mm with negative ulceration (stage IA) should be treated with wide local excision alone, whereas patients with stage IB (<0.8 mm with ulceration, and 0.8–1.0 mm with or without ulceration) should be treated with wide local excision, but SLNB may be considered.[28] This discussion should be centered on tumor characteristics that may increase the risk of a positive SLNB, countered by patient comorbidities, potential candidacy for adjuvant therapies, and anesthetic risk.

Intermediate-Thickness Melanomas

The MSLT-I trial provided strong evidence for the use of SLNB for prognostication in the intermediate-thickness melanoma group (1–4 mm thick).[18] Although OS was not improved for the entire cohort of patients randomized in the trial, a subgroup analysis evaluating survival in patients with intermediate-thickness melanoma indicated for patients who had a positive SLNB who underwent an immediate completion lymphadenectomy (16% of patients), 5-year survival was improved compared with those undergoing completion lymphadenectomy at the time of lymph node recurrence (72% vs 52% 5-year specific survival). With an overall risk of positive SLNB of approximately 15% to 20%, an SLNB may be appropriate in many patients with intermediate-thickness melanoma; however, a thorough discussion, in particular for patients with significant comorbidities and potential limited lifespan for nonmelanoma reasons is warranted.

Thick Melanomas

Contrary to intermediate-thickness melanomas, the benefit of prognostic information from SLNB for melanomas >4 mm deep is less clear. With an SLNB positivity rate of 35% to 40% in these patients, the risk recurrence and distant metastatic disease in this patient group remains very high. Despite this, in the MSLT-I trial, patients with melanomas more than 3.5 mm thick did show prognostic significance of a positive SLNB in terms of 10-year survival (65% in SLNB negative, 48% in SLNB positive, $P = .03$). The OS benefit seen in the subgroup of patients with intermediate-thickness melanoma could not be demonstrated for thick melanomas. In this situation, it is recommended to highly consider preoperative imaging to assist in patient selection (including computed tomography [CT], MRI, and PET scan, as appropriate) to identify patients with distant or bulky nodal metastatic disease at presentation, who would thus be inappropriate candidates for SLNB. Even in the setting of negative preoperative imaging, frank discussions regarding prognosis specific to the primary tumor features, balancing this with patient comorbidities and anesthesia risk, is warranted. **Table 1** depicts a summary of evidence regarding the use of SLNB in thin, intermediate, and thick melanomas.

Some other special situations that may require additional discussion with a patient before offering SLNB deserve mention. First, some patients have an initial wide local excision with delayed referral for SLNB, and closure of the defect requires large advancement flaps or complex closures may significantly affect lymphatic drainage. In general, false-negative SLNB rates have been cited with a range of 5%[29] to 19% in the MSLT-I[13]; in this situation, that number may be higher. In addition, primary site of the melanoma, in particular with more complex drainage patterns, such as the head and neck, can increase false-negative rates.[30] Another uncommon presentation is distant metastatic disease in SLNB-negative patients. This "skip-pattern" disease encompasses 16% to 21% of the SLNB-negative population, most noticeable in the elderly population (>65 years old) or high-risk tumor features (eg, thick melanoma, nodular type, and ulceration).[31] Although the elderly population typically harbors poor prognosis melanoma, comorbid disease confounds OS and outcomes.[32]

Although SLNB remains the standard of care for prognostication for many patients with primary cutaneous melanoma, specific situations including patient choice may result in surgeons forgoing the procedure and using an alternative to nodal evaluation at the time of diagnosis. With respect to the option of cross-sectional imaging before initial surgery including SLNB, no consensus exists.[33] For nodal disease between retrospective radiology studies and the MSLT-II, ultrasonography of nodal basins carried a sensitivity of 8% to 24%.[34] Similarly based on retrospective studies of T2-T4 tumors, CT fluoro-deoxyglucose positron emission tomography (FDG-PET)-CT has fairly poor sensitivity in identifying nodal disease (10%–21%[35,36]). Recently, the hybrid single-photon emission CT (SPECT)/CT has gained popularity particularly in head and neck melanoma, in deciphering drainage SLN patterns based on dynamic imaging. In a retrospective multicenter study of 600, SPECT/CT detected drainage field mismatch in 11.1% of melanoma cases, facilitating surgical adjustment for SLNB.[37]

RADICAL LYMPH NODE DISSECTION AND ALTERNATIVES

Considering our knowledge of SLNB mostly for prognostication and only for therapeutic reasons in select patients, can the same be said for complete lymph node dissection (CLND) following positive SLNB? Since the 1980s, elective CLND has been controversial, as it has not shown any survival benefit when compared with observation in context of positive SLN.[38] In light of the preceding, the MSLT-I was

Table 1
Summary of evidence with respect to thin, intermediate, and thick melanomas, both prognostic information gained and therapeutic benefit

Key Considerations	Thin (<1.2 mm)	Intermediate (1.2–3.5 mm)	Thick (>3.5 mm)
Risk of positive SLN	11.7% (0.75–1 mm) 4.6% (<0.75 mm)[79]	15%–20%[13]	35%–40%
Prognostic information	5-y MSS: 94% for T1 negative SLN (69% if positive SLN)[80]	5-y MSS: 89.8% with negative SLN (vs 69.8% with positive SLN)	5-y MSS: 70.2% with negative SLN (vs 60.8% with positive SLN)
Survival benefit (MSLT-1)	15-y DDFS: 95.6% (96.1% if stage IA vs 85% if stage IB)[81]	5-y DDFS: 54.8% in + SLNB vs 35.6% in observation	No survival benefit. 5-y DDFS: 45.3% in + SLNB vs 43.8% in observation
Current guidelines (NCCN)	Stage IA (<0.8 mm): WLE Stage IB (T2a) with high risk features[a] or II (>1 mm): WLE ± SLNB	Stage II: WLE + SLNB Stage III (positive SLN): CLND vs ultrasound surveillance ± adjuvant therapy	Preoperative imaging (CT, MRI, and PET): identify bulky/distant metastatic disease Stage II: WLE + SLNB Stage III (microscopic positive SLN): CLND vs ultrasound surveillance ± adjuvant therapy Stage III (clinically bulky disease, in-transit or satellite): CLND vs neoadjuvant therapy Stage IV (metastatic): neoadjuvant therapy

Abbreviations: CLND, complete lymph node dissection; CT, computed tomography; DDFS, distant disease-free survival; MSS, melanoma-specific survival; SLN, sentinel lymph node; SLNB, SLN biopsy; WLE, wide local excision.

[a] Factors predisposing to positive SLN: male gender, Clark level >IV, presence of ulceration, lymphovascular invasion, and increasing mitotic index ($>1/mm^2$), deep positive margins, and increasing Breslow thickness.[5]

not powered to decipher the effect of CLND on disease-free or OS when compared with observation because of the dilutional effect. Only 16% in the SLNB group had positive SLN, of which 24% at most carried a positive CLND, thereby corresponding to only 3.8% of the patients.[19] Subsequently, 2 publications led by the Memorial Sloan Kettering Cancer Center compared CLND with observation. Wong and colleagues[39] (n = 134) identified an improved recurrence-free survival (RFS) in the CLND group but no difference in disease-free survival (DFS). Following this, Kingham and colleagues[40] (n = 313) showed no difference between CLND and observation in RFS and OS, although the non-CLND group tended to represent older patients with thicker melanomas. Unfortunately, both studies did not account for the degree of SLN tumor burden. Adding more complexity, Akkooi and colleagues[41] identified that among patients with positive SLN, the SLN tumor burden is the most critical prognostic factor for DFS and OS. In the very same study, SLN micrometastases smaller than 0.1 mm were established as effectively equivalent to negative SLN and did not require CLND.

In 2012, the European Organisation for the Research and Treatment of Cancer (EORTC) group showed no 5-year DFS or OS difference between observation and immediate CLND. Although matched in nodal tumor burden, the observation group was felt not to be representative of the population, as they tended to have lower nodal tumor burden and thinner primaries.[42] In 2014, Satzger and colleagues[43] showed in a retrospective series of patients that in the case of positive SLN with small tumor burden (<0.1 mm diameter according to the Rotterdam criteria), there was no difference in RFS and OS between observation and CLND. In the studies of the EORTC group and Satzger and colleagues,[43] low tumor burden SLN was associated with low probability of positive non-SLNs (NSLNs) (2%–4%).

In 2016, the DeCOG-SLT (Complete lymph node dissection versus no dissection in patients with sentinel lymph node biopsy positive melanoma) study from Germany revealed no difference in 3-year metastasis-free survival (MFS), RFS, and OS between the observation and CLND groups (OS: 81.2% vs 81.7% [P = 0.87] in 240 vs 233 patients).[44] However, there was slightly improved regional nodal disease control in the CLND group (20 [8%] vs 34[15%] in the observation group), but this was not statistically significant. Noting positive SLN heterogeneity, the DeCOG-SLT study affirmed that the preceding findings were most consistent in and applied to the SLN micrometastases ≤1 mm in size. Surprisingly, overall, there were 25% (43 of 181) positive NSLNs in the CLND group, a proportion much higher than the 15% in the observation group. This possibly supports the hypothesis that intact lymph nodes can limit disease dissemination by an immune-surveillance mechanism. Because of the small sample size (n = 483), the study was lacking power to assess significance of CLND for SLN metastases >1 mm. Recently, the 5-year follow-up results were reported at the American Society of Clinical Oncology 2018 Annual Meeting. There continued to be no difference in DFS, RFS, and regional LN metastasis.[45]

With a body of evidence debating the utility of CLND in therapy and prognostication, the MSLT-II was designed as a large study to make more definitive conclusions. The MSLT-II was a multicenter, phase 3 trial that randomized 1755 patients with positive SLN to either CLND (n = 824) or nodal observation (n = 931).[34] The patients within the observation group were monitored by physical examination and ultrasonography every 4 months during the first 2 years and every 6 months during years 3 through 5. Moehrle and colleagues[46] described characteristics of malignant nodal appearance as length to depth ratio of less than 2, hypoechoic center, absence of hilar blood vessel, and focal nodularity with increased vascularity. The presence of any 2 of these characteristics had 100% sensitivity and 96% specificity. In light of the preceding, the MSLT-II has established the following key findings:

1. No survival benefit for immediate CLND after SLNB, irrelevant of number or tumor burden of the positive nodes. However, therapeutic effect may be diluted, as only 19.9% had positive NSLN at 5 years (26.1% in the observation group).
2. Enhanced locoregional nodal disease control in the CLND group (69% lower in the CLND group vs the observation group: hazard ratio, 0.31; 95% confidence interval [CI] 0.24–0.41; P<.001).
3. Enhanced staging in the CLND group: the pathologic status of the NSLN, rather than the number of SLNs, is a critical prognostication factor in melanoma-specific survival (hazard ratio for death, 1.78; P = .005).
4. Increased morbidity with CLND (24% in CLND vs 6% in observation).

Explaining the contrast to the MSLT-I, the lack of a survival benefit with CLND in patients of the MSLT-II indicates that increased survival with early CLND noted in MSLT-I is inherent to an early melanoma limited to SLN. Patients with non-SN metastases may have salvage treatment with CLND for locoregional control, but the timing is irrelevant.

The benefit of CLND remains controversial in the following 2 patient populations: (1) Extremely early melanoma with positive SLN (0–3.5-mm thickness, with <1 mm micrometastases in SLNB), and (2) the more advanced melanomas (more than 1.2-mm thickness, with >1 mm micrometastases in SLNB). The former because the SLNB serves as both diagnostic and therapeutic thus omission of CLND is unlikely to change the patient's survival; the latter because the disease is likely already past the SLN and additional surgery is primarily locoregional control rather than curative.[44] The DeCOG-SLT study included mostly patients with positive SLNB micrometastases of <1 mm (331 <1 mm vs 142 >1 mm) and hence showed that there was no improved MFS, RFS, or OS with CLND. In addition, the MSLT-II trial included a subgroup analysis of SLNB micrometastases >1 mm in size, with conclusions favoring nodal observation over CLND considering the high risk of systemic disease in such cohort.[34]

The opponents of the MSLT-II rightly highlight that forgoing CLND means (1) not knowing the pathology of NSLNs, which makes complete staging more difficult; and (2) the risk of losing regional disease control. In this same vein, as only 20% of patients with positive SLNB have positive NSLNs, 2 retrospective studies showed that CLND rarely leads to upstaging, in an estimated 6% of cases.[47,48] From a regional disease control perspective, the MSLT-II has clearly emphasized the regional relapse is not the same as loss of regional control. When compared with observation, CLND does not affect RFS but improves regional control.[34] A summary of outcomes with CLND can be found in **Table 2**.

Considering the preceding dilemma, the uncommon NSLN involvement of the SLNB-positive melanomas (only 10%–20%) and increased morbidity with CLND, there has been a general movement in literature toward identifying clinical prognosticators of advanced disease that would guide the application of CLND using primary tumor and SLNB characteristics. Murali and colleagues[49] used a cohort of 409 SLNB-positive patients (309 undergoing CLND) to design a score based on clinic-pathological features of their melanomas, stratifying the risk of NSLN in that same nodal basin. The predisposing risk factors of NSLN positivity included in the N-SNORE were male gender, regression of primary melanoma, percent of LNs containing melanoma, perinodal lymphatic invasion, and size of largest nodal deposit (see **Table 1**). Corroborating the N-SNORE, both MSLT-II and DeCOG-SLT revealed no association between number of positive SLNs and survival. Similar to the work of Murali and colleagues,[49] multiple studies have shown variable factors to predict NSLN involvement, including age, multifocal SLN tumor deposits, subcapsular and parenchymal SLN involvement, diameter more than 0.75 mm (2 mm, associated with 25% positive NSLN), presence of tumor-infiltrating lymphocytes, and primary tumor thickness >2 to 3 mm.[50–52] Thus, the high end of such scoring systems serves as an indication for CLND but further studies are needed for validation before routine clinical use.

Furthermore, there remain a few logistical indications for CLND use.[53] First, forgoing CLND only can be replaced by frequent follow-ups including ultrasound surveillance (every 4 months for 3 years, then every 6 months for 5 years). If follow-up is not feasible or there is concern for compliance, CLND is advised. Second, two-thirds of the DeCOG-SLT and MSLT-II populations had SLNB tumor burden ≤1 mm, which are populations with low likelihood of NSLN involvement. Thus, selection bias and lack of true population representation limit the recommendations of observation (over CLND) to primarily low tumor burden SLN ≤1 mm. Third, our prediction scores are inadequate still, as recent studies are correlating improved RFS/OS with immunologic markers like CD3+, 4+, and 8+ lymphocytes in the affected LNs among others.

Table 2
Results of trials of CLND following SLNB

Clinical Trial	MSLT-I	MSLT-II	DeCOG-SLT
Trial design	Prospective, randomized, multicenter	Prospective, randomized, multicenter	Prospective, randomized, multicenter
Inclusion criteria	• Localized cutaneous melanoma • Clark level III and Breslow thickness >1 mm or Clark level IV/V with any Breslow thickness • Life expectancy >10 y	• Localized cutaneous melanoma • Tumor-positive SN (H&E, IHC, or RT-PCR) • Life expectancy >10 y	• Localized cutaneous melanoma • Tumor thick >1 mm • SN micrometastases
Exclusion criteria	• Melanomas of the ear • Any operative procedure that could have disrupted lymphatic drainage patterns • Previous or concurrent melanoma or other malignancy • Immunosuppression or pregnancy	• Previous or concurrent melanoma or any solid tumor in past 5 y • Satellite, in-transit, regional, or metastatic disease • Extracapsular extension • Immunosuppression	• Head/neck melanoma • Previous or concurrent melanoma or other malignancy • Satellite, in-transit, regional, or metastatic disease • Macrometastasis (>2 mm) or extracapsular extension • Immunosuppression
Trial size	1191 intention-to-treat 225 Early CLND 132 Delayed CLND	1934 intention-to-treat 967 CLND	473 intention-to-treat 242 CLND
Intervention	Wide excision + SLNB vs wide excision + observation	Immediate CLND vs nodal observation with ultrasound	Immediate CLND vs nodal observation with ultrasound
Median follow-up, mo	54	43	35
Median Breslow depth, mm	1.9	2.1	2.4
Non–sentinel LN positive, %	10	11	24
Primary endpoint	Intermediate: 69.6% ± 4.4% vs 56.5% ± 5.5% (5 y) Thick: 60.6% ± 6.6% vs 53.8% ± 7.6% (5 y)	Melanoma-specific survival (86% vs 86%, $P = .42$)	Distant metastasis-free survival (75% vs 77%, $P = .87$)

Disease-free survival	Intermediate: 78.0% ± 1.6% vs 72.7% ± 2.0% (P = .0074) at 5 y Thick: 56.0% ± 3.0% vs 43.5% ± 4.7% (P = .0358) at 5 y	68% vs 63%, P = .05, at 3 y	67% vs 67%, P = .75, at 3 y
Nodal disease control	Same-basin recurrence (6.3% vs 18.1%)	92% vs 77% (P = .001) nodal basin control rate at 3 y	8% vs 15% regional nodal recurrence
Morbidity 1. Lymphedema 2. Wound infection	1. 12.4% (early) vs 20.4% (delayed) 2. 15.8% (CLND)	1. 24.1% (n = 23) 2. Not recorded	1. 8% (n = 20) 2. 1.2% (n = 3)

Abbreviations: CLND, complete lymph node dissection; DeCOG-SLT, Complete lymph node dissection versus no dissection in patients with sentinel lymph node biopsy positive melanoma; H&E, hematoxylin-eosin; IHC, immunohistochemistry; LN, lymph node; MSLT, Multicenter Selective Lymphadenectomy Trial; RT-PCR, reverse-transcriptase polymerase chain reaction; SN, sentinel node; SLNB, sentinel lymph node biopsy.

Using the data of MSLT-I, early (n = 225) and delayed CLND (n = 132) essentially had no difference in morbidity.[54] Essentially early and delayed CLND had equivalent rates of wound dehiscence (3% vs 6%), seroma/hematoma (18% vs 24%), hemorrhage (2.2% vs 3%), surgical site infection (12% in both), weakness (3.1% vs 2.25%), and dysesthesia (5.2% vs 2.2%). Unrelated of the nodal basin (inguinal vs axillary), only chronic lymphedema was more prominent in delayed CLND (20.4% vs 12.4%, $P = .04$) with mild predilection to higher body mass index (BMI).

Stepwise logistic regression analysis examined age at CLND, BMI, basin site, number of nodes evaluated, and type of CLND (delayed vs early), identifying basin site (groin vs other) as the most powerful factor (odds ratio 3.64, 95% CI 1.93–6.86, $P<.001$). Both BMI (odds ratio 1.06, 95% CI 1.00–1.13, $P = .069$) and delayed CLND (odds ratio 1.74, 95% CI 0.93–3.25, $P = .083$) had the highest rates of chronic lymphedema.[54] Other risk factors associated with increased complications included age older than 55, diabetes, smoking, extremity primary, and adjuvant radiation.[55]

Radical Lymph Node Dissection or Neoadjuvant Approaches to Bulky Nodal Disease

Although historically, advanced yet resectable melanoma was treated aggressively with primary resection and radical lymphadenectomy, removing all palpable and potentially occult disease, recent evidence shows associated increased morbidity without improved survival.[56–58] In the era of new and effective systemic therapies, the option of preoperative therapy to reduce nodal bulk and potentially reduce morbidity associated with radical lymphadenectomy has been postulated.

Amaria and colleagues[59] published results of a phase II trial in 23 patients with surgically resectable but high-risk stage III melanoma who received either neoadjuvant nivolumab or ipilimumab and nivolumab. The combined regimen did have a high response rate (Response evaluation in solid tumors 73%, Pathologic complete response rate (pCR) 45%), but unfortunately a high toxicity rate, with 73% of patients experiencing grade 3 adverse effects. Similarly, Blank and colleagues[60] completed a phase II trial of 20 patients receiving either neoadjuvant (2 courses preoperative and 2 courses postoperative) or adjuvant ipilimumab (3 mg/kg) and nivolumab (1 mg/kg). All 10 of the neoadjuvant patients did have surgery at the planned time point, but 9 of 10 of these patients had 1 or more grade 3 toxicities.

What is very clear from the neoadjuvant studies is that patient selection, balancing treatment benefit and toxicity, is of utmost importance. Pathology reporting guidelines and extent of response information has been recently published for reference.[61] In this same manner, Barbour and colleagues[62] evaluated a subgroup of patients presenting with stage III melanoma with bulky lymph nodes at time of primary diagnosis. BRAF status was available in 124 patients and showed that BRAF mutants (46%) had higher 3-year recurrence (77 vs 54%, hazard ratio 1.8, $P = .008$) and worse RFS and DSS (7, 16 months relative to 19 months). Considering the preceding, BRAF immunohistochemistry or pyrosequencing is indicated in stage III/IV melanoma for prognostication and potentially therapy.

In 2017, an open-label, single arm, dual-center, phase II study in Belgium rechallenged stages III/IV, previously treated with BRAF inhibitors, with dabrafenib plus trametinib, attaining partial response in 32% (8/25) with good tolerance.[63] Czirbesz and colleagues[64] retrospectively reviewed 43 BRAF-mutated metastatic melanomas revealing objective response in 51.0% with 79.0% disease control and 11.6% complete response to BRAF inhibitor vemurafenib. A recent systematic review of 15 randomized controlled trials on either targeted anti-BRAF or immunotherapy[65] revealed the following:

1. Improved OS with either BRAF/MEK and PD-1 relative to other therapies
2. Significant PFS with BRAF/MEK compared with all other treatment strategies
3. Higher overall response rate (ORR) (odds ratio 2.00%; 95% credible interval (CrI), 1.64–2.45) with BRAF/MEK relative to BRAF alone

Although BRAF mutation carries poor prognosis, further research is needed into the (1) utility of BRAF sequencing among others in possibly replacing SLNB in melanoma, as well as the (2) therapeutic role of BRAF inhibitors in melanoma management.

Finally, the question of "down-staging" patients with unresectable stage III melanoma with bulky nodal metastatic disease to resectable stage III disease has been investigated. In fact, a retrospective study from the Mayo Clinic of 23 patients with advanced melanoma revealed that neoadjuvant therapies (off-label ipilimumab) down-staged 5 of 7 unresectable to resectable with no progression of patients with resectable disease.[66] The 5-year OS was 84%. At the present time, although neoadjuvant approaches to bulky nodal disease in melanoma seem promising, treatment is recommended in the setting of a clinical trial.

LYMPH NODE EVALUATION AND SIGNIFICANCE IN RECURRENT MELANOMA AND IN-TRANSIT MELANOMA

Local recurrence (LR) in melanoma is fairly uncommon, with an incidence of approximately 3% to 7% of patients. Similarly in-transit (IT) melanoma is uncommon, and both LR and IT melanoma are often considered to be a precursor to systemic metastatic disease.[67–70] Roses and colleagues[71] noted that time to systemic metastases was fairly short, appearing at an average of 9.7 months following LR diagnosis. In this same study, 90% of patients with LR and 71% of patients with IT melanoma developed systemic metastases at a median follow-up of 45 months.

A select group of patients developing an isolated melanoma LR or limited IT disease have been postulated to benefit from lymph node evaluation, in the form of an SLNB. Most of these studies are retrospective cohorts, albeit from multiple centers. Beasley and colleagues[72] report on 107 patients, 52% of whom had previously had an SLNB for initial disease evaluation. In the cohort, SLNB was performed for limited IT disease in 45%, with the remainder being completed for LR. Although the SLNB was successful in 96% of patients, 40% had a positive SLNB result, with 88% of those patients undergoing CLND. Of those CLND patients, 37% had positive non-SLN. The conclusions of this multicenter study included that the time to progression after recurrence was 1.4 years in patients with a positive SLNB, versus 5.9 years for those with a negative SLNB. The investigators felt these results added prognostic information about the disease process for these patients.

Gonzalez and colleagues[73] retrospectively evaluated patients with IT melanoma with no clinical evidence of nodal disease. At the time of surgical excision of the IT lesions, 58% underwent observation of the nodal basin, whereas 41% underwent surgical nodal evaluation: 36% of that surgical group were found to have occult nodal metastatic disease. The distant MFS was found to be 71 months for surgically managed node-negative patients, and 19 months for surgically managed node-positive patients. For those patients who presented with no clinical evidence of node involvement and followed by clinical examination only, the regional nodal basin was the first site of failure in one-quarter of patients.

Although the status of the SLNB does appear to offer some prognostic information for patients with isolated LR or IT melanoma, the use of the SLNB procedure with respect to patient selection remains unclear. If the result of the SLNB does affect choice to pursue adjuvant therapies, then the procedure may be justified. However, the use of CLND in this group of patients, in particular when considering the study by Gonzalez and colleagues[73] that showed that the first site of failure in clinically node-negative patients was the regional nodal basin in only one-quarter of patients, is certainly controversial.

FUTURE DIRECTIONS
Gene Profiling in Melanoma

Despite histology-based prognostication for SLNB-negative patients related to initial biopsy results, many of these patients will experience disease recurrence. There has been interest in the development of specialized molecular testing options from paraffin-embedded slides, to improve prognostication based on histology or clinical data.

The 31-genetic expression profile test, DecisionDx Melanoma (Castle Biosciences Inc., Friendswood, TX) was designed to augment the risk stratification of patients with primary cutaneous melanoma. Based on the primary cutaneous melanoma expression levels of this profile, a patient's melanoma can be classified as low or high risk for metastases. This 31-gene expression profile was developed based on variation noted between metastatic versus nonmetastatic melanoma. The initial study to validate gene expression profile followed 104 patients, noting metastatic disease in 35 patients at a median follow-up of 7 years. The DFS at 5 years was 97% for patients with the low-risk gene expression, versus 31% for those with high-risk gene expression.[74] One criticism of this study was the high rate of metastatic disease in the SLNB cohort, which was cited as approximately 30% higher than expected.

With respect to the ability of this test to change clinical management, a study of more than 150 patients with melanoma tested with the 31-gene expression profile and managed by dermatologists and surgical oncologists at 6 centers evaluated the use and frequency of clinical evaluations, use of imaging, other surgical procedures, referrals to other providers, and laboratory testing. For the high-risk group based on the 31-gene expression profile, three-quarters of patients had some management changes compared with one-third of patients in the low-risk group, with most of these changes being increased frequency and intensity of follow-up.[75] Despite this, the effect of the more intense follow-up strategy, given that most melanoma recurrences in this group are patient-identified and reported, did not improve outcomes. In this regard, the use of the 31-gene expression profile has not been included into any clinical practice guideline.[76]

The Use of Intravital Microscopy in the Evaluation of Lymph Node Metastases

Presently the evaluation of lymph nodes in the draining nodal basin involves surgical removal and histologic evaluation, which contributes to the morbidity associated with the SLNB procedure. A study from Roswell Park Comprehensive Cancer Institute provides a fascinating alternative to SLNB, wherein intravital microscopy with fluorescein has been successfully used to identify abnormal nodes, corresponding to a positive SLNB. However, mapped lymph nodes by lymphoscintigraphy do not require excision, but can be evaluated in vivo, thus eliminating the morbidity of seroma formation, lymphedema, and nerve damage. This technique shows promise for the future evaluation of lymph nodes in patients with melanoma who are candidates for SLNB.[77,78]

SUMMARY

Management of lymph node basins in melanoma poses a clinical challenge. With an (1) unpredictable and, at times, aggressive pathology, (2) imperfect prognostic scoring systems, and (3) no highly sensitive cross-sectional imaging modality, nonsurgical management of melanoma nodal basins remains controversial.

Based on current literature, a few broad recommendations can be made. For thin melanomas (<1 mm), SLNB should be considered for high-risk histology and the intent should be curative, balancing associated morbidity. On the other hand, for thick melanomas, SLNB carries a prognostic utility. Hence, preoperative staging cross-sectional imaging is highly recommended before surgical decision making, because of the high metastatic risk. CLND remains most controversial for early melanoma with positive SLNB and advanced melanomas with no associated improved survival benefit. CLND is most useful in locoregional disease control, but in some situations, replaced by intense clinical and radiologic follow-up.

In bulky nodal metastatic melanoma, neoadjuvant therapy has emerged as a possible option, as radical resection carries significant morbidity with limited survival benefit; however, candidates should be enrolled as part of a clinical trial. In IT and LR melanomas, SLNB showed prognostic utility and can be used for stratification of neoadjuvant therapies.

Further research is required to optimize nonsurgical management of the melanoma lymph node basins, including validating stratification scoring systems, imaging modalities, genetic sequencing, in vivo microscopy, and safe neoadjuvant or adjuvant therapies.

DISCLOSURE STATEMENT

The authors have nothing to disclose.

REFERENCES

1. Rigel DS, Carucci JA. Malignant melanoma: prevention, early detection, and treatment in the 21st century. CA Cancer J Clin 2000;50(4):215–36.
2. Kosary CL, Altekruse SF, Ruhl J, et al. Clinical and prognostic factors for melanoma of the skin using SEER registries: collaborative stage data collection system, version 1 and version 2. Cancer 2014;120(Suppl 23):3807–14.
3. Linos E, Swetter SM, Cockburn MG, et al. Increasing burden of melanoma in the United States. J Invest Dermatol 2009;129(7):1666–74.
4. Erdei E, Torres SM. A new understanding in the epidemiology of melanoma. Expert Rev Anticancer Ther 2010;10(11):1811–23.
5. Morton DL, Hoon DSB, Cochran AJ, et al. Lymphatic mapping and sentinel lymphadenectomy for early-stage melanoma: therapeutic utility and implications of nodal microanatomy and molecular staging for improving the accuracy of detection of nodal micrometastases. Ann Surg 2003;238(4):538–50.
6. Snow H. Melanotic cancerous disease. Lancet 1892;2:872.
7. Veronesi U, Adamus J, Bandiera DC, et al. Inefficacy of immediate node dissection in stage I melanoma of the limbs. N Engl J Med 1977;297:627–30.
8. Cascinelli N, Morabito A, Santinami M, et al. Immediate or delayed dissection of regional nodes in patients with melanoma of the trunk: a randomized trial. Lancet 1998;351:793–6.
9. Balch CM, Soong S, Ross MI, et al. Long term results of a multi-institutional randomized trial comparing prognostic factors and surgical results for intermediate thickness melanomas (1.0 to 4.0 mm). Ann Surg Oncol 2000;7:87–97.
10. Sim FH, Taylor WF, Ivins JC, et al. A prospective randomized study of the efficacy of routine elective lymphadenectomy in management of malignant melanoma: preliminary results. Cancer 1978;41:948–56.

11. Lane N, Lattes R, Malm J. Clinicopathological correlations in a series of 117 malignant melanomas of the skin of adults. Cancer 1958;11(5):1025–43.

12. Southwick HW, Slaughter DP, Hinkamp JF, et al. The role of regional node dissection in the treatment of malignant melanoma. Arch Surg 1962;179(1):105–8.

13. Mundth ED, Guralnick EA, Raker JW. Malignant melanoma: a clinical study of 427 cases. Ann Surg 1965;162:15–28.

14. Cochran AJ, Wen DR, Herschman HR. Occult melanoma in lymph nodes detected by antiserum to S-100 protein. Int J Cancer 1984;34:159–63.

15. Cochran AJ, Pihl E, Wen DR, et al. Zoned immune suppression of lymph nodes draining malignant melanoma: histologic and immunohistologic studies. J Natl Cancer Inst 1987;78:399–405.

16. Morton DL, Wen DR, Wong JH, et al. Technical details of intraoperative lymphatic mapping for early stage melanoma. Arch Surg 1992;127:392–9.

17. Thompson JF, McCarthy WH, Bosch CM, et al. Sentinel lymph node status as indicator of the presence of metastatic melanoma in regional lymph nodes. Melanoma Res 1995;5:255–60.

18. Morton DL, Thompson JF, Cochran AJ, et al. Sentinel-node biopsy or nodal observation in melanoma. N Engl J Med 2006;355:1307–17.

19. Morton DL, Cochran AJ, Thompson JF, et al. Sentinel-node biopsy for early-stage melanoma: accuracy and morbidity in MSLT-I, an international multicenter trial. Ann Surg 2005;242(3):302–11.

20. Zogakis TG, Essner R, Wang HJ, et al. Melanoma recurrence patterns after negative selective lymphadenectomy. Arch Surg 2005;140:865–72.

21. Whiteman DC, Baade PD, Olsen CM. More people die from thin melanomas (1 mm) than from thick melanomas (> 4mm) in Queensland, Australia. J Invest Dermatol 2015;135(4):1190–3.

22. Karakousis GC, Gimotty PA, Botbyl JD, et al. Predictors or regional nodal disease in patients with thin melanomas. Ann Surg Oncol 2006;13(4):533–41.

23. Karakousis GC, Gimotty PA, Czerniecki BJ, et al. Regional nodal metastatic disease is the strongest predictor of survival in patients with thin vertical growth phase melanomas: a case for SLN staging biopsy in these patients. Ann Surg Oncol 2007;14(5):1596–603.

24. Murali R, Haydu LE, Quinn MJ, et al. Sentinel lymph node biopsy in patients with thin primary cutaneous melanoma. Ann Surg 2012;255(1):128–33.

25. Cecchi R, Buralli L, Innocenti S, et al. Sentinel lymph node biopsy in patients with thin melanomas. J Dermatol 2007;34(8):512–5.

26. Han D, Zager JS, Shyr Y, et al. Clinicopathologic predictors of sentinel lymph node metastasis in thin melanoma. J Clin Oncol 2013;31(35):4387–93.

27. Kunte C, Geimer T, Baumert J, et al. Prognostic factors associated with sentinel lymph node positivity and effect of sentinel status on survival: an analysis of 1049 patients with cutaneous melanoma. Melanoma Res 2010;20(4):330–7.

28. Melanoma guidelines. National Comprehensive Cancer Center. Available at: www.nccn.org. Accessed March 9, 2019.

29. Sinnamon AJ, Neuwirth MG, Bartlett EK, et al. Predictors of false negative sentinel lymph node biopsy in trunk and extremity melanoma. J Surg Oncol 2017;116(7):848–55.

30. Chao C, Wong SL, Edwards MJ, et al. Sentinel lymph node biopsy for head and neck melanomas. Ann Surg Oncol 2003;10(1):21–6.

31. Erdmann M, Sigler D, Uslu U, et al. Risk factors for regional and systemic metastases in patients with sentinel lymph node-negative melanoma. Anticancer Res 2018;38(11):6571–7.

32. Rees MJ, Liao H, Spillane J, et al. Localized melanoma in older patients, the impact of increasing age and comorbid medical conditions. Eur J Surg Oncol 2016;42(9):1359–66.
33. Deschner B, Wayne J. Follow-up of the melanoma patient. J Surg Oncol 2019; 119:262–8.
34. Faries MB, Thompson JF, Cochran AJ, et al. Completion dissection or observation for sentinel-node metastasis in melanoma. N Engl J Med 2017;376(23):2211–22.
35. Wagner JD, Schauwecker D, Davidson D, et al. Inefficacy of F-18 fluorodeoxy-D-glucose-positron emission tomography scans for initial evaluation in early-stage cutaneous melanoma. Cancer 2005;104:570–9.
36. Clark PB, Soo V, Kraas J, et al. Futility of fluoro-deoxyglucose F 18 positron emission tomography in initial evaluation of patients with T2 to T4 melanoma. Arch Surg 2006;141:284–8.
37. Jimenez-Heffernan A, Ellmann A, Sado H, et al. Results of a prospective multi-center International Atomic Energy Agency sentinel node trial on the value of SPECT/CT over planar imaging in various malignancies. J Nucl Med 2015;56: 1338–44.
38. Balch CM. The role of elective lymph node dissection in melanoma: rationale, results, and controversies. J Clin Oncol 1988;6:163–72.
39. Wong SL, Morton DL, Thompson JF, et al. Melanoma patients with positive sentinel nodes who did not undergo completion lymphadenectomy: a multi-institutional study. Ann Surg Oncol 2006;13:809–16.
40. Kingham TP, Panageas KS, Ariyan CE, et al. Outcome of patients with a positive sentinel lymph node who do not undergo completion lymphadenectomy. Ann Surg Oncol 2010;17:514–20.
41. Akkooi AC, Verhoef C, Eggermont AM. Importance of tumor load in the sentinel node in melanoma: clinical dilemmas. Nat Rev Clin Oncol 2010;7:446–54.
42. van der Ploeg AP, van Akkooi AC, Rutkowski P, et al. Prognosis in patients with sentinel node-positive melanoma without immediate completion lymph node dissection. Br J Surg 2012;99:1396–405.
43. Satzger I, Meier A, Zapf A, et al. Is there a therapeutic benefit of complete lymph node dissection in melanoma patients with low tumor burden in the sentinel node? Melanoma Res 2014;24:454–61.
44. Leiter U, Stadler R, Mauch C, et al. Complete lymph node dissection versus no dissection in patients with sentinel lymph node biopsy positive melanoma (DeCOG-SLT): a multicentre, randomised, phase 3 trial. Lancet Oncol 2016;17: 757–67.
45. Leiter UM, Stadler R, Mauch C, et al. Final analysis of DeCOG-SLT trial: survival outcomes of complete lymph node dissection in melanoma patients with positive sentinel node. J Clin Oncol 2018;36(15_suppl):9501.
46. Moehrle M, Blum A, Rassner G, et al. Lymph node metastases of cutaneous melanoma: diagnosis by B-scan and color Doppler sonography. J Am Acad Dermatol 1999;41:703–9.
47. Madu MF, Franke V, Bruin MM, et al. Immediate completion lymph node dissection in stage IIIA melanoma does not provide significant additional staging information beyond EORTC SN tumour burden criteria. Eur J Cancer 2017;87:212–5.
48. Verver D, van Klaveren D, van Akkooi ACJ, et al. Risk stratification of sentinel node-positive melanoma patients defines surgical management and adjuvant therapy treatment considerations. Eur J Cancer 2018;96:25–33.
49. Murali R, Desilva C, Thompson JF, et al. Non-sentinel node risk score (N-SNORE): a scoring system for accurately stratifying risk of non-sentinel node positivity in

patients with cutaneous melanoma with positive sentinel lymph nodes. J Clin Oncol 2010;28:4441–9.

50. Gershenwald JE, Scolyer RA, Hess KR, et al. Melanoma staging: evidence-based changes in the American Joint Committee on cancer eighth edition cancer staging manual. CA Cancer J Clin 2017;67(6):472–92.

51. Bhutiani N, Egger ME, Stromberg AJ, et al. A model for predicting low probability of non-sentinel lymph node positivity in melanoma patients with a single positive sentinel lymph node. J Surg Oncol 2018;118(6):922–7.

52. Sinnamon AJ, Song Y, Sharon CE, et al. Prediction of residual nodal disease at completion dissection following positive sentinel lymph node biopsy for melanoma. Ann Surg Oncol 2018;25(12):3469–75.

53. Masoud SJ, Perone JA, Farrow NE, et al. Sentinel lymph node biopsy and completion lymph node dissection for melanoma. Curr Treat Options Oncol 2018;19(11):55.

54. Faries MB, Thompson JF, Cochran A, et al. The impact on morbidity and length of stay of early versus delayed complete lymphadenectomy in melanoma: results of the Multicenter Selective Lymphadenectomy Trial (I). Ann Surg Oncol 2010; 17(12):3324–9.

55. Postlewait LM, Farley CR, Seamens AM. Morbidity and outcomes following axillary lymphadenectomy for melanoma: weighing the risk of surgery in the era of MSLT-II. Ann Surg Oncol 2018;25(2):465–70.

56. Foote M, Burmeister B, Dwyer P, et al. An innovative approach for locally advanced stage III cutaneous melanoma: radiotherapy, followed by nodal dissection. Melanoma Res 2012;22:257–62.

57. Gibbs P, Anderson C, Pearlman N, et al. A phase II study of neoadjuvant biochemotherapy for stage III melanoma. Cancer 2002;94:470–6.

58. Kounalakis N, Gao D, Gonzalez R, et al. A neoadjuvant biochemotherapy approach to stage III melanoma: analysis of surgical outcomes. Immunotherapy 2012;4:679–86.

59. Amaria RN, Reddy SM, Tawbi HA, et al. Neoadjuvant immune checkpoint blockade in high-risk resectable melanoma. Nat Med 2018;24(11):1649–54.

60. Blank CU, Rozeman EA, Fanchi LF, et al. Neoadjuvant versus adjuvant ipilimumab plus nivolumab in macroscopic stage III melanoma. Nat Med 2018;24(11):1655–61.

61. Tetzlaff MT, Messina JL, Stein JE, et al. Pathological assessment of resection specimens after neoadjuvant therapy for metastatic melanoma. Ann Oncol 2018;29(8):1861–8.

62. Barbour AP, Tang YH, Armour N, et al. BRAF mutation status is an independent prognostic factor for resected stage IIIB and IIIC melanoma: implications for melanoma staging and adjuvant therapy. Eur J Cancer 2014;50(15):2668–76.

63. Schreuer M, Jansen Y, Planken S, et al. Combination of dabrafenib plus trametinib for BRAF and MEK inhibitor pre-treated patients with advanced BRAFV600 mutant melanoma: an open-label, single arm, dual-center, phase 2 clinical trial. Lancet Oncol 2017;18(4):464–72.

64. Czirbesz K, Gorka E, Bataloni T, et al. Efficacy of vemurafenib treatment in 43 metastatic melanoma patients with BRAF mutation. single-institute retrospective analysis, early real-life survival data. Pathol Oncol Res 2019;25(1):45–50.

65. Devji T, Levine O, Neupane B, et al. Systemic therapy for previously untreated advanced braf-mutated melanoma: a systematic review and network meta-analysis of randomized clinical trials. JAMA Oncol 2017;3(3):366–73.

66. Dong XD, Tyler D, Johnson JL, et al. Analysis of prognosis and disease progression after local recurrence of melanoma. Cancer 2000;88:1063–71.
67. Jakub JW, Racz JM, Hieken TJ, et al. Neoadjuvant systemic therapy for regionally advanced melanoma. J Surg Oncol 2018;117:1164–9.
68. Cohn-Cedermark G, Mansson-Brahme E, Rutqvist LE, et al. Outcomes of patients with local recurrence of cutaneous malignant melanoma. Cancer 1997;80:1418–25.
69. Urist MM, Balch CM, Soong S, et al. The influence of surgical margins and prognostic factors predicting the risk of local recurrence in 3445 patients with primary cutaneous melanoma. Cancer 1985;55:1398–402.
70. Wildemore JK, Schuchter L, Mick R, et al. Locally recurrent malignant melanoma characteristics and outcomes: a single institution study. Ann Plast Surg 2001;46:488–94.
71. Roses DF, Harris MN, Rigel D, et al. Local and in-transit metastases following definitive excision for primary cutaneous malignant melanoma. Ann Surg 1988;198:65–9.
72. Beasley GM, Hu Y, Youngwirth L, et al. Sentinel lymph node biopsy for recurrent melanoma: a multicenter study. Ann Surg Oncol 2017;24(9):2728–33.
73. Gonzalez AB, Jakub JW, Harmsen WS, et al. Status of the regional nodal basin remains highly prognostic in melanoma patients with in-transit disease. J Am Coll Surg 2016;223(1):77–85.
74. Gerami P, Cook RW, Wilkinson J, et al. Development of a prognostic genetic signature to predict the metastatic risk associated with cutaneous melanoma. Clin Cancer Res 2015;21(1):175–83.
75. Berger AC, Davidson RS, Poitras JK, et al. Clinical impact of a 31-gene expression profile test for cutaneous melanoma in 156 prospectively and consecutively tested patients. Curr Med Res Opin 2016;32(9):1599–604.
76. Farberg AS, Glazer AM, White R, et al. Impact of a 31-gene expression profiling test for cutaneous melanoma on dermatologists' clinical management decisions. J Drugs Dermatol 2017;16(5):428–31.
77. Fisher DT, Muhitch JB, Kim M, et al. Intraoperative intravital microscopy permits the study of human tumor vessels. Nat Commun 2016;7:10684.
78. Gabriel EM, Fisher DT, Evans S, et al. Intravital microscopy in the study of the tumor microenvironment: from bench to human application. Oncotarget 2018;9(28):20165–78.
79. Maurichi A, Miceli R, Camerini T. Prediction of survival in patients with thin melanomas: results from a multi-institution study. J Clin Oncol 2014;32(23):2479–85.
80. Hieken TJ, Grotz TE, Comfere NI, et al. The effect of the AJCC 7th edition change in T1 melanoma substaging on national utilization and outcomes of sentinel lymph node biopsy for thin melanoma. Melanoma Res 2015;25(2):157–63.
81. Gimothy P, Guerry D. Prognostication in thin cutaneous melanomas. Arch Pathol Lab Med 2010;134:1758–63.

Management of Locoregionally Advanced Melanoma

David T. Pointer Jr, MD[a,b], Jonathan S. Zager, MD[a,b],*

KEYWORDS

- Melanoma • Metastatic melanoma • Intralesional therapy • Locoregional metastasis
- T-VEC • Satellite recurrence • Oncolytic therapy • In-transit recurrence

KEY POINTS

- Melanoma has a unique propensity for locoregional metastasis secondary to intralymphatic transit not seen in other cutaneous or soft tissue malignancies.
- Novel intralesional therapies using oncolytic immunotherapy exhibit increasing response rates with observed bystander effect.
- Intralesional modalities in combination with systemic immunotherapy are the subject of ongoing clinical trials.
- Regional therapy is used in isolated limb locoregional metastasis whereby chemotherapy is delivered to an isolated limb avoiding systemic side effects.
- Multimodal treatment strategy is imperative in the treatment of locoregionally advanced melanoma. One must be versed on these quickly evolving therapeutic options.

INTRODUCTION

Satellite and in-transit metastasis are classified as lesions arising between a primary melanoma and the lymph node basin. These lesions demonstrate melanoma's unique propensity for locoregional metastasis and are thought to develop from intralymphatic recurrence.[1] Commonly appearing as darkly pigmented nodules or papules on the skin, satellite or in-transit disease alone is classified as N1 disease by the American Joint Committee on Cancer 8th Edition. The delineation between these satellite and in-transit lesions is based on proximity to the site of the primary lesion (satellite ≤2 cm, in-transit >2 cm).[2,3] Resection is still the primary treatment modality in the setting of recurrent melanoma, with neoadjuvant systemic therapy strategies now

Relevant Disclosures: J.S. Zager – Consulting for Amgen and Philogen. Speakers Bureau for Amgen, Research funding from Amgen, Provectus and Philogen.
[a] Department of Cutaneous Oncology, Moffitt Cancer Center, 10920 McKinley Drive, Tampa, FL, 33612; [b] Department of Surgery, University of South Florida Morsani College of Medicine, 13220 USF Laurel Dr., Tampa, FL 33612
* Corresponding author.
E-mail address: jonathan.zager@moffitt.org

being explored off protocol or on clinical trials more widely. Unfortunately, locoregional disease is often diffuse and deemed unresectable. Substantial progress has been made in the management of unresectable locoregional melanoma. With advances in intralesional and intraarterial therapies, significant clinical response and survival advantage has become a reality for this subset of patients.

SURGICAL RESECTION OF LOCOREGIONAL DISEASE

Surgical resection rests at the core of treatment of malignant melanoma. In locoregionally advanced or recurrent disease, resection remains the primary treatment modality and is considered the standard of care. This is true when disease presentation is amenable to complete resection, operative morbidity is minimal, and there is no evidence of distant disease.[4] In a 2000 retrospective analysis of disease progression and prognosis after locoregional recurrence, Dong and colleagues evaluated more than 600 patients with local recurrence of melanoma treated with reresection. Nineteen percent of patients were disease free at a median 8-year follow-up demonstrating clear advantages to reresection in this patient cohort.[5] Locoregional recurrence does have the propensity to present in patterns precluding surgical resection. These challenges include disease involving a significant surface area and recurrence after short disease-free intervals. Second-line therapies such as intralesional, intraarterial, or systemic therapies must be considered in these scenarios, with many demonstrating promising response rates and survival benefits.

INTRALESIONAL THERAPIES

The locoregional presentation of metastatic disease along with its distinctive relationship with the immune system has provided the framework for intralesional treatment in the control of locoregional melanoma.[6,7] When disease burden precludes surgical resection due to associated morbidity of functional deficits, intralesional therapy may be considered. Treatment with concentrated delivery of agent, stimulation of systemic immune response, and minimization of systemic toxicity are the cornerstones of intralesional therapy in melanoma. The concept of intralesional treatment of malignancy was first described in 1893 by Coley, using erysipelas injections in the treatment of inoperable sarcoma and carcinoma.[8] Since this initial description, many intralesional agents and techniques have been explored for the treatment of locoregional melanoma with varying degrees of success. The following discussion reviews these agents and techniques with focus on supporting evidence, efficacy, safety, and mechanism of action.

BACILLE CALMETTE-GUERIN

Derived from *Mycobacterium bovis*, Bacille Calmette-Guerin (BCG) is a live, attenuated strain historically with a wide spectrum of uses in the medicine. Its antitumor effect on cancer was first described in the 1970s by Zbar and Rapp, with their work focusing on tumor immunity in guinea pigs.[9,10] Application of BCG to human models followed soon after with response in patients with melanoma injected with agent demonstrated by Karakousis 1976 and again by Mujagic a few years later.[11,12]

Early excitement surrounded this treatment modality leading to deeper investigation into its use and efficacy in patients with melanoma. Morton and colleagues[13] described their 7-year experience treating patients with malignant melanoma with BCG immunotherapy alone or as a surgical adjunct. Ninety percent of injected lesions in their series experienced complete response (CR), with observed regression in 17%

of uninjected lesions. Response was also durable with a reported 31% remaining disease free for up to 6 years.[13] Response to BCG was also reported in a series of 15 patients by Mastrangelo and colleagues,[14] where 5 patients experienced significant objective improvement of their injected lesions. Other reports of BCG efficacy in locally recurrent melanoma of the lower extremity and in pulmonary metastasis established early promise in the use of BCG in malignant melanoma.[15,16]

As investigation of BCG progressed, ensuing studies failed to demonstrate similar outcomes. Moreover, no survival benefit had been associated with intralesional BCG. A phase III randomized trial was conducted in 2004 (E1673) by the Eastern Cooperative Oncology Group in an effort to comprehensively evaluate the adjuvant effect of BCG on resected stage I to III melanoma.[17] From 1974 to 1978, a total of 734 patients were randomized into 2 cohorts comparing BCG with observation and BCG with BCG + dacarbazine, respectively. No significant difference in disease-free or overall survival (OS) was observed after final analysis. Furthermore, no benefit was observed with the addition of dacarbazine.[17]

Concern has also been placed on BCG-associated toxicity in the literature. Ranging from injection site induration to severe disseminated intravascular coagulation and death, BCG therapy is associated with a 12% complication rate and requires close monitoring and prophylaxis with antihistamine and isoniazid treatment.[7] With little evidence to support survival benefit and increasing concern over BCG-associated side effects, its use has declined.

INTERLEUKIN-2

Produced by T lymphocytes, interleukin-2 (IL-2) is a glycoprotein first described in 1976.[18] Its immune functions are far reaching, affecting growth, proliferation, and activation of cytotoxic T lymphocytes, natural killer, and lymphokine-activated killer cells.[18,19] Antitumor effects of IL-2 have been reported, with renal cell carcinoma and malignant melanoma being most sensitive. IL-2 was initially approved for systemic administration in the setting of metastatic renal cell carcinoma and melanoma in the mid 90s; its administration limited to low-dose regimens with unknown efficacy or combined with interferon. Although response rates ranged from 10% to 15%, severe toxicity was associated with systemic IL-2 therapy often leading to cessation of therapy.[20,21]

Promise for intralesional IL-2 has been demonstrated in 2 phase II trials. In 2003, Radny and colleagues[22] evaluated 24 patients with stage III or IV melanoma. Intralesional IL-2 injections were administered weekly for 1 to 12 weeks. CR and partial response (PR) was observed in 62.5% and 21% of patients, respectively. Importantly, toxic effects were limited when compared with systemic administration of IL-2. Weide and colleagues[23] built on these results in their study of 51 patients with metastasized melanoma. CR was reported in 69% of patients and 70% of injected metastases exhibited a durable response of 6 months or more. Distant metastases were not found to experience any objective response in this study and again, toxic effects from intralesional injection were minimal with only grade 1/2 events reported.[23]

Intralesional injection with IL-2 has proved efficacious in several smaller cohorts including a systematic review article where 2182 lesions in 140 patients were analyzed across 6 observational studies. Collective analysis demonstrated 78% CR in injected lesions, with 50% of treated patients achieving CR. Again, treatment was well-tolerated with similar previously described side effects.[24] Although results of intralesional IL-2 show impressive response rates and the potential for durable effect, cost of therapy, treatment regimen, and optimal dosing are significant barriers to its success. In addition, unlike several other intralesional therapies, there has been no observed effect on distant or uninjected metastatic lesions (bystander effect).

GRANULOCYTE-MACROPHAGE COLONY-STIMULATING FACTOR

Granulocyte-macrophage colony-stimulating factor (GM-CSF) regulates activation and production of granulocytes, monocytes, and macrophages. GM-CSF plays an important role in both innate and acquired immunity, controlling and regulating T- and dendritic cell function.[25,26] Interest in antitumor effects of GM-CSF was born out of these unique immune properties. Early investigation of this topic was undertaken by Dranoff and colleagues.[27] In a murine model, B16-F10 melanoma cells infected with a retroviral vector expressing GM-CSF demonstrated systemic anti-tumor immunity when challenged with injection of wild-type B16 cells. Ninety percent protection was noted in formulated injections containing GM-CSF expressing tumor, compared with no protection demonstrated in other cytokine expressing groups.[27]

Encouraging preclinical data led to further investigation into intralesional injection of GM-CSF. In a phase I trial, 13 patients with locoregional metastasis were enrolled. Two subcutaneous nodules were injected with GM-CSF. Lesions were excised after up to 6 months of therapy. Partial regression was seen in only 3 patients.[28] A subsequent study with 16 patients demonstrated equally disappointing results with no objective tumor response after 10 days of treatment at 4 dose levels.[29] Although objective response was not associated with GM-CSF administration, these studies did demonstrate recruitment of T-cell and dendritic cell infiltrates proposing a role for GM-CSF use in vaccine preparation.[28,29]

Although as single-agent therapy, GM-CSF has not resulted in objective tumor response, GM-CSF in combination with other agents has also been explored in an attempt to exploit its ability to recruit lymphoid infiltrates and stimulate antitumor response. Combination with IL-2 and viral transfection (discussed later in chapter) are some of the novel approaches GM-CSF is being used in the treatment of malignant melanoma today.

ALLOVECTIN-7

Velimogene aliplasmid (Allovectin-7) uses the principle of direct gene transfer to upregulate expression of HLA-B7 and beta-2 microglobulin, components of major histocompatibility complex I (MHC-I). Upregulation of MHC-I reverses the proliferative effects of cancer progression, inducing a proimflammatory reaction increasing immune response to tumor cells.[6,30] Early clinical studies presented promising results with allogenic MHC-I gene transfer within a DNA-liposome complex leading to local inhibition of tumor growth and immune stimulation with observed T-cell migration into injected lesions.[31,32] A phase I study by Stopeck and colleagues[33] demonstrated a 93% success rate in direct gene transfer of human leukocyte antigen-B7 and a 50% tumor response rate, with well-tolerated toxicitiy.[33]

Two phase II trials assessed the safety and efficacy of intralesional Allovectin-7 in patients with stage II to IV melanoma.[34,35] Gonzalez and colleagues[34] reported an overall response rate (ORR) of 9.1% after 6 weekly injections of 10 ug Allovectin-7. Median duration of response of 4.8 months and median survival of 14 months was also reported. Bedikian and colleagues'[35] analysis included 133 patients treated with escalating doses (0.5–2 mg) of Allovectin-7. An objective response was observed in 11.8% of patients with a median duration of response of 13.8 months. Toxicity was found to be minimal and treatment well tolerated in both phase II studies.[34,35]

Unfortunately, Allovectin-7 has failed to demonstrate consistent results in phase III studies. Trials comparing dacarbazine alone with dacarbazine plus intralesional Allovectin-7, and Allovectin-7 with dacarbazine or temozolomide, failed to show benefit of Allovectin-7 on objective response rate or OS.[36,37] Shortcomings in these phase III trials have led to Allovectin-7 falling out of favor in the treatment of malignant melanoma.

PV-10 (ROSE BENGAL)

Historically used as a diagnostic solution for liver function, Rose Bengal disodium is a xanthene dye used in present day medicine in the detection of ophthalmic injury.[38] Use in melanoma was demonstrated in early studies with induction of preferential cell death in melanoma cell lines, sparing normal fibroblasts.[39] Efficacy of intralesional administration in the form of PV-10 (10% Rose Bengal solution) in humans was first established by Thompson and colleagues[40] in their 2008 phase I trial. Eleven patients with locoregionally recurrent melanoma were injected with PV-10. Up to 3 lesions were injected and up to 3 lesions were identified as nontarget lesions (not injected) and observed for response. CR and PR occurred in 36% and 12% injected lesions, respectively. Nontarget lesions experienced 15% CR and 12% PR, with a strong correlation between target and nontarget lesion response, suggesting a bystander effect.[40]

Antitumor immune response secondary to PV-10 injection has been described as a mechanism for observed response in injected and noninjected lesions. In a murine model using B16 melanoma cell lines, PV-10 was shown to stimulate tumor-specific T-cell–mediated immunity leading to regression of treated and untreated lesions.[41] The described bystander in both preclinical animal models and early human studies led to further investigation of PV-10 as a primary agent and as combination therapy with chemotherapy, talimogene laherparepvec (T-VEC), and immunotherapy.

A phase II study evaluated intralesional PV-10 in the treatment of patients with refractory metastatic melanoma. Analysis of 80 patients who received up to 4 intralesional injections in target lesions revealed CR and PR of 26% and 25%, respectively. A bystander effect was again observed in untreated lesions with 33% of patients experiencing a CR or PR and correlation was again shown between target and nontarget lesion response. Treatment was also found to be well tolerated with reported grade I to III adverse events, all resolving without lasting effects.[42]

TALIMOGENE LAHERPAREPVEC

Talimogene laherparepvec (T-VEC, Amgen) is the only Food and Drug Administration (FDA)-approved oncolytic viral therapy for the treatment of locoregionally advanced melanoma. This treatment is derived from genetically modified herpes simplex virus (HSV-1) with 2 specific mechanisms of action: first to selectively infect tumor cells and second to promote their immune-mediated destruction.[43] More specifically, genetic modification of HSV-1 involves the deletion of infected cell protein 34.5 (ICP34.5). With this deletion, protein kinase R important in the inhibition of unregulated proliferation is only activated in healthy human cells prohibiting successful infection, mitigating viral pathogenicity. Infected malignant cells fail to activate PKC leading to replication within cancer cells alone. Deletion of ICP47 and insertion of cDNA coding for GM-CSF increases antigen presentation of infected tumor cells and promotes antitumor immunity associated with GM-CSF,[43–45] described earlier in this article. With these specific modifications of HSV-1, a prevalent viral infection most known for causing fever blister and rash is transformed into an oncolytic immunotherapy.

Safety of genetically engineered HSV-1 under the name OncoVEX[GM-CSF] was evaluated in a phase I study published in 2006. Intratumeral virus was administered to 26 patients using dose escalation in single and multidosing groups. Main side effects included fever, erythema, and local inflammation, and short-interval follow-up revealed viral replication, tumor necrosis, and GM-CSF expression.[46] Phase II results evaluating 50 patients with stage IIIc/IV melanoma injected with T-VEC showed ORR of 26% (CR = 8, PR = 5) by RECIST criteria including both injected and noninjected lesions. Durable response was observed with 92% of responses maintained for 7 to 31 months.[47]

Andtbacka and colleagues were first to successfully demonstrate therapeutic benefit of oncolytic therapy in a 2015 phase III clinical trial OncoVex Pivotal trial in Melanoma (OPTiM).[48] Four hundred and thirty-six patients were randomized to receive intratumeral injections of T-VEC or GM-CSF. Durable response rate ($\geq$6 months) was found to be significantly higher in the T-VEC group (16.3%; 95% confidence interval [CI], 12.1% to 20.5%) when compared with the GM-CSF group (2.1%; 95% CI, 0% to 4.5%). Moreover, prolonged median OS was also observed: 23.3 months versus 18.9 months in T-VEC versus GM-CSF, respectively ($P = .051$).[48] Results of this trial ultimately led to FDA approval of T-VEC. Bystander effect and systemic immunotherapeutic effects of T-VEC were further elucidated on the patients enrolled in the OPTiM trial mentioned earlier. Analyzing 2116 injected lesions and 981 uninjected lesions, response by greater than or equal to 50% decrease in size was seen in 64% of injected, 34% of uninjected nonvisceral, and 15% of visceral lesions. CR was observed in 47%, 22%, and 9% of injected, uninjected, nonvisceral, and visceral lesions, respectively.[49]

With the success of intralesional T-VEC, further investigation has focused on the timing of its use and its use in combination with other treatment modalities. A clinical trial exploring the use of T-VEC in the neoadjuvant setting is currently under investigation with interim results presented in abstract form at the 2019 Society of Surgical Oncology Annual Meeting. Patients with resectable stage IIIB/C/IVM1a melanoma with greater than or equal to 1 injectable lesion were randomized to T-VEC + surgery versus surgery alone. Interim analysis reported R0 resection rates greater in the neoadjuvant T-VEC group and polymerase chain reaction greater than the observed ORR in the neoadjuvant T-VEC group.[50]

Oncolytic viral immunotherapy has led to significant advances in the treatment of locoregionally advanced melanoma. With its demonstrable efficacy, possible bystander effect, and tolerable adverse event profile, T-VEC is the most effective intralesional therapy and has become the standard for intralesional treatment of unresectable cutaneous, subcutaneous, and nodal lesions recurrent after initial surgical resection (**Fig. 1**).

OTHER ONCOLYTIC VIRAL THERAPIES

The success of T-VEC has led to the development of subsequent oncolytic viral therapies in an effort to better response rates and expand therapeutic indications. Developed vectors currently under investigation in the treatment of melanoma and other malignancies include Cavatak (CVA21, coxsackievirus A21),[51,52] Pexa-Vec (JX-594, vaccinia),[53] Reolysin (Pelareorep, reovirus),[54,55] HF10 (HSV-1),[56,57] and Telomelysin (OBP-301, adenovirus).[58,59] Some, as with T-VEC, are genetically modified with transformed pathogenicity, whereas others are naturally nonpathogenic to normal human cells.

CVA21, an immunotherapeutic strain of coxsackievirus A21, demonstrated 38.6% 6-month immune-related progression-free survival (PFS), 28.1% ORR, and greater

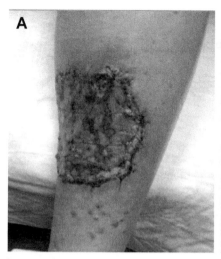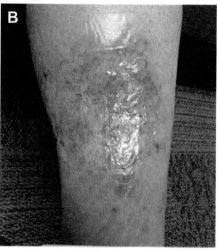

Fig. 1. A clinical example of a patient treated with T-VEC. This is a 58-year-old man with stage IIIB in-transit melanoma recurrent after initial resection on his left lower extremity in 2009. (A) Depicts in-transit disease before T-VEC treatment. There are 6 lesions ranging from 0.4 to 1.5 cm in diameter. (B) Clinical response after 5 weeks of treatment with no clearly palpable or visible disease. (Courtesy of J. Zager, MD, Tampa, FL.)

than 6 month durable response rate of 19.3% in the multiinstitutional CVA21 in Late Stage Melanoma trial.[51] Pelareorep, a strain of reovirus, showed promise in early phase trials across various malignancies,[55] later failing in a phase II trial to yield response in patients with metastatic melanoma.[54] As with many of the previously described intralesional therapies, combination with systemic immunotherapy and chemotherapy is also the subject of ongoing trails and investigation.[60–64] HF10, attenuated HSV-1, was investigated in combination with intravenous ipilimumab in stage IIIB to IV unresectable melanoma patients. In this phase II study, best ORR was reported at 41% and PFS and median OS of 19 and 21.8 months.[62] Pelareorep in conjunction with systemic carboplatin and paclitaxel improved on response rates previously reported with pelareorep alone, showing 21% ORR, PFS of 5.2 months, and OS of 10.9 months.[64] Although in-depth discussion regarding mechanism and evolution of these vectors is out of the scope of this article, it is important to note the broad and rapid development of this modality demonstrating great promise for intralesional treatment of locoregionally advanced melanoma.

INTRAARTERIAL THERAPIES
Hyperthermic Isolated Limb Perfusion

Regional perfusion with the use of an extracorporeal circuit was first described by Creech and colleagues in 1958. In an effort to limit systemic toxicity of chemotherapy, hyperthermic isolated limb perfusion (HILP) was initially used in the treatment of a myriad of malignant neoplasms with notable response in patients with melanoma where specific extremities could be isolated.[65] The technique involves surgical dissection and cannulation of the iliac or femoral vessels (lower extremity) and axillary vessels (upper extremity). A tourniquet is then placed at the base of the extremity excluding it from systemic circulation. Chemotherapy is circulated through the extremity in circuit driven by a cardiopulmonary bypass machine at flow rates ranging from 300 to 500 mL/min, heated to 38 to 42°C. Melphalan-based chemotherapy is most commonly used, often coupled with tumor necrosis factor-alpha (TNF-α) in Europe.[66,67]

Outcomes in HILP have been measured based on clinical response, limb salvage, and survival. Clinical response rates across multiple observational studies and randomized controlled trials have been reported between 64% to 100% (median 90.35%), with CR rate ranging from 25% to 89% (median 58.2%). Limb salvage rates of 95% and median OS of 36.5% with a median OS interval of 36.7 months was reported by Moreno-Ramirez and colleagues in their meta-analysis of 22 studies, 2018 HILPs from 1990 to 2008.[68]

The addition of TNF-α to melphalan perfusate has shown improved response rates across many observational studies. This was addressed in a 2006 phase III trial (ACO-SOG Trial Z0020) where 124 patients were randomized into melphalan alone or melphalan + TNF-α arms. At 3 months, no statistically significant difference was appreciated in ORR (64% vs 69%, $P = .44$) or CR (25% vs 26%, $P = .89$) in melphalan alone and melphalan + TNF-α, respectively. The melphalan + TNF-α arm experienced 17% grade 4 adverse events, compared with 5% in the melphalan alone arm ($P = .28$).[69]

HILP, although effective in the treatment of unresectable locoregional melanoma, comes with considerable potential morbidity. Complications may arise secondary to chemotherapeutic toxicity, thermal perfusate, surgical dissection, or vascular cannulation.[70] Local toxicity is graded on a scale first described by Wieberdink and colleagues, measuring clinical change in the affected limb.[71] Local toxicity can range from no change (Grade I) to severe tissue damage requiring amputation (Grade V). Most of the patients undergoing HILP experience Grade III toxicity or less. Acute vascular complication has been reported in up to 10% of cases. Compartment syndrome requiring fasciotomy and limb loss occur in 1% to 5% and 0% to 3.3%, respectively.[72] Long-term morbidity following HILP has been reported as high as 44%, with lasting effects including limb edema, muscle atrophy, stiffness, and functional impairment.[72,73]

Isolated Limb Infusion

First described by Thompson and colleagues in 1998, isolated limb infusion (ILI) was developed as a minimally invasive approach to HILP whereby smaller catheters are inserted into major inflow and outflow vessels of the extremity percutaneously.[74] ILI, similar to HILP, uses the circulation of chemotherapy through an isolated circuit involving an affected limb for the treatment on unresectable melanoma in-transit. Melphalan-based chemotherapy dosed at 75 μg/L for lower extremity and 100 μg/L for upper extremity is circulated through the limb manually, heated to 40°C. A tourniquet is used at the base of the extremity to prevent systemic leakage of chemotherapy.[75] ILI differs from HILP both in technique and logistics. ILI spares patients from potential morbidity associated with surgical exposure and cannulation of large extremity vessels. Infusion is performed in an acidotic and hypoxic environment. Moreover, the technique does not require equipment or personnel required for cardiopulmonary bypass machinery.[70,74,75]

Kroon and colleagues reported on their 14-year experience with ILI from prospectively collected data. In their analysis of 185 patients, ORR of 84% was reported with 38% CR and 46% PR. Median OS was 38 months and response to treatment was shown to be a predictor of survival with median survival of 53 months in patients with CR versus 25 months in those not achieving CR ($P = .005$).[76] A multiinstitutional series published in 2009 demonstrated CR and PR of 31% and 33%, respectively, in patients with unresectable in-transit melanoma. A single center analysis from Moffitt

Cancer Center evaluated ILI outcomes in 200 patients across 4 malignancies. In patients with melanoma, ORR of 59% (CR 25.7%, PR 33.3%) was reported. ORR was significantly higher in upper (76.9%) versus lower (55.1%) extremity ILI ($P = .04$) and responses had longer in-field PFS, distant metastatic-free survival, and OS.[77]

Acceptable regional toxicity has been achieved with reported 97% of patients experiencing less than or equal to grade III toxicity, suggesting ILI as a reasonable alternative to HILP.[76,78] Predictive factors of regional toxicity were investigated by Santillan and colleagues in their review of 171 patients undergoing ILI for melanoma. Toxicity was measured using the previously described Wieberdink limb toxicity scale and creatinine phosphokinase levels. Higher Wieberdink grade was associated with elevated creatine kinase levels, papaverine use, and female gender where melphalan adjusted for ideal body weight was associated with decreased toxicity grade.[70]

The largest and most recent ILI review comprised 687 patients across 9 tertiary referral centers in the United States and Australia. Miura and colleagues reported in stage 3B and 3C melanoma an ORR of 64.1% (CR 28.9%, PR 35.2%). Durable response was demonstrated with reported statistically significant in-field PFS, distant PFS, and OS in cohort responders. A similar toxicity profile was described where 94.8% of patients experienced Wieberdink grade III toxicity score or less. There were no reported amputations associated with treatment.[79]

In comparison with HILP, ILI has demonstrated decreased toxicity profiles and is associated with decreased overall morbidity. Its minimally invasive technique, comparative ease of execution, and no demonstrable difference in OS when compared with HILP have led to an increase in its use at centers worldwide.[78] Repeat regional perfusion with ILI or HILP has proved feasibility with comparable response rates to initial procedures.[80,81] Further advantage in ILI lies in the ease and ability to perform repeat infusion in the affected limb secondary to the decreased complexity and invasive nature of the procedure. Treatment algorithm recommendations for repeat infusion were proposed by Chai and colleagues. When possible, small volume recurrence should by excised. Unresectable disease should proceed to ILI as initial regional chemotherapy. HILP may be considered in high-volume or nodal disease, where node dissection could be coupled with perfusion. Repeat regional chemotherapy is recommended for recurrence following initial regional therapy based on initial response and disease-free interval. HILP is recommended for recurrence within 3 months and repeat ILI or HILP may be used in the setting of initial response lasting greater than 3 months.[81]

SYSTEMIC THERAPY AND COMBINATION THERAPY IN LOCOREGIONALLY ADVANCED MELANOMA

Over the past 10 years, the application of systemic therapies has changed the landscape in the treatment of metastatic melanoma. Current systemic immunomodulatory therapies include ipilimumab, nivolumab, and pembrolizumab, and targeted therapies toward BRAF and MEK inhibition include vemurafenib, dabrafenib, and tramerinib.[82–86] Starting with the validation of ipilimumab in 2010, immunomodulatory and targeted agents have demonstrated response rates and survival advantages in metastatic, unresectable melanoma never before seen with systemic therapy. The number of patients with stage III disease on these trials is unknown but their use in locoregionally advanced melanoma should be considered on an individualized basis as monotherapy or in combination with other modalities.

With the success of intralesional and intraarterial therapies, recent studies have evaluated methods to enhance treatment response in combination with systemic chemotherapy and immunotherapy (**Tables 1** and **2**). PV-10 in comparison or

Table 1
Select publications of intralesional and combination therapies

Author	Study Design	Injection Agent	No. of Participants	Injected Lesions				Uninjected Lesions
				CR (%)	PR (%)	SD (%)	PD (%)	
Intralesional Therapies								
Karakousis et al,[11] 1976	Observational	BCG	8	75	0	0	25	No response
Storm et al,[15] 1979	Prospective	BCG	27	74a (CR/PR)		NR	26	No response
Weide et al,[23] 2010	Phase II	IL-2	48	79	0.7	16.3	4.3	No response
Radny et al,[22] 2003	Phase II	IL-2	24	85	6	6	3	No response
Byers et al,[24] 2014	Systematic review	IL-2	140	78	2.5	19.6a (SD/PD)	NR	No response
Bedikian et al,[35] 2010	Phase II	Allovectin-7	127	3	9	25	63	No response
Gonzalez et al,[34] 2006	Phase II	Allovectin-7	77	3	7	23	68	Response in 21% of pts with stage IV disease
Thompson et al,[40] 2008	Phase I	PV-10	11	36	12	28	24	No response
Thompson et al,[42] 2015	Phase II	PV-10	80	26	25	18	31	Response in 27% of lesions
Senzer et al,[47] 2009	Phase II	T-VEC	50	16	10	24	50	Response in 33% of lesions
Andtbacka et al,[48] 2015	Phase III	T-VEC Vs GM-CSF	295 vs 141	11 / 1	16 / 5	73 (SD/PD) / 94 (SD/PD)	T-VEC: response in 34% nonvisceral and 15% visceral	Response

Study	Phase	Treatment						Response
Andtbacka et al,[51] 2015	Phase II	CVA21	57	14	14	-	-	
NCT03190824	Phase IIa	Telomelysin	Ongoing					
NCT02211131[50]	Phase II	Neotx T-VEC	Ongoing					
Combination Therapies								
Puzanov et al,[90] 2016	Phase Ib	T-VEC + Ipi	19	22	28	22	28	Response in 54% nonvisceral and 50% visceral lesions
Chesney et al,[89] 2018	Phase II	T-VEC + Ipi Vs Ipi	98 vs 100	13 / 7	26 / 11	19 / 24	32 / 33	Response in 57% nonvisceral and 52% visceral lesion in the T-VEC + Ipi Arm
Long et al[91]	Phase Ib	T-VEC + Pembro	21	24	33	14	29	No comment
Mahalingam et al,[64] 2017	Phase II	Pelareorep Vs. Pelareorep + carboplatin and paclitaxel	14	0	21	64	15	No comment
NCT02272855[62]	Phase II	HF10 + Ipi	44	16	25	27	-	No comment
NCT02263508[78]	Phase III	T-VEC + Pembro Vs Pembro	Ongoing					
NCT02557321[73]	Phase Ib/II	PV-10 + Pembro	Ongoing					
NCT02288897	Phase III	PV-10 vs dacarbazine/ temozolomide/T-VEC	Ongoing					

Abbreviations: Bleo, Bleomycin; ECT, electrochemotherapy; Ipi, ipilimumab; Neotx, neoadjuvant PD, progression of disease; Pembro, pembrolizumab; PR, partial response; SD, stabile disease.
  [a] Preliminary results.

Table 2
Select publications of intraarterial therapies

Author	Study Design	Therapy	No. of Participants	CR (%)	PR (%)	SD (%)	PD (%)
Intraarterial Therapies							
Cornett et al,[69] 2006	Phase III	HILP Melphalan vs HILP Melphalan + TNF-α	65 68	25 26	39 43	28 22	11 9
Thompson et al,[74] 1998	Retrospective	Single ILI vs Double ILI	44 38	39 45	52 42	-	-
Kroon et al,[76] 2008	Retrospective	ILI	185	38	46	10	6
Miura et al,[79] 2019	Retrospective	ILI	687	29	35	15	20

combination with systemic, oncolytic vital therapy and immunotherapy are current topics of investigation in on-going clinical trials. A phase III randomized controlled trial comparing PV-10 with dacarbazine/temozolomide and talimogene laherparepvec (NCT02288897) is underway. PV-10 in combination with anti-PD-1 pembrolizumab is now being evaluated in a phase 1b/2 study (NCT02557321). Patients received combination therapy every 3 weeks for 5 cycles, followed by up to 2 years of anti-PD-1 therapy alone. Preliminary results recently reported at the 15th International Congress of the Society for Melanoma Research demonstrated an ORR of 50% and a CR of 10%.[87] Ipilimumab, immunoglobulin G1 anti-CTLA4 antibody, has been studied in combination with ILI in a phase II trial out of Memorial Sloan Kettering.[88] Ipilimumab in conjunction with T-VEC has also been investigated in unresectable stage IIIB to IV melanoma.[89,90] In a phase II study, combination therapy yielded superior objective response rates when compared to ipilimumab alone (39% vs 18%, $P = .002$), with no added safety concerns.[89] A second study evaluated the efficacy of T-VEC + pembrolizumab (anti-PD1 checkpoint inhibitor). Similar to the above ipilimumab study, this phase 1b trial reported increased ORR and CR rates in the combination group suggesting clinical benefit to combination therapy.[91] This combination is under further investigation in a randomized, phase III trial comparing pembrolizumab + placebo versus pembrolizumab + T-VEC with PFS and OS as primary endpoints (NCT02263508).[92] Enrollment has recently closed and completion is estimated by April 2023.

REFERENCES

1. Pawlik TM, Ross MI, Johnson MM, et al. Predictors and natural history of in-transit melanoma after sentinel lymphadenectomy. Ann Surg Oncol 2005;12:587–96.

2. Wolf IH, Richtig E, Kopera D, et al. Locoregional cutaneous metastases of malignant melanoma and their management. Dermatol Surg 2004;30:244–7.

3. Amin M, Edge S, Greene F, et al, editors. AJCC cancer staging manual. 8th edition. Chicago: Springer International Publishing: American Joint Commission on Cancer; 2017.

4. Squires MH, Delman KA. Current treatment of locoregional recurrence of melanoma. Curr Oncol Rep 2013;15:465–72.

5. Dong XD, Tyler D, Johnson JL, et al. Analysis of prognosis and disease progression after local recurrence of melanoma. Cancer 2000;88:1063–71.
6. Agarwala SS. Intralesional therapy for advanced melanoma: promise and limitation. Curr Opin Oncol 2015;27:152–6.
7. Miura JT, Zager JS. Intralesional therapy as a treatment for locoregionally metastatic melanoma. Expert Rev Anticancer Ther 2018;18:399–408.
8. Coley WB. The classic: the treatment of malignant tumors by repeated inoculations of erysipelas. Clin Orthop Relat Res 1991;262:3–11.
9. Zbar B, Rapp HJ. Immunotherapy of guinea pig cancer with BCG. Cancer 1974;34(suppl):1532–40.
10. Zbar B, Bernstein ID, Rapp HJ. Suppression of tumor growth at the site of infection with living Bacillus Calmette-Guerin. J Natl Cancer Inst 1971;46:831–9.
11. Karakousis CP, Douglass HOJ, Yeracaris PM, et al. BCG immunotherapy in patients with malignant melanoma. Arch Surg 1976;111:716–8.
12. Mujagic H, Kolaric K, Malenica B, et al. BCG immunotherapy in previously treated malignant melanoma patients. Biomedicine 1979;30:95–102.
13. Morton DL, Eilber FR, Holmes EC, et al. BCG immunotherapy of malignant melanoma: summary of a seven-year experience. Ann Surg 1974;180:635–41.
14. Mastrangelo MJ, Sulit HL, Prehn LM, et al. Intralesional BCG in the treatment of metastatic malignant melanoma. Cancer 1976;37:684–92.
15. Storm FK, Sparks FC, Morton DL. Treatment for melanoma of the lower extremity with intralesional injection of bacille Calmette Guerin and hyperthermic perfusion. Surg Gynecol Obstet 1979;149:17–21.
16. Mastrangelo MJ, Bellet RE, Berkelhammer J, et al. Regression of pulmonary metastatic disease associated with intralesional BCG therapy of intracutaneous melanoma metastases. Cancer 1975;36:1305–8.
17. Agarwala SS, Neuberg D, Park Y, et al. Mature results of a phase III randomized trial of bacillus Calmette–Guerin (BCG) versus observation and BCG plus dacarbazine versus BCG in the adjuvant therapy of American Joint Committee on Cancer Stage I–III melanoma (E1673). Cancer 2004;100:1692–8.
18. Morgan DA, Ruscetti FW, Gallo R. Selective in vitro growth of T lymphocytes from normal human bone marrows. Science 1976;193:1007–8.
19. Liao W, Lin J-X, Leonard WJ. Interleukin-2 at the Crossroads of Effector Responses, Tolerance, and Immunotherapy. Immunity 2013;38:13–25.
20. Eklund JW, Kuzel TM. A review of recent findings involving interleukin-2-based cancer therapy. Curr Opin Oncol 2004;16:542–6.
21. Temple-Oberle CF, Byers BA, Hurdle V, et al. Intra-lesional interleukin-2 therapy for in transit melanoma. J Surg Oncol 2014;109:327–31.
22. Radny P, Caroli UM, Bauer J, et al. Phase II trial of intralesional therapy with interleukin-2 in soft-tissue melanoma metastases. Br J Cancer 2003;89:1620–6.
23. Weide B, Derhovanessian E, Pflugfelder A, et al. High response rate after intratumoral treatment with interleukin-2. Cancer 2010;116:4139–46.
24. Byers BA, Temple-Oberle CF, Hurdle V, et al. Treatment of in-transit melanoma with intra-lesional interleukin-2: a systematic review. J Surg Oncol 2014;110:770–5.
25. Hercus TR, Thomas D, Guthridge MA, et al. The granulocyte-macrophage colony-stimulating factor receptor: linking its structure to cell signaling and its role in disease. Blood 2009;114:1289–98.
26. Kaufman HL, Ruby CE, Hughes T, et al. Current status of granulocyte–macrophage colony-stimulating factor in the immunotherapy of melanoma. J Immunother Cancer 2014;2. https://doi.org/10.1186/2051-1426-2-11.

27. Dranoff G, Jaffee E, Lazenby A, et al. Vaccination with irradiated tumor cells engineered to secrete murine granulocyte-macrophage colony-stimulating factor stimulates potent, specific, and long-lasting anti-tumor immunity. Proc Natl Acad Sci U S A 1993;90:3539–43.
28. Si Z, Hersey P, Coates AS. Clinical responses and lymphoid infiltrates in metastatic melanoma following treatment with intralesional GM-CSF. Melanoma Res 1996; 6:247–55.
29. Nasi ML, Lieberman P, Busam K, et al. Intradermal injection of granulocyte-macrophage colony-stimulating factor (GM-CSF) in patients with metastatic melanoma recruits dendritic cells. Cytokines Cell Mol Ther 1999;5:139–44.
30. Plautz GE, Nabel GJ. Immunotherapy of malignancy by in vivo gene transfer into tumors. Proc Natl Acad Sci U S A 1993;90:4645–9.
31. Nabel GJ, Nabel EG, Yang ZY, et al. Direct gene transfer with DNA-liposome complexes in melanoma: expression, biologic activity, and lack of toxicity in humans. Proc Natl Acad Sci U S A 1993;90:11307–11.
32. Nabel GJ, Gordon D, Bishop DK, et al. Immune response in human melanoma after transfer of an allogeneic class I major histocompatibility complex gene with DNA-liposome complexes. Proc Natl Acad Sci U S A 1996;93:15388–93.
33. Stopeck AT, Hersh EM, Akporiaye ET, et al. Phase I study of direct gene transfer of an allogeneic histocompatibility antigen, HLA-B7, in patients with metastatic melanoma. J Clin Oncol 1997;15:341–9.
34. Gonzalez R, Hutchins L, Nemunaitis J, et al. Phase 2 trial of Allovectin-7 in advanced metastatic melanoma. Melanoma Res 2006;16:521–6.
35. Bedikian AY, Richards J, Kharkevitch D, et al. A phase 2 study of high-dose allovectin-7 in patients with advanced metastatic melanoma. Melanoma Res 2010; 20:218–26.
36. Richards J, Thompson J, Atkins M. A controlled, randomized Phase III trial comparing the response to dacarbazine with and without Allovectin-7 in patients with metastatic melanoma. Proc Am Soc Clin Oncol [abstract]. Orlando, FL, May 18–21, 2002.
37. Andtbacka RHI, Gonzalez R, Wloch MK. A Phase 3 Clinical Trial to Evaluate the Safety and Efficacy of Treatment with 2 mg Intralesional Allovectin-7® Compared to Dacarbazine (DTIC) or Temozolomide (TMZ) in Subjects with Recurrent Metastatic Melanoma. International Meeting of the Society for Melanoma Research [abstract]. Philadelphia, November 17–20, 2013.
38. Liu H, Weber A, Morse J, et al. T cell mediated immunity after combination therapy with intralesional PV-10 and blockade of the PD-1/PD-L1 pathway in a murine melanoma model. PLoS One 2018;13:1–15.
39. Mousavi H, Zhang X, Gillespie S, et al. Rose Bengal induces dual modes of cell death in melanoma cells and has clinical activity against melanoma. [abstract]. Melanoma Res 2006;16:pS8.
40. Thompson JF, Hersey P, Wachter E. Chemoablation of metastatic melanoma using intralesional Rose Bengal. Melanoma Res 2008;18:405–11.
41. Toomey P, Kodumudi K, Weber A, et al. Intralesional injection of rose bengal induces a systemic tumor-specific immune response in murine models of melanoma and breast cancer. PLoS One 2013;8:1–6.
42. Thompson JF, Agarwala SS, Smithers BM, et al. Phase 2 study of intralesional PV-10 in refractory metastatic melanoma. Ann Surg Oncol 2015;22:2135–42.
43. Kohlhapp FJ, Kaufman HL. Molecular pathways: mechanism of action for talimogene laherparepvec, a new oncolytic virus immunotherapy. Clin Cancer Res 2016;22:1048–54.

44. Liu BL, Robinson M, Han Z-Q, et al. ICP34.5 deleted herpes simplex virus with enhanced oncolytic, immune stimulating and anti-tumour properties. Gene Ther 2003;10:292–303.
45. He B, Chou J, Brandimarti R, et al. Suppression of the phenotype of gamma(1) 34.5- herpes simplex virus 1: failure of activated RNA-dependent protein kinase to shut off protein synthesis is associated with a deletion in the domain of the alpha47 gene. J Virol 1997;71:6049–54.
46. Hu JCC, Coffin RS, Davis CJ, et al. A phase I Study of OncoVEXGM-CSF, a second-generation oncolytic herpes simplex virus expressing granulocyte macrophage colony-stimulating factor. Clin Cancer Res 2006;12:6737–47.
47. Senzer NN, Kaufman HL, Amatruda T, et al. Phase II clinical trial of a granulocyte-macrophage colony-stimulating factor–encoding, second-generation oncolytic herpesvirus in patients with unresectable metastatic melanoma. J Clin Oncol 2009;27:5763–71.
48. Andtbacka RHI, Kaufman HL, Collichio F, et al. Talimogene laherparepvec improves durable response rate in patients with advanced melanoma. J Clin Oncol 2015;33:2780–8.
49. Andtbacka RHI, Ross M, Puzanov I, et al. Patterns of clinical response with talimogene laherparepvec (T-VEC) in patients with melanoma treated in the OPTiM phase III clinical trial. Ann Surg Oncol 2016;23:4169–77.
50. Andtbacka R, Dummer R, Gyorki D, et al. Interim analysis of a randomized, Open-Label phase II study of talimogene laherparepvec neoadjuvant treatment plus surgery versus surgery for resectable stage IIIB-IVM1a melanoma. Society of Surgical Oncology 2019 Annual Meeting [abstract]. San Diego, CA, March 27–30, 2019.
51. Andtbacka RHI, Curti BD, Kaufman H, et al. Final data from CALM: A phase II study of Coxsackievirus A21 (CVA21) oncolytic virus immunotherapy in patients with advanced melanoma. JCO 2015;33:9030.
52. Andtbacka RH, Curti BD, Hallmeyer S, et al. Phase II calm extension study: Coxsackievirus A21 delivered intratumorally to patients with advanced melanoma induces immune-cell infiltration in the tumor microenvironment. J Immunother Cancer 2015;3:P343.
53. Anthoney A, Samson A, West E, et al. Single intravenous preoperative administration of the oncolytic virus Pexa-Vec to prime anti-tumor immunity. JCO 2018;36: 3092.
54. Galanis E, Markovic SN, Suman VJ, et al. Phase II trial of intravenous administration of reolysin® (reovirus serotype-3-dearing strain) in patients with metastatic melanoma. Mol Ther 2012;20:1998–2003.
55. Vidal L, Pandha HS, Yap TA, et al. A phase I study of intravenous oncolytic reovirus type 3 dearing in patients with advanced cancer. Clin Cancer Res 2008;14:7127–37.
56. Ferris RL, Gross ND, Nemunaitis JJ, et al. Phase I trial of intratumoral therapy using HF10, an oncolytic HSV-1, demonstrates safety in HSV+/HSV- patients with refractory and superficial cancers. JCO 2014;32:6082.
57. Eissa IR, Naoe Y, Bustos-Villalobos I, et al. Genomic signature of the natural oncolytic herpes simplex virus HF10 and its therapeutic role in preclinical and clinical trials. Front Oncol 2017;7:149.
58. Kishimoto H, Urata Y, Tanaka N, et al. Selective metastatic tumor labeling with green fluorescent protein and killing by systemic administration of telomerase-dependent adenoviruses. Mol Cancer Ther 2009;8:3001–8.

59. Nemunaitis J, Tong AW, Nemunaitis M, et al. A phase I study of telomerase-specific replication competent oncolytic adenovirus (telomelysin) for various solid tumors. Mol Ther 2010;18:429–34.

60. Curti B, Shafren D, Richards J, et al. The MITCI (phase 1b) study: a novel immunotherapy combination of coxsackievirus A21 and ipilimumab in patients with advanced melanoma. Ann Oncol 2016;27. https://doi.org/10.1093/annonc/mdw378.06.

61. Silk AW, Kaufman H, Gabrail N, et al. Abstract CT026: Phase 1b study of intratumoral Coxsackievirus A21 (CVA21) and systemic pembrolizumab in advanced melanoma patients: Interim results of the CAPRA clinical trial. Cancer Res 2017;77:CT026.

62. Andtbacka RHI, Ross MI, Agarwala SS, et al. Final results of a phase II multicenter trial of HF10, a replication-competent HSV-1 oncolytic virus, and ipilimumab combination treatment in patients with stage IIIB-IV unresectable or metastatic melanoma. JCO 2017;35:9510.

63. Karapanagiotou EM, Roulstone V, Twigger K, et al. Phase I/II trial of carboplatin and paclitaxel chemotherapy in combination with intravenous oncolytic reovirus in patients with advanced malignancies. Clin Cancer Res 2012;18:2080–9.

64. Mahalingam D, Fountzilas C, Moseley J, et al. A phase II study of REOLYSIN((R)) (pelareorep) in combination with carboplatin and paclitaxel for patients with advanced malignant melanoma. Cancer Chemother Pharmacol 2017;79:697–703.

65. Creech O, Krementz ET, Ryan RF, et al. Chemotherapy of cancer: regional perfusion utilizing an extracorporeal circuit. Ann Surg 1958;148:616–32.

66. Fraker DL. Hyperthermic regional perfusion for melanoma and sarcoma of the limbs. Curr Probl Surg 1999;36:842–908.

67. Fraker DL. Management of in-transit melanoma of the extremity with isolated limb perfusion. Curr Treat Options Oncol 2004;5:173–84.

68. Moreno-Ramirez D, de la Cruz-Merino L, Ferrandiz L, et al. Isolated limb perfusion for malignant melanoma: systematic review on effectiveness and safety. Oncologist 2010;15:416–27.

69. Cornett WR, McCall LM, Petersen RP, et al. Randomized multicenter trial of hyperthermic isolated limb perfusion with melphalan alone compared with melphalan plus tumor necrosis factor: American College of Surgeons Oncology Group Trial Z0020. J Clin Oncol 2006;24:4196–201.

70. Santillan AA, Delman KA, Beasley GM, et al. Predictive factors of regional toxicity and serum creatine phosphokinase levels after isolated limb infusion for melanoma: a multi-institutional analysis. Ann Surg Oncol 2009;16:2570–8.

71. Wieberdink J, Benckhuysen C, Braat RP, et al. Dosimetry in isolation perfusion of the limbs by assessment of perfused tissue volume and grading of toxic tissue reactions. Eur J Cancer Clin Oncol 1982;18:905–10.

72. Möller MG, Lewis JM, Dessureault S, et al. Toxicities associated with hyperthermic isolated limb perfusion and isolated limb infusion in the treatment of melanoma and sarcoma. Int J Hyperthermia 2008;24:275–89.

73. Vrouenraets BC, Klaase JM, Kroon BB, et al. Long-term morbidity after regional isolated perfusion with melphalan for melanoma of the limbs. The influence of acute regional toxic reactions. Arch Surg 1995;130:43–7.

74. Thompson JF, Kam PC, Waugh RC, et al. Isolated limb infusion with cytotoxic agents: a simple alternative to isolated limb perfusion. Semin Surg Oncol 1998;14:238–47.

75. Kroon HM, Huismans A, Waugh RC, et al. Isolated limb infusion: technical aspects. J Surg Oncol 2014;109:352–6.
76. Kroon HM, Moncrieff M, Kam PCA, et al. Outcomes following isolated limb infusion for melanoma. a 14-year experience. Ann Surg Oncol 2008;15:3003–13.
77. O'Donoghue C, Perez MC, Mullinax JE, et al. Isolated limb infusion: a single-center experience with over 200 infusions. Ann Surg Oncol 2017;24:3842–9.
78. Dossett LA, Ben-Shabat I, Olofsson Bagge R, et al. Clinical response and regional toxicity following isolated limb infusion compared with isolated limb perfusion for in-transit melanoma. Ann Surg Oncol 2016;23:2330–5.
79. Miura JT, Kroon HM, Beasley GM, et al. Long–term oncologic outcomes after isolated limb infusion for locoregionally metastatic melanoma: an international multicenter analysis. Ann Surg Oncol 2019. https://doi.org/10.1245/s10434-019-07288-w.
80. Noorda EM, Vrouenraets BC, Nieweg OE, et al. Repeat isolated limb perfusion with TNFα and melphalan for recurrent limb melanoma after failure of previous perfusion. Eur J Surg Oncol 2006;32:318–24.
81. Chai CY, Deneve JL, Beasley GM, et al. A multi-institutional experience of repeat regional chemotherapy for recurrent melanoma of extremities. Ann Surg Oncol 2012;19:1637–43.
82. Hodi FS, O'Day SJ, McDermott DF, et al. Improved survival with ipilimumab in patients with metastatic melanoma. N Engl J Med 2010;363:711–23.
83. Robert C, Schachter J, Long GV, et al. Pembrolizumab versus ipilimumab in advanced melanoma. N Engl J Med 2015;372:2521–32.
84. Postow MA, Chesney J, Pavlick AC, et al. Nivolumab and Ipilimumab versus Ipilimumab in Untreated Melanoma. N Engl J Med 2015;372:2006–17.
85. Weber JS, D'Angelo SP, Minor D, et al. Nivolumab versus chemotherapy in patients with advanced melanoma who progressed after anti-CTLA-4 treatment (CheckMate 037): a randomised, controlled, open-label, phase 3 trial. Lancet Oncol 2015;16:375–84.
86. Chapman PB, Hauschild A, Robert C, et al. Improved survival with vemurafenib in melanoma with BRAF V600E mutation. N Engl J Med 2011;364:2507–16.
87. Agarwala S, Ross M, Zager J, et al. Interim results of a Phase 1b/2 study of PV-10 and anti-PD-1 in advanced melanoma. International Meeting of the Society of Melanoma Research [abstract]. Manchester, England, October 24–27, 2018.
88. Ariyan CE, Brady MS, Siegelbaum RH, et al. Robust antitumor responses result from local chemotherapy and CTLA-4 blockade. Cancer Immunol Res 2018;6:189–200.
89. Chesney J, Puzanov I, Collichio F, et al. Randomized, open-label phase ii study evaluating the efficacy and safety of talimogene laherparepvec in combination with ipilimumab versus ipilimumab alone in patients with advanced, unresectable melanoma. J Clin Oncol 2018;36:1658–67.
90. Puzanov I, Milhem MM, Minor D, et al. Talimogene Laherparepvec in combination with ipilimumab in previously untreated, unresectable stage IIIB-IV melanoma. J Clin Oncol 2016;34:2619–26.
91. Long G, Dummer R, Ribas A, et al. Efficacy analysis of MASTERKEY-265 Phase 1b study of talimogene laherparepvec and pembrolizumab for unresectable stage IIIB-IV melanoma. [abstract]. J Clin Oncol 2016;34(15):9568–9568.
92. Long GV, Dummer R, Ribas A, et al. A phase 1/3 multicenter trial of talimogene laherparepvec in combination with pembrolizumab for unresected, stage IIIB-IV melanoma (MASTERKEY-265). JCO 2016;34:TPS9598.

Role of Surgery for Metastatic Melanoma

Laura M. Enomoto, MSc, MD*, Edward A. Levine, MD, Perry Shen, MD, Konstantinos I. Votanopoulos, MD, PhD

KEYWORDS

- Metastatic melanoma • Metastasectomy • Stage IV melanoma
- Oligometastatic melanoma

KEY POINTS

- Metastatic melanoma has an overall poor prognosis, but long-term survival is not uncommon in patients responding to immunotherapy.
- Metastasectomy should be considered for local control in oligometastatic disease if a complete macroscopic resection can be obtained while any remaining distant disease is stable on immunotherapy.
- Clinical trial results are awaited to help further delineate the sequence and combination of systemic therapy and surgery.

INTRODUCTION

More than 96,000 new cases of melanoma are estimated in 2019 in the United States alone, with more than 7000 patients ultimately succumbing to the disease.[1] Historically, treatment options for those with metastatic melanoma were limited, with complete surgical resection reserved as the only meaningful option for patients with limited disease who could tolerate surgery,[2] mainly due to largely ineffective previous systemic therapies. Survival outcomes were poor, with an estimated median overall survival (OS) barely reaching 6 months.[3] In the past decade, however, the management of metastatic melanoma has rapidly evolved with the introduction of new therapeutic drug classes, such as BRAF and MEK pathway targeted inhibitors and immune checkpoint inhibitors consisting of monoclonal antibodies against cytotoxic T-lymphocyte-associated protein 4 (CTLA-4) and programmed cell death protein 1 (PD-1). Dramatic improvements in survival outcomes have been demonstrated, with 1-year OS rates of 72% with combined targeted inhibitors and a median OS greater than 30 months with the use of immune checkpoint inhibitors.[4,5] Accordingly, clinical decision making in patients with metastatic melanoma has become increasingly complex, with multiple

Department of Surgery, Wake Forest Baptist Medical Center, Medical Center Boulevard, Winston Salem, NC 27157, USA
* Corresponding author.
E-mail address: lenomoto@utmck.edu

Surg Clin N Am 100 (2020) 127–139
https://doi.org/10.1016/j.suc.2019.09.011
0039-6109/20/© 2019 Elsevier Inc. All rights reserved.

surgical.theclinics.com

current clinical trials evaluating the sequence and combination of systemic treatment and surgery. This article discusses the evolving role of surgical resection and integration of targeted therapies and immune checkpoint inhibitors in the management of stage IV cutaneous melanoma.

RATIONALE FOR SURGERY

Resection of metastatic disease in the absence of effective systemic treatment previously seemed counterintuitive, because it is a local treatment of a systemic problem (**Box 1**). Several large clinical trials, however, have demonstrated the benefit of metastasectomy over systemic treatment alone. The international, randomized, phase 3 trial, Malignant Melanoma Active Immunotherapy Trial for Stage IV Disease (MMAIT-IV), evaluated patients after complete resection of metastatic disease who underwent adjuvant treatment with bacillus Calmette-Guérin (BCG) and a melanoma vaccine Canavaxin (CancerVax Corp., Carlsbad, CA) compared with adjuvant BCG and a placebo.[6] Although the study did not demonstrate a benefit in the vaccine arm, the 5-year OS rate was approximately 40% in both arms, which was significantly higher than expected for patients treated with only systemic therapies available at that time. The Southwest Oncology Group (SWOG) phase 2, randomized, multicenter trial also demonstrated a survival benefit with complete resection compared with systemic treatment alone in patients with resectable metastatic melanoma.[7] Three-year and 4-year OS rates in patients who underwent complete resection were 36% and 31%, respectively. Although the relapse-free survival was only 5 months, of those who recurred, more than a third were able to undergo subsequent resection. In a retrospective analysis of patients included in the first Multicenter Selective Lymphadenectomy Trial (MSLT-1) who developed distant metastases, surgery conferred a significant survival advantage over systemic therapy alone.[3] Median OS was 15.8 months for patients who underwent surgery for their distant metastases at any point during treatment, which was significantly better than the 6.9-month median OS for patients who received only systemic treatment. All 3 of these trials, however, were performed prior to the introduction of targeted therapies or immune checkpoint inhibitors and their widespread use as systemic treatment.

The biologic mechanisms underlying improved survival in patients with distant metastatic melanoma who undergo complete resection are not well understood. In metastatic disease, tumor cells must escape the primary lesion and gain hematogenous access. They must then avoid stimulating a host immune response, adhere to the metastatic site, penetrate the basement membrane, and subsequently promote enough growth factors and angiogenesis to proliferate.[8,9] Oligometastatic disease thus may represent only the small percentage of circulating tumor cells with the capability of forming metastatic tumor deposits, and the resection of these cell populations with

---

Box 1
Rationale for surgery

- The MMAIT-IV demonstrated 40% 5-year OS rate after surgical resection, significantly higher than expected with systemic treatment alone.

- The SWOG trial showed 3-year and 4-year OS rates of 36% and 31%, respectively, with complete surgical resection (gross resection of all disease).

- The MSLT-1 demonstrated a 15.8-month median OS after complete metastasectomy compared with 6.9 months with systemic treatment.

the proved ability to form metastatic lesions may provide a local therapy for what is an otherwise systemic process.

Currently the authors approach metastatic melanoma through the concept of clonality. These patients for various reasons have more than 1 distinct cell population with specific biologic behavior and variable response to immunotherapy. It is possible that, by resecting a resistant clonal population, the remaining of disease will continue to respond to immunotherapy in conjunction with the patient's own immune system. One of the escape mechanisms for new melanoma clones is the loss of class I major histocompatibility complex that makes an immune response impossible.[10] Multiple studies have demonstrated that malignant cells either manufacture or induce surrounding tissue to produce immune factors that suppress the host's antitumor immune response.[2] Complete surgical resection of all disease provides a reduction in the immunosuppressive factors created by tumor deposits and their microenvironment, potentially restoring the patient's immune function to a level that controls the progression of residual occult metastases.[11–13] The correlation with the development of an endogenous immune response to a melanoma-associated tumor antigen after distant metastasectomy supports the importance of the patient's immune system as a determinant of OS and its likely contribution to the improved survival found after complete metastasectomy.[13,14]

CONSIDERATIONS FOR SURGERY

Appropriate selection of candidates for metastasectomy can be challenging, especially in the era of improved systemic therapies. With 3-year OS rates greater than 50% with combination immunotherapy,[4] the morbidity of surgery must be carefully balanced against the side effects and tolerance of systemic treatment. In order for surgical resection to even be considered a therapeutic option, however, the number of disease sites, projected ability to achieve complete resection, tumor doubling time (TDT), disease-free interval (DFI), serum lactate dehydrogenase (LDH), and response to systemic medical treatment all must be carefully weighed (**Box 2**).

Number of Metastatic Sites

The number of metastases is a well-recognized determinant of OS in melanoma.[3,15,16] Patients with a single-organ site metastasis are the ideal candidates for resection, with OS estimates significantly decreasing with increasing sites of metastases.[2,3] Essner and colleagues[2] found a 5-year OS rate of 29% for patients with a solitary metastasis compared with an 11% 5-year OS for patients with 4 or more metastases. Likewise, Howard and colleagues[3] demonstrated that OS

Box 2
Considerations for surgical resection

- Number of metastases
- Ability to achieve complete resection
- TDT
- DRI
- Serum LDH level
- Response to immunotherapy

significantly decreased as the number of organ sites increased. Median OS for patients undergoing a single metastasectomy was 17.6 months, compared with 13.4 months with resection of 2 organ sites. The median OS of 4.5 months with 3 or more organ sites resected was essentially the same as the 4.8-month median OS of patients undergoing systemic treatment alone.

Resectability

The completeness of resection of disease has also been consistently shown to affect OS.[6,17,18] Meyer and colleagues[17] demonstrated a significant improvement in survival in patients who underwent curative resection of their distant disease compared with patients who underwent incomplete, palliative cytoreduction, with a median OS of 17 months and 6 months, respectively. Similarly, Wood and colleagues[18] found a median OS of 27.6 months in patients who underwent complete metastasectomy, compared with a median OS of 8.4 months in the group who had incomplete or palliative resection. Over a 20-year period, the same group showed similar survival outcomes with liver metastasectomy, with completeness of surgical resection independently predictive of OS on multivariate analysis (hazard ratio 3.4; 95% CI, 1.4–8.1).[19]

Selecting those patients in whom a complete cytoreduction is possible can be challenging. The SWOG trial demonstrated that of 72 patients with presumed resectable metastatic melanoma on preoperative work-up, 64 (89%) were completely resected.[7] Thus, even in an experienced center, 10% of patients considered resectable preoperatively did not undergo a complete resection. Surgical experience and careful deliberation of the potential morbidity and mortality of metastasectomy balanced against its benefit is critical.

Tumor Doubling Time and Disease-Free Interval

In addition to the number of disease sites and the ability to achieve complete resection, the biological aggressiveness of the metastatic melanoma also must be considered. Patients with indolent, slow-growing disease are optimal candidates for resection, whereas those with rapidly progressive metastatic lesions are not likely to benefit from resection. Although there is no current biologic marker to measure the aggressiveness of disease, TDT serves as an indirect indicator of the disease process. Described by Ollila and colleagues,[20] the TDT is calculated by measuring changing diameters of each nodule, with serial measurements providing an assessment of the speed of growth. For pulmonary metastases, a TDT greater than 2 months was associated with a 5-year OS rate of 20.7% and median OS of 29 months, compared with a 0% 5-year OS rate and 16-month median OS when the TDT was less than 2 months. The investigators argue that TDT is a highly significant prognostic factor and that pulmonary metastasectomy should not be attempted if the TDT cannot be increased to greater than 2 months with systemic treatment.[20]

DFI, or interval between initial diagnosis of melanoma and development of stage IV disease, is another indirect indicator of aggressiveness. Howard and colleagues[3] demonstrated significantly improved OS in patients undergoing surgical resection with a DFI greater than 12 months compared with those with a DFI less than 12 months (17.8 vs 9.3 months, respectively). Likewise, Essner and colleagues[2] had previously shown an improved median OS of 30 months with a DFI greater than 36 months compared with those patients with a DFI less than 36 months who experienced an 18-month median OS. For patients with a short DFI considered indicative of more aggressive disease, the benefit of systemic treatment outweighs the potential morbidity of surgical resection.

Serum Lactate Dehydrogenase

Serum LDH is a well-known prognostic factor in metastatic melanoma and since 2009 has been included in the staging guidelines from the American Joint Committee on Cancer (AJCC).[21–24] In the 7th edition of the AJCC, an elevated LDH was considered such a poor prognostic factor that any distant metastases combined with an elevated serum LDH was classified as M1c disease.[23,25–27] This has since been changed in the 8th edition of the AJCC staging guidelines so that an elevated LDH no longer independently defines M1c disease, but elevated LDH now has its own subcategory designation.[24] Regardless of its classification, however, elevated levels of serum LDH are indicative of poor prognosis, and attempts at curative metastasectomy should take this into consideration.[28]

Response to Systemic Treatment

Historically, the lack of effective systemic treatment limited the ability to use response to systemic medical therapy as a prognostic factor. With the improved OS seen with targeted therapies and immune checkpoint inhibitors, however, the response to systemic medical therapy has become an important selection tool for metastasectomy. Faries and colleagues[19] reported significantly better OS for patients who had stabilization of disease (complete response, partial response, or stable disease) during systemic medical therapy prior to hepatic resection compared with those who did not have stable disease prior to surgery. On multivariate analysis, stabilization of disease on systemic therapy was found independently predictive of OS.[19] Evaluating the response to medical therapy can provide powerful selection criteria for metastasectomy.

SITE-SPECIFIC SURGICAL TREATMENT

In 2017, the AJCC issued a 8th edition of the melanoma staging system that divided metastatic melanoma into 4 subcategories based on anatomic location.[24] Patients with distant metastases to skin, subcutaneous tissue, muscle, or distant lymph nodes were categorized as M1a disease. M1b disease included any pulmonary metastases, and M1c disease included metastases to any other visceral site, excluding the central nervous system (CNS). New to the 8th edition, patients with metastases to any component of the CNS, including brain, spinal cord, and leptomeninges, were designated M1d disease. Using this framework, resections of M1a, M1b, M1c, and M1d diseases are discussed separately (**Box 3**).

M1a Disease

Metastases to the skin, subcutaneous tissue, muscle, or distant lymph nodes is the second most common presentation of metastatic melanoma, representing approximately 20% of patients with metastatic disease.[29] One-year OS for all M1a disease is 62%[23] but may be improving with more effective systemic treatments.[29]

Box 3
Site-specific metastasectomy

- M1a disease: skin, subcutaneous tissue, muscle, distant lymph nodes
- M1b disease: lung
- M1c disease: any visceral site excluding the CNS
- M1d disease: any component of the CNS

Patients who are able to undergo complete metastasectomy have improved survival outcomes. Howard and colleagues[3] found a median OS of greater than 60 months for patients with M1a disease metastases who undergo surgery compared with a median OS of 12.4 months with systemic treatment alone. The 4-year OS was 69% in patients undergoing metastasectomy,[3] whereas other studies report 5-year OS rates of 25% and 30% after complete resection.[2,9]

Within the M1a disease subcategory, skin and soft tissue metastases have a better prognosis compared with distant nodal metastases.[9,15] There are no high-quality data addressing margins or extent of lymph node dissection.[28–30] Aggressive resection with 2-cm margins is recommended by some investigators due to the known propensity of melanoma to infiltrate along tissue planes beyond macroscopic tumor mass,[9] whereas others determine margins of resection based on extent of disease, morbidity of required operation, prognosis, and functional status of the patient. Nodal disease also should be aggressively excised with complete nodal basin dissection. Axillary nodal dissection should include levels I to III, and cervical lymph node metastases requires modified radical neck dissection.[9,28] Parotid metastases requires both superficial and deep parotidectomy as well as a modified radical neck dissection. Inguinal nodal disease may be excised with a superficial groin dissection, but if superficial nodes are palpable or contain multiple metastases, a deep groin dissection is recommended.[9]

M1b Disease

The lung is the most common site of distant metastasis for melanoma, comprising 15% to 40% of stage IV disease.[9,29,31] Compared with metastases in other visceral sites, patients with pulmonary disease have improved OS at 1 year but no difference in 2-year survival.[32] In patients with resected pulmonary metastases, Howard and colleagues[3] found a median OS of 17.9 months compared with a 15-month median OS in patients with resected metastases of other visceral organs.

Specific factors influencing pulmonary resection were reported by Leo and colleauges[33] using data from the International Registry of Lung Metastases. Time to pulmonary metastases (TPM), number of metastases, and completeness of resection were considered significant. Patients with a single metastatic lesion that was completely resected and TPM greater than 36 months had the best outcomes, with a 5-year OS rate of 29% and 10-year OS rate of 26%.[33] OS significantly worsened with a TPM less than 36 months, multiple metastases, and incomplete resection, with no 5-year survivors with an incomplete metastasectomy. Other studies have found similar results, with TDT, prior response to systemic treatment, and extrathoracic metastatic disease also providing prognostic information.[9,20]

Pulmonary metastases can be resected using a minimally invasive video-assisted thoracoscopic surgery approach. Most pulmonary lesions occur just below the pleura, and wedge resection of surrounding tissue ensures adequate local tumor control.[9] Complete metastasectomy can be performed with a wedge resection 85% of the time, with only a minority of patients requiring an anatomic lobectomy.[34] Preoperative imaging may underestimate, however, the true number of pulmonary lesions. Kidner and colleagues[35] found that manual palpation of the subpleural parenchyma revealed lesions not identified on preoperative imaging in 26% of patients who underwent pulmonary resection. Currently, most agree that lung metastasectomy should be entertained in a multidisciplinary environment after metastases exhibit clinical stability on immunotherapy without progression of disease at other sites.

M1c Disease

M1c disease represents a diverse group of patients, because it includes metastases to any visceral organ excluding the CNS. As such, the presentation of disease can be widely variable, ranging from an incidental finding on imaging to clinically apparent bleeding. Similar to other metastastic sites, patients who underwent complete metastasectomy had an improved OS compared with patients who received systemic therapy only, with median OSs of 15 months and 6.3 months, respectively.[3] These figures should be interpreted with caution, however, because they include patients with CNS metastases, which has recently been redesignated as M1d disease due to associated poor prognosis.[24] Median OS of patients with currently defined M1c disease is potentially higher without the inclusion of CNS metastases and again persistent or stable disease after initial response to immunotherapy is a major determinant in proceeding with metastasectomy in M1c disease patients.

Gastrointestinal tract

Although melanoma metastasizes to the gastrointestinal (GI) tract in only 2% to 4% of patients,[9] autopsy studies show that approximately 50% of patients who die of metastatic melanoma have GI involvement.[36] The most common site of involvement is the small bowel (75%), followed by colon (25%) and stomach (16%).[9] Metastases often are symptomatic, with patients presenting with pain (29%–55%), obstruction (27%), bleeding (27%), palpable mass (12%), or weight loss (9%).[9] Even if complete resection is not possible, palliative intervention may be undertaken to relieve obstruction or bleeding.[9,37,38]

The median OS of patients undergoing palliative resection or systemic therapy only is poor. Ollila and colleagues[37] reported their series of patients with GI tract metastases who underwent surgery with curative intent, palliative resection, and systemic treatment alone. Median OS was 48.9 months for those who underwent complete metastasectomy and only 5.4 months and 5.7 months for palliation and systemic treatment, respectively. Spread to contiguous organs and high serum LDH levels also have been shown to predict a worse prognosis.[9,37,39]

Liver

Melanoma metastasizes to the liver in 15% to 20% of patients with metastatic disease.[9] Similar to other sites, hepatic metastasectomy should be offered only if complete resection can be obtained. Selecting patients for metastasectomy, however, can be challenging. Rose and colleagues[40] reported their series of patients with hepatic metastases from 2 high-volume melanoma centers. Of 1750 patients, only 34 (2%) were considered surgical candidates. Of those, 24 patients ultimately underwent surgical resection, and at exploration only 18 patients underwent a complete resection. Median OS was 28 months for the 1% of patients who underwent complete resection and only 4 months for those who underwent exploration only.[40]

In the era of more effective systemic therapies, Faries and colleagues[19] examined their series of patients undergoing hepatic resection, ablation, or combined treatment. They demonstrated a median OS of 24.8 months for patients undergoing complete metastasectomy compared with 8 months for those receiving systemic therapy alone. Outcomes were not significantly different among the resection, ablation, and resection/ablation groups. OS was independently related to the completeness of surgical treatment and to the stabilization of disease on medical therapy.[19]

Adrenal, pancreas, and spleen

Metastases to other solid organs, such as the adrenals, pancreas, and spleen, are uncommon, and the literature contains largely case reports. The largest series of adrenal metastases from melanoma included 154 patients, and only 22 underwent adrenalectomy.[41] Similar to other sites of disease, patients who underwent metastasectomy compared with systemic treatment alone had a significantly longer median OS (20.7 months vs 6.8 months),[41] and similar results have been demonstrated by other investigators.[18,42,43]

Pancreatic and splenic metastases from melanoma are exceedingly rare. Wood and colleagues[18] examined their 30-year experience and found only 20 and 53 patients with pancreatic and splenic metastases, respectively. In 1 of the largest series, Reddy and Wolfgang[44] reported a 14-month median OS in 11 patients who underwent pancreatic metastasectomy. A 23-month median OS in patients who underwent splenectomy for a solitary metastatic lesion was reported by de Wilt and colleagues.[45]

Bones

Osseous metastases are rare, occurring in up to 6.9% of metastatic melanoma patients,[46] and the prognosis is extremely poor.[30,45,47] In their 30-year experience, DeBoer and colleagues[48] reported 14 patients with isolated skeletal metastases. They found that metastases to the extremities had a better outcome compared with those with metastases to the axial skeleton, but OS was only 3 months to 7 months.[48] There is a paucity of literature regarding curative intent surgery for bone metastases because the prognosis is so poor that resection is almost never indicated.

M1d Disease

The revision in the 8th edition of the AJCC staging guidelines to designate CNS metastases as M1d disease, irrespective of metastases at other sites, reflects the generally overall poor prognosis of patients with CNS metastases.[24] Moreover, most contemporary clinical trial eligibility includes the presence or absence of CNS disease, and the M1d disease designation better reflects this practice.[24]

Unfortunately, CNS metastases, in particular brain metastases, are common. More than 50% of patients with metastatic disease at other sites develop brain metastases,[9] and autopsy reports show even higher rates, ranging from 50% to 70% of patients with metastatic melanoma.[9,30] Prognosis is poor, with a median OS of 4 months with systemic treatment alone.[9,49,50] Surgical resection, whole-brain radiation, and stereotactic radiosurgery can provide more durable options, extending median OS to 6 months to 22 months.[30] The number of brain metastases and serum LDH levels are independent prognostic factors for survival.[51]

Metastases to the spinal cord are rare and difficult to manage, and the literature consists largely of case reports.[9,52] Surgical decompression may be offered, because patients treated with surgery retain the ability to walk significantly longer than those treated with radiotherapy alone and have improved urinary continence and less steroid use.[53] Even with surgery, however, prognosis remains poor, and OS is typically less than 1 year.[54]

REPEAT METASTASECTOMY

Recurrence after surgical resection of distant metastases is unfortunately relatively common,[55,56] but additional metastasectomy is still a valuable option. Ollila and colleagues[55] examined 211 patients who were disease-free after surgical resection of distant metastases and found 131 patients (62%) who developed recurrent distant metastases. Those patients who were able to undergo another metastasectomy had a median OS of 18.2 months compared with the 12.5 months or 5.9 months median OS after palliative resection or nonoperative management, respectively. Moreover, complete surgical resection was found independently predictive of survival on multivariate analysis.[55] Thus, metastasectomy of distant disease can prolong survival even in those patients who require addition resection for recurrence after a DFI.

FUTURE DIRECTIONS

With the dramatic improvements in survival seen with the introduction of targeted therapies and immune checkpoint inhibitors, multiple clinical trials currently are evaluating the sequence and combination of systemic treatment and surgery. In a phase 2 trial (Combi-Neo [Neoadjuvant and Adjuvant Dabrafenib and Trametinib in Patients with Clinical Stage III Melanoma]), patients with surgically resectable stage III or oligometastatic stage IV BRAF V600–emutated or BRAF V600K–emutated melanoma were randomly assigned to upfront surgery and adjuvant systemic therapy (standard of care) or neoadjuvant plus adjuvant dabrafenib and trametinib.[57] The trial was stopped after only a quarter of the patients had been accrued because early analysis showed a significantly longer event-free survival in patients who received neoadjuvant plus adjuvant targeted therapy that with standard of care (19.7 months vs 2.9 months, respectively). The study is still accruing as a single-arm study for neoadjuvant and adjuvant dabrafenib and trametinib.

Based on the results of the Combi-Neo trial and previous studies demonstrating feasibility in non–small cell lung cancer, the same group conducted another phase 2 trial to evaluate nivolumanb and ipilimumab in the neoadjuvant setting.[58] Patients with resectable stage III or oligometastatic stage IV melanoma were randomized to neoadjuvant and adjuvant nivolumab or neoadjuvant ipilimumab plus nivolumab and adjuvant nivolumab. Combined ipilimumab plus nivolumab showed high overall response rates (ORRs) and pathologic complete response rates (pCRs) of 73% and 45%, respectively, but patients experienced substantial toxicity (73% grade 3 adverse events [AEs]). Nivolumab alone had inferior response rates (ORR 25% and pCR 25%) but lower toxicity (8% grade 3 AEs). Alternative dosing strategies are currently being investigated to preserve efficacy but limit toxicity (NCT02977052 and NCT03068455).[58]

Other systemic neoadjuvant therapy combinations for metastatic melanoma currently are being investigated. Early data from Tarhini and colleauges[59] investigating neoadjuvant pembrolizumab plus high-dose interferon alfa-2b have shown a pCR of 35% at a median follow-up of 11 months, but long-term results are still maturing. A phase 2 trial of neoadjuvant nivolumab with or without ipilimumab or relatlimab, a monoclonal antibody blocking lymphocyte-activation gene 3, currently is recruiting (NCT02519322).

Although early reports of systemic targeted therapy and checkpoint inhibitors in conjunction with surgical resection are promising, there are limited long-term survival data. Response and failure patterns need to be fully characterized in order to determine appropriate cohorts of patients eligible for treatment. The authors anticipate, however, increased use of neoadjuvant treatment combined with surgical metastasectomy in the future.

SUMMARY

With the introduction of targeted therapies and immune checkpoint inhibitors, the landscape for management of metastatic melanoma has changed dramatically. Systemic medical therapy no longer is only for those patients who are unable to undergo surgical resection but is now a complementary treatment modality. As long-term survival outcomes from trials of neoadjuvant treatment combinations and timing become available, use of targeted therapies and immune checkpoint inhibitors are likely to become more intertwined than ever with surgical resection. The care of patients with metastatic melanoma remains complex in a field of evolving treatments, and multidisciplinary care will continue to play a crucial role in guiding treatment decisions.

DISCLOSURE

None of the authors has any relationship with a commercial company that has a direct financial interest in subject matter or materials discussed in the article or with a company making a competing product.

REFERENCES

1. Key Statistics for Melanoma Skin Cancer, American Cancer Society. Available at: https://www.cancer.org/cancer/melanoma-skin-cancer/about/key-statistics.html#references. Accessed March 19, 2019.
2. Essner R, Lee JH, Wanek LA, et al. Contemporary surgical treatment of advanced-stage melanoma. Arch Surg 2004;139(9):961–6 [discussion: 966–7].
3. Howard JH, Thompson JF, Mozzillo N, et al. Metastasectomy for distant metastatic melanoma: analysis of data from the first Multicenter Selective Lymphadenectomy Trial (MSLT-I). Ann Surg Oncol 2012;19(8):2547–55.
4. Wolchok JD, Chiarion-Sileni V, Gonzalez R, et al. Overall survival with combined nivolumab and ipilimumab in advanced melanoma. N Engl J Med 2017;377(14):1345–56.
5. Robert C, Karaszewska B, Schachter J, et al. Improved overall survival in melanoma with combined dabrafenib and trametinib. N Engl J Med 2015;372(1):30–9.
6. Faries MB, Mozzillo N, Kashani-Sabet M, et al. Long-term survival after complete surgical resection and adjuvant immunotherapy for distant melanoma metastases. Ann Surg Oncol 2017;24(13):3991–4000.
7. Sosman JA, Moon J, Tuthill RJ, et al. A phase 2 trial of complete resection for stage IV melanoma: results of Southwest Oncology Group Clinical Trial S9430. Cancer 2011;117(20):4740–6.
8. Ollila DW, Laks S, Hsueh EC. Surgery for Stage IV Metastatic Melanoma. In: Riker AI, editor. Melanoma: A Modern Multidisciplinary Approach. Switzerland: Springer International Publishing; 2018. p. 467–81.
9. Leung AM, Hari DM, Morton DL. Surgery for distant melanoma metastasis. Cancer J 2012;18(2):176–84.
10. Rodig SJ, Gusenleitner D, Jackson DG, et al. MHC proteins confer differential sensitivity to CTLA-4 and PD-1 blockade in untreated metastatic melanoma. Sci Transl Med 2018;10(450) [pii:eaar3342].
11. Roth JA, Grimm EA, Osborne BA, et al. Suppressive immunoregulatory factors produced by tumors. Lymphokine Res 1983;2(2):67–73.
12. Avradopoulos K, Mehta S, Blackinton D, et al. Interleukin-10 as a possible mediator of immunosuppressive effect in patients with squamous cell carcinoma of the head and neck. Ann Surg Oncol 1997;4(2):184–90.
13. Hsueh EC, Gupta RK, Yee R, et al. Does endogenous immune response determine the outcome of surgical therapy for metastatic melanoma? Ann Surg Oncol 2000;7(3):232–8.

14. Morton DL, Foshag LJ, Hoon DS, et al. Prolongation of survival in metastatic melanoma after active specific immunotherapy with a new polyvalent melanoma vaccine. Ann Surg 1992;216(4):463–82.
15. Karakousis CP, Velez A, Driscoll DL, et al. Metastasectomy in malignant melanoma. Surgery 1994;115(3):295–302.
16. Petersen RP, Hanish SI, Haney JC, et al. Improved survival with pulmonary metastasectomy: an analysis of 1720 patients with pulmonary metastatic melanoma. J Thorac Cardiovasc Surg 2007;133(1):104–10.
17. Meyer T, Merkel S, Goehl J, et al. Surgical therapy for distant metastases of malignant melanoma. Cancer 2000;89(9):1983–91.
18. Wood TF, DiFronzo LA, Rose DM, et al. Does complete resection of melanoma metastatic to solid intra-abdominal organs improve survival? Ann Surg Oncol 2001;8(8):658–62.
19. Faries MB, Leung A, Morton DL, et al. A 20-year experience of hepatic resection for melanoma: is there an expanding role? J Am Coll Surg 2014;219(1):62–8.
20. Ollila DW, Stern SL, Morton DL. Tumor doubling time: a selection factor for pulmonary resection of metastatic melanoma. J Surg Oncol 1998;69(4):206–11.
21. Eton O, Legha SS, Moon TE, et al. Prognostic factors for survival of patients treated systemically for disseminated melanoma. J Clin Oncol 1998;16(3):1103–11.
22. Weide B, Elsasser M, Buttner P, et al. Serum markers lactate dehydrogenase and S100B predict independently disease outcome in melanoma patients with distant metastasis. Br J Cancer 2012;107(3):422–8.
23. Balch CM, Gershenwald JE, Soong SJ, et al. Final version of 2009 AJCC melanoma staging and classification. J Clin Oncol 2009;27(36):6199–206.
24. Gershenwald JE, Scolyer RA, Hess KR, et al. Melanoma staging: Evidence-based changes in the American Joint Committee on Cancer eighth edition cancer staging manual. CA Cancer J Clin 2017;67(6):472–92.
25. Nosrati A, Tsai KK, Goldinger SM, et al. Evaluation of clinicopathological factors in PD-1 response: derivation and validation of a prediction scale for response to PD-1 monotherapy. Br J Cancer 2017;116(9):1141–7.
26. Long GV, Grob JJ, Nathan P, et al. Factors predictive of response, disease progression, and overall survival after dabrafenib and trametinib combination treatment: a pooled analysis of individual patient data from randomised trials. Lancet Oncol 2016;17(12):1743–54.
27. Kelderman S, Heemskerk B, van Tinteren H, et al. Lactate dehydrogenase as a selection criterion for ipilimumab treatment in metastatic melanoma. Cancer Immunol Immunother 2014;63(5):449–58.
28. Lasithiotakis K, Zoras O. Metastasectomy in cutaneous melanoma. Eur J Surg Oncol 2017;43(3):572–80.
29. Deutsch GB, Kirchoff DD, Faries MB. Metastasectomy for stage IV melanoma. Surg Oncol Clin N Am 2015;24(2):279–98.
30. Martinez SR, Young SE. A rational surgical approach to the treatment of distant melanoma metastases. Cancer Treat Rev 2008;34(7):614–20.
31. Raigani S, Cohen S, Boland GM. The role of surgery for melanoma in an era of effective systemic therapy. Curr Oncol Rep 2017;19(3):17.
32. Balch CM, Soong SJ, Gershenwald JE, et al. Prognostic factors analysis of 17,600 melanoma patients: validation of the American Joint Committee on Cancer melanoma staging system. J Clin Oncol 2001;19(16):3622–34.
33. Leo F, Cagini L, Rocmans P, et al. Lung metastases from melanoma: when is surgical treatment warranted? Br J Cancer 2000;83(5):569–72.

34. Neuman HB, Patel A, Hanlon C, et al. Stage-IV melanoma and pulmonary metastases: factors predictive of survival. Ann Surg Oncol 2007;14(10):2847–53.
35. Kidner TB, Yoon J, Faries MB, et al. Preoperative imaging of pulmonary metastases in patients with melanoma: implications for minimally invasive techniques. Arch Surg 2012;147(9):871–4.
36. Ollila DW, Gleisner AL, Hsueh EC. Rationale for complete metastasectomy in patients with stage IV metastatic melanoma. J Surg Oncol 2011;104(4):420–4.
37. Ollila DW, Essner R, Wanek LA, et al. Surgical resection for melanoma metastatic to the gastrointestinal tract. Arch Surg 1996;131(9):975–9, 979–80.
38. Gutman H, Hess KR, Kokotsakis JA, et al. Surgery for abdominal metastases of cutaneous melanoma. World J Surg 2001;25(6):750–8.
39. Agrawal S, Yao TJ, Coit DG. Surgery for melanoma metastatic to the gastrointestinal tract. Ann Surg Oncol 1999;6(4):336–44.
40. Rose DM, Essner R, Hughes TM, et al. Surgical resection for metastatic melanoma to the liver: the John Wayne Cancer Institute and Sydney Melanoma Unit experience. Arch Surg 2001;136(8):950–5.
41. Mittendorf EA, Lim SJ, Schacherer CW, et al. Melanoma adrenal metastasis: natural history and surgical management. Am J Surg 2008;195(3):363–8 [discussion: 368–9].
42. Haigh PI, Essner R, Wardlaw JC, et al. Long-term survival after complete resection of melanoma metastatic to the adrenal gland. Ann Surg Oncol 1999;6(7):633–9.
43. Flaherty DC, Deutsch GB, Kirchoff DD, et al. Adrenalectomy for metastatic melanoma: current role in the age of nonsurgical treatments. Am Surg 2015;81(10):1005–9.
44. Reddy S, Wolfgang CL. The role of surgery in the management of isolated metastases to the pancreas. Lancet Oncol 2009;10(3):287–93.
45. de Wilt JH, McCarthy WH, Thompson JF. Surgical treatment of splenic metastases in patients with melanoma. J Am Coll Surg 2003;197(1):38–43.
46. Stewart WR, Gelberman RH, Harrelson JM, et al. Skeletal metastases of melanoma. J Bone Joint Surg Am 1978;60(5):645–9.
47. Barth A, Wanek LA, Morton DL. Prognostic factors in 1,521 melanoma patients with distant metastases. J Am Coll Surg 1995;181(3):193–201.
48. DeBoer DK, Schwartz HS, Thelman S, et al. Heterogeneous survival rates for isolated skeletal metastases from melanoma. Clin Orthop Relat Res 1996;(323):277–83.
49. Ollila DW. Complete metastasectomy in patients with stage IV metastatic melanoma. Lancet Oncol 2006;7(11):919–24.
50. Fife KM, Colman MH, Stevens GN, et al. Determinants of outcome in melanoma patients with cerebral metastases. J Clin Oncol 2004;22(7):1293–300.
51. Eigentler TK, Figl A, Krex D, et al. Number of metastases, serum lactate dehydrogenase level, and type of treatment are prognostic factors in patients with brain metastases of malignant melanoma. Cancer 2011;117(8):1697–703.
52. Gokaslan ZL, Aladag MA, Ellerhorst JA. Melanoma metastatic to the spine: a review of 133 cases. Melanoma Res 2000;10(1):78–80.
53. Patchell RA, Tibbs PA, Regine WF, et al. Direct decompressive surgical resection in the treatment of spinal cord compression caused by metastatic cancer: a randomised trial. Lancet 2005;366(9486):643–8.
54. Connolly ES Jr, Winfree CJ, McCormick PC, et al. Intramedullary spinal cord metastasis: report of three cases and review of the literature. Surg Neurol 1996;46(4):329–37 [discussion 337–8].

55. Ollila DW, Hsueh EC, Stern SL, et al. Metastasectomy for recurrent stage IV melanoma. J Surg Oncol 1999;71(4):209–13.
56. Friedman EB, Thompson JF. Continuing and new roles for surgery in the management of patients with stage IV melanoma. Melanoma Manag 2018;5(1):MMT03.
57. Amaria RN, Prieto PA, Tetzlaff MT, et al. Neoadjuvant plus adjuvant dabrafenib and trametinib versus standard of care in patients with high-risk, surgically resectable melanoma: a single-centre, open-label, randomised, phase 2 trial. Lancet Oncol 2018;19(2):181–93.
58. Amaria RN, Reddy SM, Tawbi HA, et al. Neoadjuvant immune checkpoint blockade in high-risk resectable melanoma. Nat Med 2018;24(11):1649–54.
59. Tarhini A, Lin Y, Drabick JJ, et al. Neoadjuvant combination immunotherapy with pembrolizumab and high dose IFN-α2b in locally/regionally advanced melanoma. J Clin Oncol 2018;36(5 supplement):181.

Surgical Considerations and Systemic Therapy of Melanoma

Adriana C. Gamboa, MD[a], Michael Lowe, MD, MA[a],
Melinda L. Yushak, MD, MPH[b], Keith A. Delman, MD[a],*

KEYWORDS

- Adjuvant therapy • Neoadjuvant therapy • Immunotherapy • Targeted therapy
- Advanced melanoma

KEY POINTS

- The management of unresectable stage III and stage IV melanoma involves a multimodal treatment, including surgery, systemic immunotherapies, and targeted therapies.
- Resection of progressive foci of disease may modulate the immunosuppressive effects of melanoma.
- Checkpoint inhibitors have dramatically improved survival for patients with metastatic melanoma. Nivolumab, pembrolizumab, and ipilimumab are currently approved for the adjuvant and metastatic setting.
- Small studies have already demonstrated the benefit of both systemic immunotherapy and targeted therapy in the neoadjuvant setting. Clinical trials are ongoing.

INTRODUCTION

The incidence of metastatic melanoma has rapidly increased over the last 3 decades with an associated increase in mortality worldwide when compared with other cancers.[1-3] Data from the US Surveillance, Epidemiology, and End Results program demonstrate that the incidence of melanoma quadrupled over the past 4 decades, increasing by 1.5% annually over the last 10 years.[4] For patients with regional or distant melanoma, the treatment armamentarium remained unchanged for the first decade of the twenty-first century. Based on advancements in the understanding of the role of the immune system, new systemic strategies have transformed the

Financial Support: Supported in part by the National Center for Advancing Translational Sciences of the National Institutes of Health under Award Number TL1TR002382 and the Katz Foundation
[a] Division of Surgical Oncology, Emory University School of Medicine, 1365B Clifton Road Northeast, Suite B4000, Atlanta, GA 30322, USA; [b] Division of Medical Oncology, Emory University School of Medicine, 1365B4 Clifton Road Northeast, Suite B4000, Atlanta, GA 30322, USA
* Corresponding author.
E-mail address: kdelman@emory.edu

therapeutic landscape and have led to survival improvements in patients with advanced melanoma. These successes have broadened the indications for surgery, and there is now an enhanced justification for resecting oligometastatic disease as either first-line treatment or salvage therapy.

The eighth edition of the American Joint Committee on Cancer (AJCC) stratifies stage III melanoma into 4 categories based on histopathologic factors, whereas stage IV disease is distinctly classified into 4 categories based on metastatic location, including distant cutaneous, subcutaneous, or nodal disease (M1a), lung (M1b), noncentral nervous system visceral (M1c), and central nervous system metastasis with or without metastasis at other sites (M1d). These anatomic sites can be further substratified based on serum lactate dehydrogenase levels. In this article, the authors outline available evidence supporting resection of metastatic disease for both stage III and IV melanoma in the context of currently available systemic therapeutic options. They additionally review the evidence supporting the use of adjuvant systemic therapies and other treatment modalities, including radiotherapy, chemotherapy, and vaccines in advanced melanoma. Last, the authors highlight the effort of translating the success of these therapies to the neoadjuvant setting and summarize active clinical trials.

SURGICAL MANAGEMENT OF METASTATIC DISEASE
Introduction

Approximately 9% of patients diagnosed with cutaneous melanoma in the United States present with regional disease. There is marked heterogeneity in prognosis ranging from a 10-year disease-specific survival (DSS) of 88% in stage IIIA to 24% in stage IIID. An additional 4% of patients present with synchronous distant metastatic disease, and these patients have a 5-year DSS of 10%.[5] For decades, systemic therapies with limited efficacy compelled clinicians to consider surgery in patients with good performance status and disease amenable to resection. The advent of effective systemic therapy has transformed this paradigm, and although systemic therapies are now the mainstay of treatment of stage IV melanoma, surgical resection is an appropriate adjuvant treatment for selected patients and necessary for palliation, diagnosis, and certain therapeutic regimens. Importantly, these recent advances in systemic therapy may support a rationale for a more aggressive surgical approach. The decision to resect metastatic melanoma should be based on a complete evaluation of the extent of metastasis, a thorough assessment of the patient's physiologic reserve, and an optimal estimation of the biologic behavior of the disease. Confirmation of metastatic disease in patients with clinical or radiographically identified lymphadenopathy should be obtained with fine-needle aspiration biopsy before surgical intervention. Furthermore, staging evaluation with cross-sectional imaging is warranted to ensure candidacy for surgical control of disease.

Surgery for Locoregional Disease

In the AJCC eighth edition, regional lymph node disease is further divided into clinically occult or clinically evident disease.[5] Importantly, these designations refer to the mode of detection of the nodal metastases with clinically occult disease detected by sentinel lymph node (SLN) biopsy and clinically evident disease detected by physical examination or radiographic imaging.[6] Based on the results of the Multicenter Selective Lymphadenectomy Trial-II (MSLT-II), either completion lymph node dissection (CLND) or observation may be offered to patients with a positive SLN, although most patients will not benefit from CLND.[7] However, current consensus guidelines suggest that those with high-risk features, including extracapsular spread/extension, concomitant microsatellitosis of the primary tumors, more than 3 involved nodes, or more than 2 involved nodal basins, be strongly considered for CLND.[8] For patients with clinically evident disease, once metastases have been histopathologically confirmed, and in the absence of extraregional disease, therapeutic lymph node dissection is recommended given its established association with long-term survival outcomes and the absence of evidence to the contrary. In a large retrospective series, 38% of patients with resected clinically evident nodal melanoma remained disease free after 5 years.[9] For axillary lymph node dissection, levels 1 to 3 should be excised. For inguinal lymph node dissection, controversy remains as to the extent of lymphadenectomy, although a 2011 retrospective study demonstrated that disease-free survival did not differ between patients who underwent superficial groin dissection and those who underwent superficial and deep groin dissection. Despite this finding, inguinopelvic lymphadenectomy (superficial and deep groin dissection) can be considered for patients with multiple positive lymph nodes on superficial groin dissection or abnormal pelvic nodes on cross-sectional imaging.[10] In the presence of cervical nodal disease, a modified radical neck dissection should be performed with excision of levels 2 to 5 and with consideration of levels 1 or 6, or a parotidectomy where appropriate. Following complete resection of nodal recurrence, adjuvant treatment with immunotherapy or targeted therapy is recommended as outlined in later discussion.

Nonnodal locoregional metastasis includes satellite disease and in-transit metastasis (ITM), which are associated with a prognosis similar to that of patients with clinically detected nodes.[5] By convention, satellite lesions are differentiated from ITMs by their distance from the primary site. Lesions within 2 cm of the primary melanoma are characterized as satellites, whereas ITMs are located greater than 2 cm from the primary tumor but proximal to the locoregional lymph nodes.[11] Because of the heterogeneity of this disease process, there have been few clinical trials comparing the efficacy of therapeutic options. As such, there is no classic definition of what amount of disease should be considered resectable as long as limb function can be maintained. Despite this ambiguity, definitive surgical resection with narrow negative margins remains the preferred treatment of limited satellite or ITM deposits. Although its impact remains unknown, in the absence of clinically identifiable nodal metastases, lymphatic mapping with SLN biopsy may also be considered.[12] Patients who present with both ITM and clinical regional nodal disease should be strongly considered for systemic therapy as a first-line approach given the high likelihood of subsequent distant disease. For patients in whom surgery is not feasible because of extensive lesions, evidence of distant metastatic disease, or patient-related factors, regional therapies such as isolated limb perfusion (ILP) and intralesional therapies or systemic therapies may be used to achieve disease control. These modalities are detailed later in this issue.

Surgery for Distant Metastatic Disease

Improved long-term outcomes in patients undergoing metastasectomy for melanoma have been reported in several retrospective studies, which demonstrate that 15% to 28% of patients may achieve a 5-year survival when distant metastases can be completely resected.[13–19] Despite considerable selection bias in these studies, there is evidence demonstrating that resection of distant metastases may be associated with improved survival in carefully selected patients, particularly those with long disease-free intervals and favorable performance status. These findings have been further confirmed in 2 large-scale, multicenter trials. The Southwestern Oncology Group's prospective multicenter trial of patients with surgically resectable stage IV melanoma found that despite a short relapse-free survival of 5 months, complete resection conferred a median overall survival (OS) of 21 months versus historical rates of 6 to 10 months with systemic therapy.[20] In the MSLT-I, retrospective analysis of patients who were longitudinally followed and developed distant metastases found that metastasectomy conferred a survival advantage, even in patients who developed high-risk visceral metastases. If surgery was performed, the median survival was 15.8 months compared with 6.9 months in those treated with systemic therapy alone, with an improved 4-year survival compared with systemic medical therapy alone (20.8% vs 7.0%, hazard ratio [HR] = 0.41, $P<.0001$).[21] Unfortunately, these data may have limited applicability in the current paradigm of systemic therapy.

The results of the 2006 Canvaxin trial were likely some of the most transformative data at their time in support of aggressive surgery. This phase 3 trial compared adjuvant treatment with Bacillus Calmette-Guerin (BCG) and an allogenic melanoma vaccine to BCG with placebo after complete resection of stage IV disease. Although the study did not show any benefit in the vaccine-treated arm, 5-year OS rates following complete surgical resection were approximately 40% in both groups, substantially higher than would have been expected if the patients had been treated with the systemic therapies that were available at the time.[22] Although these data provide a foundation for the application of surgery in metastatic disease, they remain limited by the facts that this was a highly selected subset of patients and that modern effective systemic therapy was not available as a comparator or adjunct.

Although only present in about 2% to 4% of patients with melanoma, gastrointestinal metastases in stage IV disease are common, accounting for up to 40% of all metastases. With appropriate patient selection, resection of gastrointestinal metastases has also been associated with improved survival.[23] A retrospective review of 1623 patients with localized intraabdominal metastases confined to the gastrointestinal tract, liver, adrenal glands, pancreas, and the spleen demonstrated an improvement in median OS of 18 months after metastasectomy compared with 7 months in those who only underwent treatment with systemic drug treatment.[24] Several other studies have recapitulated these findings with 5-year OS rates of 20.5% after resection of liver and adrenal metastases.[25,26]

The lungs are another common site of visceral metastases, comprising 15% to 35% of patients with metastatic melanoma.[18] Several studies have shown improved survival after pulmonary metastasectomy, with median survival from 10 to 28 months and 5-year survival rates up to 35%.[27,28] Selection for pulmonary metastasectomy should be based on ability to achieve complete resection, disease-free interval greater than 1 year, fewer than 3 pulmonary nodules, absence of extrathoracic and lymph node metastasis, and response to chemotherapy or immunotherapy.

The impact of metastasectomy is multifactorial. Surgical resection can render an individual disease free in a short amount of time with minimal morbidity in carefully selected patients. Furthermore, excision can yield consistent results with iterative metastasectomy. Surgery also decreases the amount of tumor-secreted immunosuppressant potentially allowing the host's immune system to generate an improved response to remaining cancer cells.[29] This concept was supported by a recent study that demonstrated that pathologic specimens from progressive foci of disease demonstrate a high percentage of T-regulatory cells and low T-effector cells, suggesting a mechanism of immune escape. Resection of these progressive foci in the setting of other stable lesions resulted in median survival of 9.5 months.[30]

Patient selection for metastasectomy is paramount and should take into consideration several factors that may give insight into tumor biology. Disease-free interval, longer tumor doubling time, number of metastatic lesions, and stabilization on systemic therapy have been shown to be favorable indicators for benefit from surgery.[31] One of the most ambiguous considerations in the current era is how to optimally interface surgery and systemic therapy. Given improvements in the armamentarium, surgery may play a larger role as "consolidative" therapy (ie, to achieve complete response when patients have largely responded but only have limited disease remaining) or more aggressive resections may be considered in otherwise healthy patients with the knowledge that adjuvant therapy has a significant impact on disease response. Although the survival benefits of tumor debulking remain unclear, there is certainly a benefit to palliative resection in symptomatic patients in whom surgery offers the potential for alleviating symptoms.

ADJUVANT THERAPY
Introduction

For decades, the management of metastatic melanoma was limited to a small number of largely ineffective drugs, including dacarbazine and high-dose interleukin-2 (IL-2). With the introduction of immune checkpoint inhibitors and targeted agents, the treatment of melanoma was revolutionized. In addition, the recent Food and Drug Administration (FDA) approval of talimogene laherparepvec (T-VEC), a genetically engineered virus that secretes granulocyte-macrophage colony-stimulating factor (GM-CSF) selectively inside the tumor cells thus initiating a tumor-directed immune response, has incited additional enthusiasm. In this section, the authors outline landmark studies in the development of adjuvant therapy, the currently accepted indications for initiation of adjuvant therapy in both surgically resected, high-risk melanoma as well as advanced, unresectable melanoma and discuss other emerging options.

Indications for Adjuvant Therapy

The goal of adjuvant therapy is to improve survival by treating occult metastatic disease after known sites of malignancy are resected or otherwise treated. Early and late adjuvant therapy has been characterized as treatment after resection of a primary lesion and its associated synchronous metastatic disease (early) or after recurrence and resection of disease, including metastasectomy (late). The differentiation of these 2 treatment groups is important because patients who undergo early adjuvant therapy are considered lower risk when evaluating long-term survival outcomes, and the risk of adverse events is higher given their longer survival.[32] At present, adjuvant therapy is approved for patients with stage IIIA disease or higher with trials currently underway investigating the role of systemic therapy in patients with resected high-risk stage IIB and C disease.

Adjuvant Immunotherapy

Immunotherapy entails the administration of monoclonal antibodies, T cells, or immunostimulatory cytokines aimed at priming the immune system and activating immune responses against residual tumor cells. The first immunomodulatory agent to be approved for the treatment of advanced melanoma was IL-2 in 1998. Subsequently, for 2 decades before FDA approval of adjuvant ipilimumab in 2015, interferon-α (IFN-α) was the only approved agent for the adjuvant treatment of high-risk cutaneous melanoma (**Table 1**). This agent had such a high rate of side effects that only 50% of patients were able to successfully complete the entire year of intended therapy.[33] In addition, on long-term follow-up, this drug had no impact on distant metastasis-free survival or OS.[34]

More recently, newer and more effective therapeutic agents have emerged. Agents targeting cytotoxic T-lymphocyte associated protein-4 (CTLA-4) and the programmed death-1 (PD-1) regulatory pathway have shown considerable success in the adjuvant and metastatic setting. Together, these therapies are known as checkpoint

Table 1
Adjuvant therapy Food and Drug Administration approval and indications

Drug Name	FDA Approval	Indication	Trial Leading to Approval	Dosing Regimen
High-dose IFN-α	1996	High-risk resected melanoma	ECOG 1684	Initiation: 20 million IU/m² for 4 wk Maintenance: 10 million IU/m² for 11 mo
Ipilimumab	2015	Resected stage III melanoma	EORTC 18071	3 mg/kg q2w for up to 2 y
Nivolumab	2017	Resected stage III or IV melanoma	Checkmate-238	3 mg/kg q2w for 4 doses, then 3 mg/kg q2w for up to 2 y
Dabrafenib + trametinib	2018	Resected stage III melanoma with BRAF V600 mutations	COMBI-AD	350 mg po daily + 2 mg po daily until disease progression
Pembrolizumab	2019	Resected stage III melanoma	EORTC 1325	2 mg/kg q3w for up to 2 y
Vemurafenib	Unknown status	Stages IIC-IIIB resected melanoma	BRIM8	960 mg bid until disease progression or unacceptable toxicity

inhibitors, because they are antibody therapies directed against negative immunologic regulators.

Ipilimumab, a monoclonal antibody against CTLA-4, was granted FDA approval in 2011 after a phase 3 clinical study by Hodi and colleagues[35] found a significant improvement in median OS in patients with unresectable stage III or IV melanoma treated with ipilimumab as compared with control (10 vs 6.4 months, respectively; HR 0.66, $P = .0026$). Its approval was subsequently expanded for use in the adjuvant setting in 2015 after the phase 3 international EORTC 18071 trial compared adjuvant high-dose ipilimumab to placebo in patients with completely resected stage III melanoma (**Table 1**). The trial demonstrated a median recurrence-free survival (RFS) of 26.1 months with ipilimumab versus 17.1 months with placebo (HR 0.75, 95% confidence interval [CI] 0.64–0.9, $P = .0013$).[36] A subsequent analysis demonstrated that ipilimumab resulted in significantly higher rates of 5-year RFS (40.8% vs 30.3%, $P<.001$), 5-year distant metastasis-free survival (48.3 vs 38.9, $P = .002$), and 5-year OS (65.4% vs 54.4%, $P = .001$) when compared with placebo.[37] Despite these improvements in RFS and OS, ipilimumab is associated with a high incidence of adverse events. Grade 3 or 4 immune-related adverse events, which include diarrhea, hepatitis, thyroiditis, and adrenal insufficiency, appear to be dose related at 10 mg/kg, and the rate of grade 3 or 4 adverse events has been reported in 43% of patients.[36] Based on these data, ipilimumab was approved for adjuvant therapy. When administered, National Comprehensive Cancer Network guidelines recommend ipilimumab monotherapy at 3 mg/kg until disease progression in patients with resected stage IIIA with metastases greater than 1 mm, resected stage IIIB-C, or resected nodal recurrence.[38] However, given its associated toxicity and the arrival of newer agents, adjuvant ipilimumab is no longer routinely administered.

Pembrolizumab and nivolumab are both antibodies that target PD-1 and received FDA approval in the metastatic setting in 2014 and 2017, respectively, initially for use in patients with disease progression after receiving first-line therapy. Two phase 3 studies demonstrated the efficacy of nivolumab in stage III or IV melanoma and further established its superiority to chemotherapy in advanced melanoma. Check-Mate 037 randomized patients with unresectable or metastatic melanoma to receive either nivolumab or chemotherapy with a primary endpoint of objective response. Results demonstrated an overall response rate (ORR) of 32% in patients from the nivolumab group as compared with 11% in the chemotherapy group.[39] CheckMate 066 was designed to analyze OS in nivolumab-treated patients and randomized patients with metastatic melanoma to treatment with nivolumab or dacarbazine. OS at 1 year was reported as 73% in the nivolumab group versus 42% in the dacarbazine group ($P<.001$).[40] The success of this agent was further established in the CheckMate 238 trial, which led to the 2017 FDA approval of nivolumab as adjuvant therapy (**Table 1**). This trial randomized patients with high-risk, completely resected stage IIIB, IIIC, or IV melanoma to receive either nivolumab or ipilimumab. RFS, the primary endpoint, was 71% at 12 months for patients assigned to adjuvant nivolumab, compared with 61% for adjuvant ipilimumab (HR 0.65, 95% CI 0.51–0.83, $P<.001$). Nivolumab also had a better safety profile, with a 14.4% incidence of grade 3 or 4 treatment related adverse events, compared with 45.9% for ipilimumab.[41] As such, adjuvant nivolumab is preferred over high-dose ipilimumab based on improved efficacy and less toxicity, even in the absence of superior survival data.

The efficacy and safety of pembrolizumab were confirmed in KEYNOTE-002, a phase 2 study that randomized patients to either 2 mg/kg pembrolizumab, 10 mg/kg pembrolizumab, or chemotherapy. Findings demonstrated a significant improvement in progression-free survival (PFS) in patients treated with either 2 mg/kg (HR 0.57, $P<.0001$) or 10 mg/kg (HR 0.5, $P<.0001$) compared with chemotherapy.[42] The 2019 FDA approval of pembrolizumab in the adjuvant setting was based on the results of the randomized, phase 3 EORTC 1325/KEYNOTE-054 trial (**Table 1**), in which pembrolizumab was compared with placebo as adjuvant therapy for patients with resected, high-risk stage III melanoma. At a median follow-up of 15 months, use of pembrolizumab resulted in a 1-year RFS of 75.4% compared with 61.0% in the placebo group (HR 0.57, 95% CI 0.43–0.74, $P<.001$).[43] The efficacy of PD-1 inhibition and CTLA-4 blockade was further compared in KEYNOTE-006, a phase 3 clinical trial for patients with advanced melanoma. Results demonstrated that response rates were significantly better in patients who received pembrolizumab every 2 weeks (34%) and every 3 weeks (33%) compared with patients who received ipilimumab (12%). In addition, pembrolizumab prolonged PFS and OS with comparatively less high-grade toxicity in patients with advanced melanoma.[44] Overall, this study led to the conclusion that anti-PD1 should be considered first-line therapy in all patients with advanced melanoma, regardless of mutation status. Similar to ipilimumab, immune-related adverse events of anti-PD-1 inhibitors include fatigue, diarrhea, nausea, anemia, and decreased appetite with a grade 3 to 4 incidence of approximately 14%.[45] However, these do not appear to be significantly affected by the dose level.

Given their different mechanisms of action, several studies assessed the synergistic effect of combining CTLA-4 and PD-1 inhibitors demonstrating significant improvements in PFS and OS in advanced melanoma.[46–48] In CheckMate 067, the combination of nivolumab and ipilimumab was compared with monotherapy in patients with unresectable stage III or stage IV disease. The combination therapy showed a significantly higher PFS of 11.2 months compared with 5.3 months with nivolumab monotherapy. Treatment-related adverse events of any grade that led to discontinuation of the study therapy occurred in 7.7% of the patients in the nivolumab group, 14.8% of patients in the ipilimumab group, and 36.4% of the patients in the combination group.[47] This trial led to FDA approval of the combination therapy of nivolumab and ipilimumab in 2015 for use in metastatic or unresectable melanoma. CheckMate 915 is currently evaluating the use of combination ipilimumab and nivolumab as adjuvant treatment for patients with fully resected stage IIIB, IIIC, IIID, or IV cutaneous melanoma, and the results of this trial are eagerly awaited. Active trials involving combination immunotherapy in the adjuvant setting are summarized in **Table 2**.

Adjuvant Targeted Therapy

The treatment of melanoma was also revolutionized with the identification of the BRAF mutation in 2002.[49] BRAF and its product, BRAF kinase, regulate the mitogen-activated protein kinase RAS-RAF-MEK-ERK pathway, which further regulates transcription and translation of proteins that promote cell division and survival. The mutated BRAF gene transcribes a constitutively activated BRAF kinase, which promotes cell proliferation and prevents apoptosis.[50,51] BRAF V600E mutations were found to be very common in melanoma, and it is estimated that nearly 40% to 50% of tumor samples of patients with metastatic melanoma contain BRAF V600E mutations.[49,52]

Vemurafenib was the first BRAF inhibitor approved by the FDA in 2011 after a phase 2 trial, which included patients with previously treated metastatic melanoma, demonstrated a response rate of 50% with a median duration of 6.7 months and median OS of 15.9 months.[53] Since that initial approval, the combination of BRAF and MEK inhibitors has proved superior to single-agent BRAF inhibitors. In the metastatic setting, there are now 3 combinations that are approved: vemurafenib and cobimetinib, dabrafenib and trametinib, and encorafenib and binimetinib. In the COMBI-AD trial, patients with BRAF V600E or V600K-mutated stage III cutaneous melanoma who had undergone complete resection were randomized to receive either combination therapy with dabrafenib plus trametinib or placebo. After a median follow-up of 2.8 years, the 3-year RFS was 58% for the combination arm versus 30% for the placebo arm with a higher rate of overall and distant metastasis-free survival. The main toxicities of treatment include pyrexia, fatigue, and nausea. Serious adverse events were noted in 36% of patients in the combination arm.[54]

BRAF inhibitors may induce acquired resistance with continuous dosing, and half of the patients treated with BRAF-targeted therapies will relapse within 6 months.[55] The challenge now is to develop therapies that may prevent this resistance, and this approach may hinge on harnessing the potential of BRAF inhibitors to alter the tumor microenvironment. Indeed, investigations studying combination therapy for BRAF inhibitors with immunotherapy or T-cell therapy are currently underway.[56]

Adjuvant Radiation Therapy

In the current era of effective systemic therapies, the role of radiation therapy (RT) remains controversial. However, there are distinct scenarios whereby adjuvant radiation should be considered. The ANZMTG trial was a prospective multicenter phase 3 study in which 250 patients with high-risk disease were randomized to either observation or regional nodal basin RT. Results demonstrated that after a median follow-up for 40 months, RT significantly reduced the risk of locoregional recurrence. However,

Table 2
Active adjuvant trials in stage III or IV melanoma

Trial	Adjuvant Treatment	N	Treatment Duration	Primary Endpoint	Estimated Completion
NCT02231775	Dabrafenib + trametinib vs standard of care	21	Neoadjuvant 8 wk, adjuvant 44 wk	Relapse-free survival	2019
NCT01274338	High-dose ipilimumab or low-dose ipilimumab vs high-dose IFN alfa-2b (HDI)	1673	Adjuvant: q3w × 4 then every 3 mo × 4 vs 1 y	RFS OS	2020
NCT02434354	Pembrolizumab	27	Neoadjuvant: 3 wk, adjuvant: 1 y	Adverse events	2022
NCT02656706	Ipilimumab + nivolumab	25	Adjuvant: 6 mo	Toxicity RFS OS	2019
NCT01502696	PEG-IFN	1200	Adjuvant: 2 y	Relapse-free survival	2019
NCT02506153	Pembrolizumab	1378	Adjuvant: 1 y	Relapse-free survival OS	2023
NCT03698019	Pembrolizumab	556	Neoadjuvant: 9 wk Adjuvant: 11–14 wk	Event-free survival	2022
NCT02231775	Dabrafenib + Trametinib	78	Neoadjuvant: 8 wk, adjuvant: 44 wk	Relapse-free survival	2019
NCT02718391	Autologous dendritic cell vaccine	120	Adjuvant: daily injection × 5 d	Relapse-free survival	2019
NCT02523313	Nivolumab + placebo or Nivolumab + Ipilimumab or double placebo control	312	Adjuvant: 1 y	PFS	2021
NCT03047928	Drug: Nivolumab Biological: PD-L1/IDO peptide vaccine	50	Drug: indefinitely Biological: 15 vaccines	Adverse events	2019
NCT03276832	Pembrolizumab + Imiquimod	10	2 y	OS PFS	2021

there was no difference in OS.[57] The North Central Cancer Center Treatment Group conducted a single-arm phase 2 trial to assess the role of adjuvant RT for patients with desmoplastic melanoma. Results demonstrated a 2-year locoregional recurrence rate of 10% and 5-year OS of 77%.[58] There is also a current randomized trial comparing adjuvant RT (48 Gy in 20 fractions) to observation for patients with primary melanoma of the head and neck region with neurotropism (NCT00975520). As results are awaited from these trials, RT holds promise and should be considered after regional lymph node dissection of macroscopic lymph node disease in patients with extracapsular extension, lymph node diameter greater than 3 cm (neck or axilla), or 4 cm (groin), or at least 1 involved lymph node in the parotid lymph node region, 2 in the neck and axillary region, or 3 in the groin region.[59] Radiation may also be considered after failure of previous regional lymph node dissection, and after resection of desmoplastic or other melanoma subtypes with neurotropism. Furthermore, stereotactic radiation surgery is gaining wider acceptance in the management of brain metastases, because several retrospective studies have demonstrated 1-year local tumor control rates of 72% to 100% for patients with limited disease.[60,61] However, prospective randomized trials are needed to determine the benefit of RT for melanoma brain tumors.

Other Adjuvant Therapeutic Options: Vaccine Strategies, Intralesional Therapies, and Isolated Limb Perfusion

Various melanoma vaccine strategies are currently under investigation. Cancer vaccines can be categorized based on the type of tumor-associated antigen involved, including whole tumor cells, cancer cell lysates, peptides, DNA/RNA strands, and stimulated dendritic cells used for antigen presentation. The antigens may be shared across many melanomas, or they may be neoantigens that are uniquely expressed through malignant transformation.

A recent publication in *Nature* described the results of a melanoma vaccine targeting up to 20 personal tumor neoantigen administered in 6 patients with resected stage III–IV melanoma. Four stage III patients had no recurrence at 25 months after vaccination, whereas the 2 patients with metastatic disease who did recur later experienced complete response when treated with anti-PD-1.[62] Similarly, Sahin and colleagues[63] developed a personalized RNA-based vaccine to treat 13 patients with stage III–IV melanoma. Among the 8 patients with no detectable disease at the time of vaccination, most experienced prolonged DFS. Importantly, among 5 patients with evident metastatic disease at the time of vaccination, 2 experienced vaccine-related objective responses. These data provide a strong rationale for further development of this approach, both alone and in combination with checkpoint blockade or other systemic therapies.

Intralesional therapies are yet another option for patients with stage III ITM. In 2015, the FDA approved the oncolytic virus (herpes simplex virus 1)-derived therapy T-VEC for the treatment of cutaneous melanoma. T-VEC replicates selectively in tumor cells and encodes GM-CSF, lysing cells in injected tumors, which are then taken up by antigen-presenting cells. The OPTiM randomized phase 3 study compared intralesional T-VEC to subcutaneous GM-CSF and demonstrated a median OS of 41 months in the T-VEC arm compared with 21.5 months in the GM-CSF arm. In addition, T-VEC had a higher durable response rate (16.3% vs 2.1%, $P<.001$) and ORR (26.4% vs 5.7%, $P<.001$). Subset analyses also demonstrated a bystander effect in 15% of non-injected visceral metastases decreasing in size by more than 50%. Common toxicities for T-VEC included fatigue, chills, flulike symptoms, and injection-site pain.[64] It has been proposed that intralesional therapies will be combined with systemic therapies to offer a synergistic effect in the mechanism of action of these 2 modalities. A double-blind, placebo-controlled phase 3 study has been designed to include 660 patients with unresectable stage III–IV melanoma who will be randomized to receive T-VEC plus pembrolizumab or placebo injections plus pembrolizumab (NCT02965716). The results of this promising trial are currently awaited.

For patients with extensive regional disease not amenable to local therapy or resection, ILP remains a viable option. This technique was introduced in 1958 by Creech and colleagues[65] and is currently a well-established treatment of ITM that develops in 6% to 10% of patients.[66] ILP entails obtaining vascular access to either axillary or femoral vessels and administering hyperthermic chemotherapy with melphalan. Moreno-Ramirez and colleagues[67] published a systematic review on ILP analyzing 22 studies, which included more than 2000 patients with primary endpoints of ORR and survival. The median complete response rate to ILP was of 58%, with a median ORR of 90%. The recurrence rate was reported as 40%, with a median survival of 10.5 months until local recurrence. Although ILP remains an option, isolated limb infusion (ILI), which was later developed in the 1990s, is generally a preferred option for managing unresectable locally advanced disease. Unlike ILP, access is obtained percutaneously, and melphalan is infused at a lower rate in combination with actinomycin D.[68] Given its less invasive nature, this remains the preferred option for patients being considered for regional therapy, especially those with a compromised performance status. In the largest study to date reporting the long-term outcomes for ILI, the complete response rate was 28.9% and ORR was 64.1%. Importantly, significant limb toxicity only developed in 3.9%.[69] In a recent study comparing 3-month response rates and regional toxicity between the 2 techniques, ILP was associated with a higher ORR of 81% compared with 57% in ILI (P<.001), and overall, both therapies were well tolerated with a less than 3% risk of major toxicity. Despite the difference in response rates, there was no significant difference in median OS (40 months vs 46 months, P = .31), which has led to the continued predilection toward the use of the less invasive technique.[70] Although effective, ILP and ILI are labor intensive and limited to centers with the expertise to perform these procedures and manage the associated potential complications.

NEOADJUVANT THERAPY
Introduction

The concept of neoadjuvant therapy is well established in many solid tumors, including breast, rectal, and gastric cancer. However, the role for neoadjuvant therapy in melanoma is not as well defined, and the current standard of care for patients with clinical stage III melanoma is surgery followed by adjuvant therapy. However, following the recent successes with adjuvant therapy in the treatment of advanced melanoma, there is evidence that a trial of preoperative therapy may be the best course of action.

Compared with adjuvant therapy, neoadjuvant therapy in stage III melanoma can provide several advantages, including determining therapy efficacy for tailoring of subsequent adjuvant treatment, reducing tumor burden before planned surgery, and eventually correlating pathologic response data to long-term outcomes, including RFS and OS.

Neoadjuvant Immunotherapy

A recent trial by Amaria and colleagues[71] sought to assess the benefit of neoadjuvant nivolumab versus combined ipilimumab with nivolumab in 23 patients with clinical stage III or oligometastatic stage IV melanoma. Unfortunately, the trial was stopped

Table 3
Active neoadjuvant melanoma clinical trials

Trial	Neoadjuvant Treatment	Treatment Duration	Primary Endpoint	Estimated Completion
Immunotherapy				
NCT02519322	Group A: Nivolumab Group B: Nivolumab + Ipilimumab	Neoadjuvant: 7 wk Adjuvant: 6 mo	Pathologic complete response	2020
NCT03259425	Nivolumab + HF 10	12 wk	Pathologic complete response	2022
NCT03313206	Pembrolizumab Procedure: Surgery Radiation: intensity-modulated radiotherapy (IMRT)	12 wk	Disease-free survival	2025
NCT02339324	Pembrolizumab and HDI	6–8 wk	Adverse events	2019
NCT02858921	Group A: Dabrafenib + Trametinib THEN Pembrolizumab Group B: Dabrafenib + Trametinib + Pembrolizumab Group C: Pembrolizumab ONLY	Neoadjuvant: 6 wk Adjuvant: 46 wk	Pathologic complete response	2019
NCT02977052	Ipilimumab + Nivolumab	6 wk	Response rate Recurrence-free survival	2020
NCT02434354	Pembrolizumab	One dose	Number of adverse events	2022
NCT03698019	Pembrolizumab	9 wk	Event-free survival	2022
NCT03769155	Group A: VX15/2503 + Nivolumab + surgery Group B: VX15/2503 + Ipilimumab + surgery Group C: VX15/2503 + Nivolumab + Ipilimumab Group D: VX15/2503 + surgery	Two doses	Extent of CD8 T-cell infiltration following treatment	2031
Targeted therapy				
NCT02036086	Drug: Vemurafenib + Cobimentinib	8 wk	Resectability rate	2022
NCT02231775	Drug: Dabrafenib + Trametinib	8 wk	Relapse-free survival	2019

NCT02303951	Drug: Vemurafenib + Cobimentinib	4 wk	Resectability rate	2019
NCT03554083	Group A: Atezolizumab + Vemurafenib + Cobimentinib Group B: Atezolizumab + Cobimentinib	12 wk	Pathologic complete response	2023
NCT02858921	Group A: Dabrafenib + Trametinib THEN Pembrolizumab Group B: Dabrafenib + Trametinib + Pembrolizumab Group C: Pembrolizumab ONLY	Neoadjuvant: 6 wk Adjuvant: 46 wk	Pathologic response rate Resectability rate	2019
Other therapies				
NCT02451488	GM-CSF	14 d	Th1/Th2 ratio	2019
NCT03567889	Daromun	4 wk	Recurrence-free survival	2020

early because of observed disease progression preventing resection in the nivolumab treatment arm and substantial toxicity in the combination arm, but results did demonstrate a 58% pathologic complete response in the combination arm with an associated longer distant metastasis-free survival. A recently published trial demonstrated a rapid response to neoadjuvant anti-PD-1 treatment in patients with stage IIIB, IIIC, or IV melanoma. All 29 patients received a single dose of pembrolizumab, followed by complete resection 3 weeks later and continued adjuvant therapy for 1 year. Approximately 30% of patients had a complete or major pathologic complete response, and all remain disease free at 24 months.[72] Although the results of these studies suggest that neoadjuvant immunotherapy offers promise in the treatment of patients with stage III–IV oligometastatic melanoma, evidence remains premature, and the optimal neoadjuvant treatment regimen is unclear for now. Notably, a recent study also demonstrated the safety of ipilimumab use in the perioperative setting with a grade 1 wound complication of 17% and no associated grade 3 to 5 complications.[30] Trials involving immunotherapy in the neoadjuvant setting are gaining attention, both with individual agents and in combination (**Table 3**).

Neoadjuvant Targeted Therapy

The high and rapid response rate and good safety profile of BRAF-targeted agents provide an unprecedented opportunity for a neoadjuvant approach in melanoma. A recent phase 2 trial by Amaria and colleagues[73] randomized 21 patients with stage IIIB, IIIC, or oligometastatic stage IV BRAF-mutated melanoma to upfront surgery and adjuvant therapy or neoadjuvant plus adjuvant dabrafenib and trametinib. After a median follow-up of 18.6 months, PFS was 71% versus 0% in the standard-of-care arm. Importantly, therapy was well tolerated with no grade 4 adverse events. In addition, a recent study demonstrated that patients presenting with stage III, BRAF V600E-positive, nonresectable melanoma can be treated with BRAF inhibitors and achieve a successful R0 resection.[74] Questions that remain in the use of neoadjuvant targeted therapy include the optimal timing of therapy, the extent of surgery after therapy, and the use of pathologic response information to help guide postoperative therapy.

SUMMARY

The management of advanced stage melanoma has changed dramatically with the development of molecularly targeted therapies and immunotherapies, both of which have demonstrated a survival benefit for patients with advanced stage III and IV melanoma. Currently, dabrafenib and trametinib are approved for use in the adjuvant setting along with nivolumab and pembrolizumab. Novel ways to further modulate the immune system are under investigation, and developing additional salvage strategies for advanced melanoma will hinge on using combination therapies and other strategies, such as T-cell therapy. Given this expanding realm of systemic therapy, indications for metastasectomy continue to expand because this can render patients disease free or can serve as a complementary treatment in patients receiving systemic therapy who demonstrate progressive lesions in the setting of otherwise stable disease. In addition, palliative surgery remains an option for patients presenting with symptomatic resectable metastases.

With this recent breakthrough in the adjuvant treatment of melanoma and the availability of multiple effective agents, efforts are now focused on translating these therapies to the neoadjuvant setting. In addition to potentially improving survival outcomes, tumor resectability, and local control, neoadjuvant therapy has the major advantage of allowing one to assess the clinical and pathologic response of treatment. Several studies of neoadjuvant combination immunotherapy are currently underway to address the choice of agent and the timing of treatment of a neoadjuvant protocol. The information presented in this article aims to integrate the latest advancements in the treatment of advanced melanoma while acknowledging that the clinical decisions should take into consideration the physician's expertise and judgment and, more importantly, be individualized to each patient's needs and wishes.

DISCLOSURE

None.

REFERENCES

1. Siegel RL, Miller KD, Jemal A. Cancer statistics, 2018. CA Cancer J Clin 2018; 68(1):7–30.
2. Ghazawi FM, Cyr J, Darwich R, et al. Cutaneous malignant melanoma incidence and mortality trends in Canada: a comprehensive population-based study. J Am Acad Dermatol 2018;80(2):448–59.
3. Whiteman DC, Green AC, Olsen CM. The growing burden of invasive melanoma: projections of incidence rates and numbers of new cases in six susceptible populations through 2031. J Invest Dermatol 2016;136(6):1161–71.
4. Cancer stat facts: melanoma of the skin. Available at: https://seer.cancer.gov/statfacts/html/melan.html. Accessed January 22, 2019.
5. Gershenwald JE, Scolyer RA, Hess KR, et al. Melanoma staging: evidence-based changes in the American Joint Committee on Cancer eighth edition cancer staging manual. CA Cancer J Clin 2017;67(6):472–92.
6. Crompton JG, Gilbert E, Brady MS. Clinical implications of the eighth edition of the American Joint Committee on Cancer melanoma staging. J Surg Oncol 2019;119(2):168–74.
7. Faries MB, Thompson JF, Cochran AJ, et al. Completion dissection or observation for sentinel-node metastasis in melanoma. N Engl J Med 2017;376(23):2211–22.
8. Wong SL, Faries MB, Kennedy EB, et al. Sentinel lymph node biopsy and management of regional lymph nodes in melanoma: American Society of Clinical Oncology and Society of Surgical Oncology Clinical Practice Guideline Update. J Clin Oncol 2018;36(4):399–413.
9. van der Ploeg AP, Haydu LE, Spillane AJ, et al. Melanoma patients with an unknown primary tumor site have a better outcome than those with a known primary following therapeutic lymph node dissection for macroscopic (clinically palpable) nodal disease. Ann Surg Oncol 2014;21(9):3108–16.
10. van der Ploeg AP, van Akkooi AC, Schmitz PI, et al. Therapeutic surgical management of palpable melanoma groin metastases: superficial or combined superficial and deep groin lymph node dissection. Ann Surg Oncol 2011;18(12):3300–8.
11. Testori A, Ribero S, Bataille V. Diagnosis and treatment of in-transit melanoma metastases. Eur J Surg Oncol 2017;43(3):544–60.
12. Yao KA, Hsueh EC, Essner R, et al. Is sentinel lymph node mapping indicated for isolated local and in-transit recurrent melanoma? Ann Surg 2003;238(5):743–7.
13. Fletcher WS, Pommier RF, Lum S, et al. Surgical treatment of metastatic melanoma. Am J Surg 1998;175(5):413–7.
14. Karakousis CP, Velez A, Driscoll DL, et al. Metastasectomy in malignant melanoma. Surgery 1994;115(3):295–302.

15. Meyer T, Merkel S, Goehl J, et al. Surgical therapy for distant metastases of malignant melanoma. Cancer 2000;89(9):1983–91.
16. Ollila DW, Essner R, Wanek LA, et al. Surgical resection for melanoma metastatic to the gastrointestinal tract. Arch Surg 1996;131(9):975–9, 979–980.
17. Agrawal S, Yao TJ, Coit DG. Surgery for melanoma metastatic to the gastrointestinal tract. Ann Surg Oncol 1999;6(4):336–44.
18. Harpole DH Jr, Johnson CM, Wolfe WG, et al. Analysis of 945 cases of pulmonary metastatic melanoma. J Thorac Cardiovasc Surg 1992;103(4):743–8 [discussion: 748–50].
19. Leo F, Cagini L, Rocmans P, et al. Lung metastases from melanoma: when is surgical treatment warranted? Br J Cancer 2000;83(5):569–72.
20. Sosman JA, Moon J, Tuthill RJ, et al. A phase 2 trial of complete resection for stage IV melanoma: results of Southwest Oncology Group Clinical Trial S9430. Cancer 2011;117(20):4740.
21. Howard JH, Thompson JF, Mozzillo N, et al. Metastasectomy for distant metastatic melanoma: analysis of data from the first Multicenter Selective Lymphadenectomy Trial (MSLT-I). Ann Surg Oncol 2012;19(8):2547–55.
22. Faries MB, Mozzillo N, Kashani-Sabet M, et al. Long-term survival after complete surgical resection and adjuvant immunotherapy for distant melanoma metastases. Ann Surg Oncol 2017;24(13):3991–4000.
23. Wei IH, Healy MA, Wong SL. Surgical treatment options for stage IV melanoma. Surg Clin North Am 2014;94(5):1075–89, ix.
24. Deutsch GB, Flaherty DC, Kirchoff DD, et al. Association of surgical treatment, systemic therapy, and survival in patients with abdominal visceral melanoma metastases, 1965-2014: relevance of surgical cure in the era of modern systemic therapy. JAMA Surg 2017;152(7):672–8.
25. Mittendorf EA, Lim SJ, Schacherer CW, et al. Melanoma adrenal metastasis: natural history and surgical management. Am J Surg 2008;195(3):363–8 [discussion: 368–9].
26. Ryu SW, Saw R, Scolyer RA, et al. Liver resection for metastatic melanoma: equivalent survival for cutaneous and ocular primaries. J Surg Oncol 2013;108(2):129–35.
27. Schuhan C, Muley T, Dienemann H, et al. Survival after pulmonary metastasectomy in patients with malignant melanoma. Thorac Cardiovasc Surg 2011;59(3):158–62.
28. Neuman HB, Patel A, Hanlon C, et al. Stage-IV melanoma and pulmonary metastases: factors predictive of survival. Ann Surg Oncol 2007;14(10):2847–53.
29. Morton DL, Ollila DW, Hsueh EC, et al. Cytoreductive surgery and adjuvant immunotherapy: a new management paradigm for metastatic melanoma. CA Cancer J Clin 1999;49(2):101–16, 165.
30. Gyorki DE, Yuan J, Mu Z, et al. Immunological insights from patients undergoing surgery on ipilimumab for metastatic melanoma. Ann Surg Oncol 2013;20(9):3106–11.
31. Faries MB, Leung A, Morton DL, et al. A 20-year experience of hepatic resection for melanoma: is there an expanding role? J Am Coll Surg 2014;219(1):62–8.
32. Grob JJ, Dreno B, de la Salmoniere P, et al. Randomised trial of interferon alpha-2a as adjuvant therapy in resected primary melanoma thicker than 1.5 mm without clinically detectable node metastases. French Cooperative Group on Melanoma. Lancet 1998;351(9120):1905–10.

33. Kirkwood JM, Strawderman MH, Ernstoff MS, et al. Interferon alfa-2b adjuvant therapy of high-risk resected cutaneous melanoma: the Eastern Cooperative Oncology Group Trial EST 1684. J Clin Oncol 1996;14(1):7–17.

34. Eggermont AM, Suciu S, Testori A, et al. Long-term results of the randomized phase III trial EORTC 18991 of adjuvant therapy with pegylated interferon alfa-2b versus observation in resected stage III melanoma. J Clin Oncol 2012; 30(31):3810–8.

35. Hodi FS, O'Day SJ, McDermott DF, et al. Improved survival with ipilimumab in patients with metastatic melanoma. N Engl J Med 2010;363(8):711–23.

36. Eggermont AM, Chiarion-Sileni V, Grob JJ, et al. Adjuvant ipilimumab versus placebo after complete resection of high-risk stage III melanoma (EORTC 18071): a randomised, double-blind, phase 3 trial. Lancet Oncol 2015;16(5):522–30.

37. Eggermont AM, Chiarion-Sileni V, Grob JJ, et al. Prolonged survival in stage III melanoma with ipilimumab adjuvant therapy. N Engl J Med 2016;375(19): 1845–55.

38. National Comprehensive Cancer Network (U.S.). The complete library of NCCN oncology practice guidelines. Rockledge (PA): NCCN; 2000.

39. Weber JS, D'Angelo SP, Minor D, et al. Nivolumab versus chemotherapy in patients with advanced melanoma who progressed after anti-CTLA-4 treatment (CheckMate 037): a randomised, controlled, open-label, phase 3 trial. Lancet Oncol 2015;16(4):375–84.

40. Robert C, Long GV, Brady B, et al. Nivolumab in previously untreated melanoma without BRAF mutation. N Engl J Med 2015;372(4):320–30.

41. Weber J, Mandala M, Del Vecchio M, et al. Adjuvant nivolumab versus ipilimumab in resected stage III or IV melanoma. N Engl J Med 2017;377(19):1824–35.

42. Ribas A, Puzanov I, Dummer R, et al. Pembrolizumab versus investigator-choice chemotherapy for ipilimumab-refractory melanoma (KEYNOTE-002): a randomised, controlled, phase 2 trial. Lancet Oncol 2015;16(8):908–18.

43. Eggermont AMM, Blank CU, Mandala M, et al. Adjuvant pembrolizumab versus placebo in resected stage III melanoma. N Engl J Med 2018;378(19):1789–801.

44. Robert C, Schachter J, Long GV, et al. Pembrolizumab versus ipilimumab in advanced melanoma. N Engl J Med 2015;372(26):2521–32.

45. Ribas A, Wolchok JD, Robert C, et al. P0116 Updated clinical efficacy of the anti-PD-1 monoclonal antibody pembrolizumab (MK-3475) in 411 patients with melanoma, vol. 51, 2015.

46. Postow MA, Chesney J, Pavlick AC, et al. Nivolumab and ipilimumab versus ipilimumab in untreated melanoma. N Engl J Med 2015;372(21):2006–17.

47. Larkin J, Chiarion-Sileni V, Gonzalez R, et al. Combined nivolumab and ipilimumab or monotherapy in untreated melanoma. N Engl J Med 2015;373(1):23–34.

48. Wolchok JD, Kluger H, Callahan MK, et al. Nivolumab plus ipilimumab in advanced melanoma. N Engl J Med 2013;369(2):122–33.

49. Davies H, Bignell GR, Cox C, et al. Mutations of the BRAF gene in human cancer. Nature 2002;417(6892):949–54.

50. Roberts PJ, Der CJ. Targeting the Raf-MEK-ERK mitogen-activated protein kinase cascade for the treatment of cancer. Oncogene 2007;26(22):3291–310.

51. Munoz-Couselo E, Garcia JS, Perez-Garcia JM, et al. Recent advances in the treatment of melanoma with BRAF and MEK inhibitors. Ann Transl Med 2015; 3(15):207.

52. Pollock PM, Harper UL, Hansen KS, et al. High frequency of BRAF mutations in nevi. Nat Genet 2003;33(1):19–20.

53. Sosman JA, Kim KB, Schuchter L, et al. Survival in BRAF V600-mutant advanced melanoma treated with vemurafenib. N Engl J Med 2012;366(8):707–14.

54. Long GV, Hauschild A, Santinami M, et al. Adjuvant dabrafenib plus trametinib in stage III BRAF-mutated melanoma. N Engl J Med 2017;377(19):1813–23.

55. Hauschild A, Grob JJ, Demidov LV, et al. Dabrafenib in BRAF-mutated metastatic melanoma: a multicentre, open-label, phase 3 randomised controlled trial. Lancet 2012;380(9839):358–65.

56. Goff SL, Rosenberg SA. BRAF inhibition: bridge or boost to T-cell therapy? Clin Cancer Res 2019;25(9):2682–4.

57. Henderson MA, Burmeister BH, Ainslie J, et al. Adjuvant lymph-node field radiotherapy versus observation only in patients with melanoma at high risk of further lymph-node field relapse after lymphadenectomy (ANZMTG 01.02/TROG 02.01): 6-year follow-up of a phase 3, randomised controlled trial. Lancet Oncol 2015; 16(9):1049–60.

58. Rule WG, Allred JB, Pockaj BA, et al. Results of NCCTG N0275 (Alliance)–a phase II trial evaluating resection followed by adjuvant radiation therapy for patients with desmoplastic melanoma. Cancer Med 2016;5(8):1890–6.

59. Burmeister B, Henderson M, Thompson J, et al. Adjuvant radiotherapy improves regional (lymph node field) control in melanoma patients after lymphadenectomy: results of an Intergroup randomized trial (TROG 02.01/ANZMTG 01.02), vol. 75, 2009.

60. Frakes JM, Figura NB, Ahmed KA, et al. Potential role for LINAC-based stereotactic radiosurgery for the treatment of 5 or more radioresistant melanoma brain metastases. J Neurosurg 2015;123(5):1261–7.

61. Christ SM, Mahadevan A, Floyd SR, et al. Stereotactic radiosurgery for brain metastases from malignant melanoma. Surg Neurol Int 2015;6(Suppl 12):S355–65.

62. Ott PA, Hu Z, Keskin DB, et al. An immunogenic personal neoantigen vaccine for patients with melanoma. Nature 2017;547(7662):217–21.

63. Sahin U, Derhovanessian E, Miller M, et al. Personalized RNA mutanome vaccines mobilize poly-specific therapeutic immunity against cancer. Nature 2017; 547(7662):222–6.

64. Andtbacka RH, Kaufman HL, Collichio F, et al. Talimogene laherparepvec improves durable response rate in patients with advanced melanoma. J Clin Oncol 2015;33(25):2780–8.

65. Creech O Jr, Krementz ET, Ryan RF, et al. Chemotherapy of cancer: regional perfusion utilizing an extracorporeal circuit. Ann Surg 1958;148(4):616–32.

66. Thompson JF. Local and regional therapies for melanoma: many arrows in the quiver. J Surg Oncol 2014;109(4):295.

67. Moreno-Ramirez D, de la Cruz-Merino L, Ferrandiz L, et al. Isolated limb perfusion for malignant melanoma: systematic review on effectiveness and safety. Oncologist 2010;15(4):416–27.

68. Kroon HM, Huismans AM, Kam PC, et al. Isolated limb infusion with melphalan and actinomycin D for melanoma: a systematic review. J Surg Oncol 2014; 109(4):348–51.

69. Miura JT, Kroon HM, Beasley GM, et al. Long-term oncologic outcomes after isolated limb infusion for locoregionally metastatic melanoma: an international multicenter analysis. Ann Surg Oncol 2019;26(8):2486–94.

70. Dossett LA, Ben-Shabat I, Olofsson Bagge R, et al. Clinical response and regional toxicity following isolated limb infusion compared with isolated limb perfusion for in-transit melanoma. Ann Surg Oncol 2016;23(7):2330–5.

71. Amaria RN, Reddy SM, Tawbi HA, et al. Neoadjuvant immune checkpoint blockade in high-risk resectable melanoma. Nat Med 2018;24(11):1649–54.
72. Huang AC, Orlowski RJ, Xu X, et al. A single dose of neoadjuvant PD-1 blockade predicts clinical outcomes in resectable melanoma. Nat Med 2019;25(3):454–61.
73. Amaria RN, Prieto PA, Tetzlaff MT, et al. Neoadjuvant plus adjuvant dabrafenib and trametinib versus standard of care in patients with high-risk, surgically resectable melanoma: a single-centre, open-label, randomised, phase 2 trial. Lancet Oncol 2018;19(2):181–93.
74. Zippel D, Markel G, Shapira-Frommer R, et al. Perioperative BRAF inhibitors in locally advanced stage III melanoma. J Surg Oncol 2017;116(7):856–61.

Principles of Immunotherapy in Melanoma

Adedayo A. Onitilo, MD, PhD, MSCR, FACP[a],*,
Jaimie A. Wittig, PharmD, BCOP[b]

KEYWORDS

- Malignant melanoma • Immunotherapy • IFNα-2b • IL-2
- Immune checkpoint inhibitors • CTLA-4 • PD-1

KEY POINTS

- Advanced/metastatic melanoma generally has a low survival rate.
- Immunotherapy is a promising treatment of advanced/metastatic melanoma.
- Immune checkpoint inhibitors, such as ipilimumab, nivolumab, and pembrolizumab, are Food and Drug Administration (FDA)–approved treatments of advanced/malignant melanoma with more immunomodulatory therapies in development.
- Immunotherapy produces a unique set of adverse side effects associated with immune system activation.
- Tumor response to immunotherapy differs from traditional agents and is measured using modified response criteria.

INTRODUCTION

Malignant melanoma is the most aggressive and deadliest form of skin cancer with an estimated 91,000 new diagnoses and 9,300 deaths in 2018.[1] Although improvements in melanoma screening have led to more cases being diagnosed in the early stages of disease, outcomes for patients diagnosed with advanced or metastatic melanoma remain poor when treated with traditional cytotoxic chemotherapy with a median overall survival (OS) of approximately 6 months to 8 months.[2] Due to poor outcomes seen with traditional cytotoxic chemotherapy agents, exploration of immunotherapy as an option to treat this disease has become a primary focus of melanoma research. Recent advancements in immunotherapy has advanced the field of oncology and increased the repertoire of treatments available for metastatic melanoma.

[a] Department of Hematology/Oncology, Marshfield Clinic – Weston Center, 3501 Cranberry Boulevard, Weston, WI 54476, USA; [b] Pharmacy Services, Marshfield Medical Center, 1000 North Oak Avenue, Marshfield, WI 54449, USA
* Corresponding author.
E-mail address: onitilo.adedayo@marshfieldclinic.org

Surg Clin N Am 100 (2020) 161–173
https://doi.org/10.1016/j.suc.2019.09.009
0039-6109/20/© 2019 Elsevier Inc. All rights reserved.

Immunotherapy as a means to treat cancer was first postulated in 1893 when William Coley[3] reported that an injection of killed bacteria into sites of sarcoma could lead to tumor shrinkage. Since this initial discovery, research has been dedicated to determining how the immune system may be harnessed and used in cancer treatment. In general, immunotherapy functions to assist the immune system in recognizing cancer cells as foreign, activate the immune system to react to these foreign cells, and reverse the inhibitory mechanisms that allow tumor cells to grow and spread unchecked. This greatly differs from the mechanisms of other types of cancer treatment, such as cytotoxic chemotherapy, which primarily functions by attacking and damaging the DNA or DNA synthesis mechanisms of rapidly dividing cells in the body; radiation therapy, which directly damages DNA of selected cells; or targeted therapies, which disrupt molecular processes necessary for cancer cell proliferation and metastasis.

IMMUNE EVASION AND SUBVERSION BY TUMOR CELLS

Cancer cells promote tumor development and metastasis by undermining immunomodulatory signaling receptors on immune cells and antigen-presenting cells (APCs) as well as hijacking preexisting immunologic functions in 1 or more ways:[4–7]

1. Blocking, altering the expression of, and/or altering the surface expression of cell recognition and/or foreign antigen-presenting receptors.
2. Preventing immune system activation.
3. Reprogramming immune cells to produce molecules that promote tumor survival and aggressiveness.
4. Enhancing activity of regulatory T-cells (T_{reg}) and other immune cells that dampen the immune response and/or induce effector T-cell ($T_{effector}$) apoptosis.

Because melanoma is an immunoreactive cancer, it is a prime target for immunotherapies.

CYTOKINES

In 1996, the cytokine interferon alpha-2b (IFNα-2b) was the first immunotherapy approved for the treatment of melanoma.[8,9] Cytokines are naturally occurring glycoproteins released by the immune system in response to infections or other antigens. Although the exact mechanism of cytokines in cancer treatment is still not well understood, cytokine effects in immunomodulation, antiproliferative activity, and inhibition of angiogenesis all likely contribute to the antitumor activity of these agents **(Fig. 1)**.[4,8–11]

Interferon Alpha-2b

Until the recent development of immune checkpoint inhibitors, high-dose interferon alpha was the only therapy that had shown improvement in OS as an adjuvant treatment of high-risk melanoma.[8,9,11,12] In 1995, the Eastern Cooperative Oncology Group (ECOG) 1684 trial demonstrated significant improvements in relapse-free survival (RFS) (5-year RFS rate of 37% compared with 26%) and OS (5-year OS rate of 46% compared with 37%) with IFNα-2b dosed at 20 million units (MU)/m^2/d intravenously 5 days per week for 4 weeks followed by 10 MU/m^2/d 3 times per week subcutaneously for 48 weeks compared with observation for patients with high-risk melanoma (defined as deep primary tumor of >4 mm in depth [T4 per TNM staging system for melanoma] and/or regional lymph node metastases) in the adjuvant setting.[12] Adverse side effects, such as myelosuppression, hepatotoxicity, and neurologic symptoms, occurred in response to high doses of IFNα-2b which required dose modifications

Systemic Cytokine Treatment

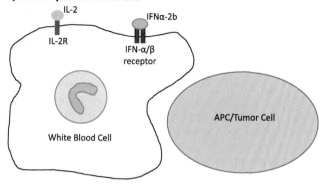

INFα-2b
- Alters immune cell function and trafficking to tumor cells.
- Alters immune cell populations.
- Alters expression of growth factors, adhesion molecules, pro- and anti-angiogenic molecules, pro- and anti-apoptotic molecules, and pro- and anti-inflammatory cytokines and chemokines.

IL-2
- Alters immune cell function.
- Generates lymphokine-activated killer cells (LAK).

Fig. 1. Schematic of systemic cytokine treatments. IFNAR-1 and -2, IFN-α/β receptor. Edit confirmed for IFN.

or discontinuation of therapy in a majority of patients in ECOG 1684. Furthermore, 2 deaths that occurred during the trial were attributed to adverse events associated with high-dose IFN-α2b therapy although close monitoring and dose adjustments based on liver enzyme levels prevented additional instances of life-threatening hepatic events. Other common adverse events that occurred during the initial clinical trials included elevations in liver enzymes, nausea, vomiting, and flulike symptoms.[8,11,12]

In an effort to decrease toxicity associated with high-dose interferon therapy, low and intermediate doses were tested in the adjuvant setting for nonmetastatic melanoma at high risk for recurrence but failed to demonstrate any consistent improvements in RFS or OS.[9] Therefore, high-dose IFN-α2b remained the standard of care adjuvant therapy for patients with high-risk nonmetastatic melanoma for close to a decade, and current National Comprehensive Cancer Network (NCCN) guidelines for melanoma treatment do not support the use of low-dose or intermediate-dose interferon due to inconsistent results.[13] NCCN guidelines for adjuvant use of high dose IFN-α2b and pegylated interferon for the treatment of complete resected stage III melanoma carries a category 2A recommendation (ie, based on lower-level evidence, there is uniform NCCN consensus that the intervention is appropriate) for patients with positive sentinel nodes or clinically positive nodes although for patients with in-transit lesions this recommendation is down-graded to category 2B (ie, based on lower-level evidence, there is NCCN consensus that the intervention is appropriate).[13] Flulike symptoms, the most common and often most disruptive set of adverse events, occurs in upward of 80% of melanoma patients treated with high-dose interferon and commonly are managed with supportive care, including antipyretics and oral hydration.[13] With long-term follow-up, interferon has failed to maintain statistically significant improvements in OS, and, with the introduction of immune checkpoint inhibitors and targeted therapies, use of interferon for the treatment of melanoma has become less prominent in recent years.[9]

Interleukin-2

The cytokine interleukin-2 (IL-2) also has been used for melanoma treatment, but, unlike interferon, IL-2 therapy has been used primarily in the setting of metastatic disease. High-dose IL-2 was the first treatment to modify outcomes of patients with metastatic melanoma by demonstrating disease cure in a small number of patients; 270 patients with metastatic melanoma were treated with 360,000 or 540,000 IU/kg/dose (Chiron-sponsored study), 600,000 IU/kg/dose (3 studies), or 720,000 IU/kg/dose (4 studies) of IL-2 as an intravenous infusion every 8 hours for up to 14 consecutive doses over 5 days with a second identical treatment cycle scheduled after 6 days to 9 days of rest and courses repeated every 6 weeks to 12 weeks.[14] Although overall response (16%), partial response (10%), and complete response rate (6%) were relatively low, long-term follow-up demonstrated that these responses were very durable because disease did not progress in any patient who achieved response for greater than 30 months. Unfortunately, toxicity of IL-2 therapy is significant and requires careful selection of patients to limit morbidity and mortality. Common serious adverse events associated with high-dose IL-2 therapy include hypotension, cardiac arrhythmias, pulmonary edema, fever, metabolic acidosis, nausea, vomiting, dyspnea, neurotoxicity, renal dysfunction, and bacterial infection.[11,14,15] Infections, in particular catheter-related sepsis, contribute significantly to the toxicity of IL-2 and treatment-related deaths although prophylactic antibiotic regimens have prevented further fatalities from sepsis, and updated treatment algorithms have improved the identification and reversal of toxicities except perhaps hypothyroidism. Due to multiorgan toxicities of high-dose IL-2 therapy, only patients with excellent baseline organ function and good performance status should be selected for this therapy.[11,15] Additionally, the NCCN guidelines recommend that only facilities with medical staff experienced in the administration and management of high-dose IL-2 therapies administer such regimens due to the severity of its toxicity profile.[13] Similar to interferon therapy, high-dose IL-2 therapy has largely been supplanted by immune checkpoint inhibitors and targeted therapy agents in the past several years. Current NCCN guidelines list high-dose IL-2 as a category 2A recommendation for metastatic or unresectable melanoma after disease progression or maximum benefit from BRAF-targeted therapy alongside checkpoint inhibitor therapies, targeted therapies, and cytotoxic chemotherapy.[13]

IMMUNE CHECKPOINT INHIBITORS

The development and approval of the first immune checkpoint inhibitor therapy in 2011 yielded the most significant advancement in melanoma treatment in more than a decade.[13] Checkpoints within the human immune system refer to various inhibitory pathways that prevent immune cells from attacking certain cells or tissues. In a healthy host, immune checkpoints are essential for prevention of autoimmunity and protection of healthy tissue from damage during an immune response to pathogens. Tumor cells, however, can exploit these immune checkpoint mechanisms as a method for evading detection and destruction by the host immune system. Immune checkpoint inhibitors act at various steps in the interaction process between APCs, T-cells, and tumor cells to enhance immune system activation and tumor cell targeting (**Fig. 2**).[5,7]

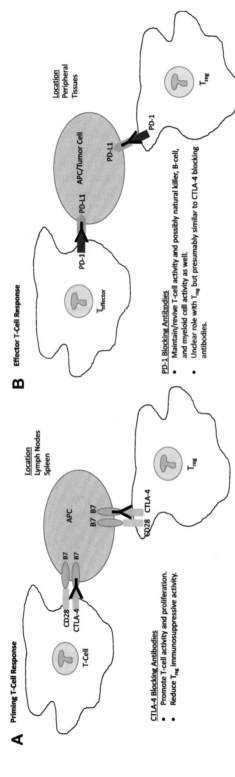

Fig. 2. Immunomodulatory effects of immune checkpoint inhibitors.

Cytotoxic T-Lymphocyte–Associated Antigen 4

The first of the immune checkpoint inhibitors to be approved by the FDA was the cytotoxic T-lymphocyte–associated antigen 4 (CTLA-4) blocking antibody ipilimumab. CTLA-4 is a T-cell–specific receptor that possesses a higher binding affinity for the B7.1 and B7.2 ligands than CD28.[5,7,16–19] Due to this higher binding affinity, it is thought that when CTLA-4 is expressed on T-cells that CTLA-4 will bind to B7.1 and B7.2 preferentially in place of CD28 which in turn decreases T-cell activation in response to CD28 binding.[5,7] As a CTLA-4 blocking antibody, ipilimumab augments T-cell activity by physically binding to and blocking the CTLA-4 receptor (see **Fig. 2**A).[5]

Ipilimumab has been studied and approved as a primary treatment of unresectable stage III or metastatic melanoma and as an adjuvant treatment of lymph node–positive stage III melanoma after complete resection. The first phase III trial to evaluate ipilimumab for the treatment of unresectable stage III or progressive metastatic melanoma used a dosing regimen of 3 mg/kg of body weight administered once every 3 weeks for 4 total doses on patients who were receiving therapy for metastatic disease compared with patients who received a glycoprotein 100 peptide vaccine (gp100).[20] The results of this trial yielded a significantly improved median duration of OS in patients treated with ipilimumab alone, 10.1 months, and ipilimumab in combination with gp100, 10.0 months, compared with patients treated with gp100 alone, 6.4 months. These responses were also found to be durable with approximately 20% of ipilimumab-only treated patients surviving at least 2 years after completion of treatment which made ipilimumab the first therapy to demonstrate a survival benefit in patients with metastatic melanoma.[20,21] Due to this efficacy of treatment of metastatic melanoma, a larger phase III trial was performed to evaluate treatment with ipilimumab (10 mg/kg every 3 weeks for 4 total doses with reinduction every 3 months for a maximum of 3 years depending on toxicity, compliance, disease recurrence, or refusal of treatment) against placebo for treatment of completely resected stage III melanoma.[22] A significantly improved median RFS of 26.1 months occurred with ipilimumab therapy compared with 17.1 months with placebo. Although these efficacy results are significant, the adverse event rate associated with ipilimumab therapy and the emergence of programmed cell death protein 1 (PD-1) blocking antibodies have greatly decreased utilization of ipilimumab although ipilimumab remains an NCCN recommended therapy for both treatment-naïve and relapsed stage III and stage IV melanoma.[13] These recommendations, however, are lower-level recommendations than those of the PD-1–blocking antibodies nivolumab and pembrolizumab as well as the BRAF-targeting tyrosine kinase inhibitors (for patients with BRAF mutated disease) for the same indications.[13]

Programmed Cell Death Protein 1

The other primary immune checkpoint target used clinically for melanoma treatment is PD-1. The PD-1 receptor is expressed on the surface of Tcells and is normally expressed in response to T-cell activation.[5,7] When the PD-1 receptor interacts with its ligand, PD-L1 or PD-L2, T-cell activation in inhibited and immune response is diminished. Tumor cells exploit the PD-1 coinhibitory pathway as a means to avoid detection and destruction by the host immune system. There are 2 currently FDA-approved PD-1 blocking antibodies for the treatment of melanoma, nivolumab and pembrolizumab, which bind to and block the interaction of the PD-1 receptor with its ligands. This restores antitumor immune responses and allows activated T cells to destroy tumor cells (see **Fig. 2**B).

Both pembrolizumab and nivolumab are viable options for adjuvant treatment of completely resected stage III melanoma based on current NCCN guidelines (category 1).[13] Nivolumab was initially studied as an adjuvant treatment of completely resected stage III or stage IV melanoma at a dose of 3 mg/kg of body weight every 2 weeks for up to 1 year compared with ipilimumab at a dose of 10 mg/kg of body weight every 3 weeks for 4 total doses then every 12 weeks for up to 1 year or until disease recurrence, toxicity, or patient withdrawal.[23] The 12-month recurrence-free survival (RFS) was significantly improved at 70.5% in nivolumab-treated patients compared with 60.8% in ipilimumab-treated patients (hazard ratio [HR] = 0.65; 97.56% confidence interval (CI), 0.51–0.83; $P<.001$). RFS improvement also was demonstrated with pembrolizumab treatment of adjuvant treatment of patients with completely resected stage III melanoma in a phase III trial where patients received pembrolizumab at a dose of 200 mg every 3 weeks or placebo for approximately 1 year (18 doses); patients could cross over or receive additional treatment as needed.[24] Twelve-month RFS was significantly improved in 75.4% of pembrolizumab-treated patients compared with 61.0% in patients who received placebo (HR 0.57; 98.4% CI, 0.43–0.74; $P<.001$). Neither trial has reported OS data at this time.

Because pembrolizumab and nivolumab had demonstrated improvement in survival compared to ipilimumab in clinical trials, these antibody-based treatments, alone or in combination with ipilimumab, also have received category 1 designation (the highest recommendation) from the NCCN for use as first-line therapy for metastatic or unresectable melanoma.[13] In the initial pembrolizumab trial, pembrolizumab was studied at a dose of 10 mg/kg given every 2 weeks or 3 weeks for 2 years or until disease progression, patient withdrawal, toxicity, or complete response compared with ipilimumab, 3 mg/kg given every 3 weeks for 4 total doses; crossover from the ipilimumab to the pembrolizumab group was permitted after results from the second interim analysis in 2015.[25] Twenty-four month OS rates were 55% (95% CI, 49–61) in the pembrolizumab every 2 weeks group, 55% (95% CI, 49–61) in the pembrolizumab every 3 weeks group, and 43% (95% CI, 37–49) in the ipilimumab group. Both pembrolizumab groups were determined to be superior to the ipilimumab group (HR 0.68; 95% CI, 0.53–0.87; $P = .0009$, every 2 weeks group; HR 0.68; 95% CI, 0.53–0.86, every 3 weeks group), and progression-free survival were improved in both pembrolizumab groups compared with ipilimumab (HR 0.61; 95% CI, 0.50–0.75; $P<.0001$).

In a similar study, the clinical efficacy of nivolumab at a dosage of 3 mg/kg every 2 weeks was compared with ipilimumab at a dosage of 3 mg/kg every 3 weeks for 4 doses and combination treatment of nivolumab (1 mg/kg for first 4 doses) and ipilimumab (3 mg/kg every 3 weeks for 4 total doses) followed by nivolumab (3 mg/kg every 2 weeks alone) for treatment of unresectable stage III and stage IV melanoma.[26] Four-year OS was greatest at 53% in the combination group followed by nivolumab (46%) and 30% in the ipilimumab monotherapy groups. HR for OS was significantly different for the combination group compared with the ipilimuab group (0.54; 95% CI, 0.44-0.67; $P<.001$) for the nivolumab versus the ipilimumab group. Due to trial results, the combination of nivolumab with ipilimumab is also a treatment option for metastatic or unresectable melanoma and is listed at the highest level of evidence in the NCCN guidelines.[13]

In the setting of metastatic melanoma, factors such as BRAF mutation status, PD-L1 expression, ulceration of the primary tumor, and central nervous system (CNS) metastases can influence treatment selection decisions. Subgroup analyses conducted in several pembrolizumab and nivolumab clinical trials have noted that patients with BRAF-mutant and BRAF wild-type tumors achieved improved outcomes with pembrolizumab or nivolumab treatment versus ipilimumab, and combination treatment with nivolumab and ipilimumab may achieve better outcomes in patients with BRAF-mutated tumors than monotherapy nivolumab.[23–26] Subgroup analyses also seem to indicate improvement in outcomes with pembrolizumab, nivolumab, or nivolumab with ipilimumab compared with ipilimumab regardless of level of PD-L1 expression. Because melanoma frequently metastasizes to the brain, the presence of CNS metastases is another important factor to assess for the utility of immune checkpoint inhibitor therapy. At this time, no specific trials have evaluated the utility of immune checkpoint inhibitors for treatment of CNS metastases, although patients with CNS metastases were included in some of the ipilimumab, pembrolizumab, and nivolumab clinical trials.

Toxicities Associated with Immune Checkpoint Inhibitors

Immune checkpoint inhibitor therapy comes with a unique toxicity profile requiring careful monitoring and management. Because immune checkpoint inhibitor therapy functions by activating the host immune system, the toxicity profile of immune checkpoint inhibitor therapies are largely autoimmune and/or inflammatory in nature and have been termed immune-related adverse events (irAEs). Due to the immune system's presence throughout the body, irAEs can affect any organ system or tissue but most commonly occur in the skin, gastrointestinal (GI) tract, liver, and endocrine system.[27–29] Overall rates of irAEs are lower with PD-1 inhibitors (73%–82% all grades, 10%–16% grade ≥3) compared with ipilimumab (73%–93% all grades, 20%–27% grade ≥3), with combination of ipilimumab and nivolumab having the highest rate of irAEs (91%–96% all grades, 54%–55% grade ≥3).[13] Although fatal irAEs remain rare, many can be serious, so vigilant monitoring and management is required for patients receiving immune checkpoint inhibitor therapies.[29]

Dermatologic and GI irAEs seem to be the most common irAEs associated with immune checkpoint inhibitor therapy for melanoma and also are some of the earliest to appear (within the first 1–2 months of therapy).[27] The most common dermatologic irAEs typically are rash, pruritus, and vitiligo.[13] Grades 1 to 2 dermatologic irAEs typically are managed with oral antihistamines, topical emollients, and moderate-potency to high-potency topical corticosteroids while continuing immune checkpoint inhibitor therapy. For the management of grades 3 to 4 dermatologic toxicities, it is recommended to hold immune checkpoint inhibitor therapy until resolution to grade 1 or less as well as initiate oral corticosteroids in addition to measures for management of grades 1 to 2 toxicity. Additionally, a dermatology consult often is recommended for dermatologic toxicities of grades 3 and higher.

In the GI tract, the most common irAEs are diarrhea and colitis.[13] Grade 1 GI irAEs (an increase of <4 stools per day) are managed with vigilant monitoring for worsening of symptoms or dehydration, and physicians may consider temporarily holding checkpoint inhibitor therapy until symptoms improve. Checkpoint inhibitor therapy should be held for any grade 2 irAEs (increase in stools by 4–6 per day) until resolution to grade 1 or less, and patients should receive a full work-up to rule out infectious processes. A gastroenterology consult also is appropriate. Once infection is ruled out, it is recommended to start oral corticosteroids, such as prednisone 1 mg/kg/d, and provide supportive care measures. If symptoms persist for more than 2 days to 5 days, corticosteroid doses may be escalated or infliximab at 5 mg/kg to 10 mg/kg may be initiated. The management for grade 3 GI irAEs is similar to that of grade 2 except that it is recommended to permanently discontinue anti–CTLA-4 therapy if used. Grade 4 toxicity should be managed in a hospital setting utilizing aggressive supportive care measures like intravenous methylprednisolone at 1 mg/kg/d to 2 mg/kg/d and consideration of use of concurrent infliximab therapy. For grade 4 GI irAEs, the offending immune checkpoint inhibitor should be permanently discontinued.[28,30]

In general, the majority of irAEs associated with immune checkpoint inhibitor therapy appears to be responsive to oral corticosteroid therapy and/or holding the offending checkpoint inhibitor until symptoms improve.[27,29] Endocrinopathies, however, seem to be the exception to this trend. Endocrinopathies associated with immune checkpoint inhibitor therapy often require hormone replacement therapy in conjunction with corticosteroid treatment and many require ongoing hormone replacement therapy even after discontinuation of antibody treatment.[13] Primary hypothyroidism, characterized by high serum thyroid-stimulating hormone levels and low thyroxine (T4) levels, occurs in approximately 3% to 13% of patients treated with immune checkpoint inhibitor therapy with the highest rates occurring in patients treated with combination therapy followed by PD-1 inhibitor monotherapy.[31] Management of asymptomatic hypothyroidism includes monitoring whereas symptomatic patients are recommended to receive levothyroxine as thyroid hormone replacement therapy. Immune checkpoint inhibitors typically are continued unless severe symptoms arise.[27,28,30] Hyperthyroidism is rare, with an estimated overall incidence of approximately 2.9% and typically is managed with β-blockers, supportive care measures, and continuation of immune checkpoint inhibitor therapy for grades 1 to 2.[30,31] If grade 2 hyperthyroidism is persistent for greater than 6 weeks, severe symptoms/thyrotoxicosis occurs, Graves disease is suspected, or any grade 3 to grade 4 hyperthyroidism develops, then immune checkpoint inhibitor therapy is held and patients referred to endocrinology for management.[28,30] Hypophysitis is estimated to occur in approximately 6.4% of patients treated with combination immune checkpoint inhibitor therapy which corresponds to 3.2% of patients treated with ipilimumab and less than 1% of patients treated with PD-1 inhibitors.[31] Management of hypophysitis for all grades includes hormone replacement as needed (ie, hydrocortisone, levothyroxine, testosterone, and estrogen) and holding immune checkpoint inhibitor therapy until resolution of hypophysitis.[28,30] For symptomatic patients, corticosteroid therapy with oral prednisone at 1 mg/kg/d to 2 mg/kg/d, is recommended. If corticosteroids are started for hypophysitis, they should be initiated several days prior to initiation of thyroid hormone therapy to prevent precipitation of adrenal crisis.[28,30]

OTHER THERAPIES

In addition to the aforementioned treatments, other therapies, alone or in combination with chemotherapy, immune checkpoint inhibitors, cytokines/chemokines, and/or vaccines, have been or are currently under study.[5,11,32,33] Atezolizumab, avelumab, and durvalumab, antibodies to the PD-1 ligand (PD-L1), currently are approved treatments for solid tumors that may have a slightly less toxic profile than PD-1 inhibitors although more data are needed to compare the safety and efficacy of these regimens.[7,33] Other immunomodulatory receptors, such as Toll-like receptors and CD40, are additional therapeutic targets under consideration for oncology trials.[32] Indoleamine 2,3-dioxygenase 1 (IDO) inhibitors, like indoximod and epacadostat, enhance immune system function by altering tryptophan metabolism in tumor cells and currently are being tested in clinical trials; these inhibitors may be a good adjuvant therapy for immune checkpoint inhibitors.[32]

INTRALESIONAL IMMUNOTHERAPY

Intralesional immunotherapy injections are used to treat advanced melanoma lesions by eliciting an antitumor immune response against a target lesion or lesions while avoiding adverse events related to systemic administration of anticancer therapy. A commonly used treatment for this administration route is talimogene laherparepvec (TVEC). TVEC is a genetically modified herpes simplex-1 virus that encodes sequences to encourage immune cell activation such as cytokine granulocyte-macrophage colony-stimulating factor.[32] The first immunotherapy used for intralesional injection for the treatment of melanoma was bacillus Calmette-Guérin (BCG), which was found to elicit complete regression in approximately 90% of injected cutaneous lesions and 45% of injected subcutaneous lesions.[34] Despite the demonstrated efficacy of intralesional BCG, serious cases of cutaneous adverse events, infections, coagulation, and anaphylaxis associated with intralesional BCG have led to its very low utilization in the treatment of melanoma lesions in the present day.[34–37]

IMMUNOTHERAPY RESPONSE ASSESSMENT

Unlike response patterns with traditional cytotoxic chemotherapies and radiation therapy, where traditional Response Evaluation Criteria in Solid Tumors (RECIST) and World Health Organization (WHO) criteria based on predefined morphologic volume changes during therapy (i.e., tumor size and/or the appearance of new lesions) are used to define progressive disease and indicate treatment failure, immunotherapy ex-hibits some unique pattern differences, and tumor progression/regression is not as easily determined as with solid tumors during immunotheraapy. Variations, such as initial increase of tumor size and/or new lesions followed by a decrease that ordinarily would meet RECIST/WHO criteria for partial or complete response in comparison with baseline, which is sometimes called pseudoprogression, may be considered stable disease with immunotherapy and are not an indicator of treatment success.[7,38] Furthermore, immunotherapeutic response is slower to manifest, and it can take longer to see tumor response to therapy compared with traditional chemotherapy.[5,38]

To account for these variations in response, 3 response methodologies have been developed over time for immunotherapies, namely immune-related response criteria (irRC), immune-related RECIST (irRECIST), and immune RECIST (iRECIST). The irRC is a modification of WHO response criteria for solid tumors where change in tumor burden is calculated as a bidimensional measurement of lesions before and after treatment with an additional term for the appearance of new lesions that occur during immunotherapy.[38,39] In 2013, revised irRC criteria using unidimensional measurements based on the original RECIST and later using RECIST 1.1 as termed irRECIST were developed and proposed in 2017.[40,41] The iRECIST standardizes and validates irRC, taking into account novel response patterns seen with immunotherapies and is a general criterion for evaluation of immunotherapy-based treatments for metastatic melanoma.[42]

DISCUSSION

Immunotherapy is one of the most fascinating advances in the past decade in the field of oncology and probably medicine at large. This research has revolutionized the treatment and prognosis for individuals with many deadly solid tumors, especially malignant melanoma. In addition to improvements in response rate and OS leading to the approval of multiple immunotherapy agents for patients with advanced and metastatic melanoma, these therapies generally are well-tolerated for many of the newer therapies, including ipilimumab, nivolumab, and pembrolizumab, compared with the original cytokine-based treatments. Immunotherapy, however, comes with its own unique toxicity and response profiles requiring careful monitoring and management. Due to the ubiquity of the immune system, immune-related adverse effects can affect practically any organ or system in the body and may lead to potentially life-threating conditions if not identified quickly. Early detection and management of immune-related adverse effects is a continual challenge for providers administering immuno-therapies; therefore, additional study is necessary to determine which patients derive maximum benefit from immunotherapies. Due to the delay in response to immuno-therapy that can occur and unique response patterns of this treatment class, modifi-cations have been made to the traditional radiologic evaluation methods of tumor response to therapy. Studies are ongoing to evaluate the role of immunotherapy as adjuvant therapy for high-risk stage I and stage II melanoma, and molecular profiling is increasingly used to select immunotherapies for patients with advanced melanoma that will maximize immune system response while limiting toxic side effects.

ACKNOWLEDGMENTS

The authors gratefully acknowledge Emily Andreae, PhD, for content addition and figure development for this article.

DISCLOSURE

The authors have no personal or financial conflicts of interest to disclose.

REFERENCES

1. Cancer Statistics Center: melanoma of the skin. American Cancer Society. Available at: https://cancerstatisticscenter.cancer.org/?_ga=2.254190927.630277394. 1543264605-226162472.1497898949#!/cancer-site/Melanoma%20of%20the%20skin. Accessed November 26, 2018.

2. Middleton MR, Grob JJ, Aaronson N, et al. Randomized phase III study of temo-zolomide versus dacarbazine in the treatment of patients with advanced metasta-tic malignant melanoma. J Clin Oncol 2000;18(1):158–66.

3. Coley WB. The treatment of malignant tumors by repeated inoculations of erysip-elas: with a report of ten original cases. Am J Med Sci 1893;105(5):487.

4. Reiman JM, Kmieciak M, Manjili MH, et al. Tumor immunoediting and immuno-sculpting pathways to cancer progression. Semin Cancer Biol 2007;17(4):275–87.

5. Pardoll DM. The blockade of immune checkpoints in cancer immunotherapy. Nat Rev Cancer 2012;12(4):252–64.

6. Frey AB. Suppression of T cell responses in the tumor microenvironment. Vaccine 2015;33(51):7393–400.

7. Buchbinder EI, Desai A. CTLA-4 and PD-1 pathways: similarities, differences, and implications of their inhibition. Am J Clin Oncol 2016;39(1):98–106.

8. Sabel MS, Sondak VK. Pros and cons of adjuvant interferon in the treatment of melanoma. Oncologist 2003;8(5):451–8.

9. Di Trolio R, Simeone E, Di Lorenzo G, et al. The use of interferon in melanoma pa-tients: a systematic review. Cytokine Growth Factor Rev 2015;26(2):203–12.

10. Yurkovetsky ZR, Kirkwood JM, Edington HD, et al. Multiplex analysis of serum cy-tokines in melanoma patients treated with interferon-alpha2b. Clin Cancer Res 2007;13(8):2422–8.

11. Buchbinder EI, McDermott DF. Interferon, interleukin-2, and other cytokines. Hematol Oncol Clin North Am 2014;28(3):571–83.

12. Kirkwood JM, Strawderman MH, Ernstoff MS, et al. Interferon alfa-2b adjuvant therapy of high-risk resected cutaneous melanoma: The Eastern Cooperative Oncology Group Trial EST 1684. J Clin Oncol 1996;14(1):7–17.

13. National Comprehensive Cancer Network. Melanoma. 2018. Available at: https://www.nccn.org/professionals/physician_gls/pdf/cutaneous_melanoma.pdf. Updated November 1, 2018. Accessed December 28, 2018.

14. Atkins MB, Lotze MT, Dutcher JP, et al. High-dose recombinant interleukin 2 therapy for patients with metastatic melanoma: analysis of 270 patients treated between 1985 and 1993. J Clin Oncol 1999;17(7):2105–16.

15. Marabondo S, Kaufman HL. High-dose interleukin-2 (IL-2) for the treatment of melanoma: safety considerations and future directions. Expert Opin Drug Saf 2017;16(12):1347–57.

16. Linsley PS, Brady W, Urnes M, et al. CTLA-4 is a second receptor for the B cell activation antigen B7. J Exp Med 1991;174(3):561–9.

17. Linsley PS, Greene JL, Brady W, et al. Human B7-1 (CD80) and B7-2 (CD86) bind with similar avidities but distinct kinetics to CD28 and CTLA-4 receptors. Immunity 1994;1(9):793–801.

18. Greene JL, Leytze GM, Emswiler J, et al. Covalent dimerization of CD28/CTLA-4 and oligomerization of CD80/CD86 regulate T cell costimulatory interactions. J Biol Chem 1996;271(43):26762–71.

19. Morton PA, Fu XT, Stewart JA, et al. Differential effects of CTLA-4 substitutions on the binding of human CD80 (B7-1) and CD86 (B7-2). J Immunol 1996;156(3):1047–54.

20. Hodi FS, O'day SJ, McDermott DF, et al. Improved survival with ipilimumab in patients with metastatic melanoma. N Engl J Med 2010;363(8):711–23.

21. McDermott D, Haanen J, Chen TT, et al. MDX010-20 Investigators. Efficacy and safety of ipilimumab in metastatic melanoma patients surviving more than 2 years following treatment in a phase III trial (MDX010-20). Ann Oncol 2013;24(10):2694–8.

22. Eggermont AMM, Chiarion-Sileni V, Grob JJ, et al. Adjuvant ipilimumab versus placebo after complete resection of high-risk stage III melanoma (EORTC 18071): a randomised, double-blind, phase 3 trial. Lancet Oncol 2015;16(5):522–30.

23. Weber J, Mandala M, Del Vecchio M, et al. Adjuvant nivolumab versus ipilimumab in resected stage III or IV melanoma. N Engl J Med 2017;377(19):1824–35.

24. Eggermont AMM, Blank CU, Mandala M, et al. Adjuvant pembrolizumab versus placebo in resected stage III melanoma. N Engl J Med 2018;378(19):1789–801.

25. Schachter J, Ribas A, Long GV, et al. Pembrolizumab versus ipilimumab for advanced melanoma: final overall survival results of a multicentre, randomised, open-label phase 3 study (KEYNOTE-006). Lancet 2017;390(10105):1853–62.

26. Hodi FS, Chiarion-Sileni V, Gonzalez R, et al. Nivolumab plus ipilimumab or nivolumab alone versus ipilimumab alone in advanced melanoma (CheckMate 067): 4-year outcomes of a multicentre, randomised, phase 3 trial. Lancet Oncol 2018;19(11):1480–92.

27. Postow MA, Sidlow R, Hellmann MD. Immune-related adverse events associated with immune checkpoint blockade. N Engl J Med 2018;378(2):158–68.

28. National Comprehensive Cancer Network. Management of immune related toxicities. 2018. Available at: https://www.nccn.org/professionals/physician_gls/pdf/immunotherapy.pdf. Updated November 14, 2018. Accessed February 19, 2019.

29. Wang DY, Salem JE, Cohen JV, et al. Fatal toxic effects associated with immune checkpoint inhibitors: a systematic review and meta-analysis. JAMA Oncol 2018; 4(12):1721–8.

30. Brahmer JR, Lacchetti C, Schneider BJ, et al. Management of immune-related adverse events in patients treated with immune checkpoint inhibitor therapy: American Society of Clinical Oncology Clinical Practice Guideline. J Clin Oncol 2018;36(17):1714–68.

31. Barroso-Sousa R, Barry WT, Garrido-Castro AC, et al. Incidence of endocrine dysfunction following the use of different immune checkpoint inhibitor regimens: a systematic review and meta-analysis. JAMA Oncol 2018;4(2):173–82.

32. Luther C, Swami U, Zhang J, et al. Advanced stage melanoma therapies: detailing the present and exploring the future. Crit Rev Oncol Hematol 2019;133: 99–111.

33. Alsaab HO, Sau S, Alzhrani R, et al. PD-1 and PD-L1 checkpoint signaling inhibition for cancer immunotherapy: Mechanism, combinations, and clinical outcome. Front Pharmacol 2017;8:561.

34. Cohen MH, Jessup JM, Felix EL, et al. Intralesional treatment of recurrent metastatic cutaneous malignant melanoma: a randomized prospective study of intralesional Bacillus Calmette-Guerin versus intralesional dinitrochlorobenzene. Cancer 1978;41(6):2456–63.

35. Sloot S, Rashid OM, Sarnaik AA, et al. Developments in intralesional therapy for metastatic melanoma. Cancer Control 2016;23(1):12–20.

36. Robinson JC. Risks of BCG intralesional therapy: an experience with melanoma. J Surg Oncol 1977;9(6):587–93.

37. Proctor JW, Zidar B, Pomerantz M, et al. Anaphylactic reaction to intralesional B.C.G. Lancet 1978;2(8081):162.

38. Hoos A, Eggermont AMM, Janetzki S, et al. Improved endpoints for cancer immunotherapy trials. J Natl Cancer Inst 2010;102(18):1388–97.

39. Wolchok JD, Hoos A, O'Day S, et al. Guidelines for the evaluation of immune therapy activity in solid tumors: immune-related response criteria. Clin Cancer Res 2009;15(23):7412–20.

40. Nishino M, Giobbie-Hurder A, Gargano M, et al. Developing a common language for tumor response to immunotherapy: immune-related response criteria using unidimensional measurements. Clin Cancer Res 2013;19(14):3936–43.

41. Bohnsack O, Ludajic K, Hoos A. Adaptation of the immune-related response criteria: irRECIST. Ann Oncol 2014;25(suppl 4):iv361, iv372.

42. Seymour L, Bogaerts J, Perrone A, et al. iRECIST: Guidelines for response criteria for use in trials testing immunotherapeutics. Lancet Oncol 2017;18(3):e143–52.

Principles of Targeted Therapy for Melanoma

James Sun, MD, Michael J. Carr, MD, Nikhil I. Khushalani, MD*

KEYWORDS

- BRAF • MEK • NRAS • KIT • Brain metastasis • Melanoma • Mutation

KEY POINTS

- The mitogen-activated protein kinase (MAPK) pathway is involved in the pathogenesis of most cutaneous melanomas.
- Up to 50% of melanomas arising in sun-damaged skin harbor a single nucleotide substitution at codon 600 in the *BRAF* oncogene (*BRAF V600*).
- *BRAF V600* mutations provide a therapeutic target with BRAF/MEK inhibitors, which provide rapid clinical results in most patients, but are also associated with high rates of treatment resistance through MAPK reactivation.
- The role of perioperative use of BRAF-targeted therapy is evolving.
- Activating *KIT* mutations are rarely found in melanomas but may be an actionable target of therapy, which is the subject of several ongoing clinical trials.

INTRODUCTION

Over the past decade, there has been significant advancement in the understanding of the pathophysiology of melanoma. These advancements have led to the systematic development of new effective therapies for advanced disease in the form of molecularly targeted therapy and immunotherapy. Randomized trials have also demonstrated efficacy in reducing relapse after complete surgical resection of stage III or stage IV melanoma, thus making modern management of melanoma a multidisciplinary endeavor. The most common activating mutations in melanoma cells are *BRAF*, *NRAS*, and *KIT* mutations.[1] These mutations cause derangements in cell signaling pathways, leading to unchecked tumor proliferation. The cell signaling pathways implicated in the progression of benign melanocytes to malignant disease are now better understood. These pathways may be the key to identifying new therapeutic targets and providing more options against this devastating disease.

Department of Cutaneous Oncology, Moffitt Cancer Center, 10920 North McKinley Drive, 4th Floor, Tampa, FL 33612, USA
* Corresponding author.
E-mail address: nikhil.khushalani@moffitt.org

Surg Clin N Am 100 (2020) 175–188
https://doi.org/10.1016/j.suc.2019.09.013
0039-6109/20/© 2019 Elsevier Inc. All rights reserved.

surgical.theclinics.com

BRAF MUTATIONS

The mitogen-activated protein kinase (MAPK) pathway is a signaling pathway that is normally responsible for intracellular processes, which include acute hormone responses, embryogenesis, cellular differentiation, cellular proliferation, and apoptosis. This pathway is activated by extracellular binding of receptor tyrosine kinases (RTK), leading to activation of the rat sarcoma (RAS) family protein, which subsequently activates intracellular serine-threonine protein kinases of the rapidly accelerated fibrosarcoma (RAF) family (ARAF, BRAF, CRAF). Activation of RAF leads to the phosphorylation of MAPK extracellular receptor kinase (MEK), which in turn phosphorylates extracellular signal-regulated kinase (ERK). ERK activation promotes cellular proliferation and activates mitochondrial proteins, which promote growth and inhibit apoptosis.[2,3] Activated ERK also provides negative feedback at various levels of the pathway.

The MAPK pathway has an important role in melanoma oncogenesis. Derangements in the MAPK pathway are most commonly caused by single nucleotide substitutions at codon 600 in the *BRAF* oncogene, which encodes the BRAF protein. This mutation is found in approximately 50% of all melanomas. *BRAF* mutations are more frequent in melanomas that develop in sun-exposed skin.[4] This mutation leads to unregulated activation of RAS independent of RTK binding, thus causing constitutive activation of MEK and ERK, resulting in unchecking cellular proliferation.[3] The most common mutation at this locus is due to a single nucleotide valine-to-glutamic acid substitution (*BRAFV600E*), which occurs in approximately 90% of *BRAF*-mutant melanomas. The second most common mutation is *BRAFV600K* (substituting lysine for valine), which accounts for another 5% to 6% of *BRAF*-mutant melanomas. Other observed, albeit less common mutations include *BRAFV600D* and *BRAFV600R*. BRAF mutations are associated with approximately 80% of melanocytic nevi, suggesting an early role oncogenesis. However, only a small portion of nevi actually progress to melanoma.[5–7]

NEUROBLASTOMA RAT SARCOMA MUTATIONS

Activating mutations within the RAS family are seen in approximately 20% of all melanomas at diagnosis and are most common in the human neuroblastoma RAS (NRAS) GTPase. *NRAS* mutations are mutually exclusive with *BRAF* mutations. The most common *RAS* mutations occur at codons 12, 61, or 13; 15% of cases have point mutations. All of these are activating mutations that exert a different effect on the NRAS protein. However, the end result is the same, leading to GTP-bound, activated RAS protein.[8] NRAS amplification and mutation cause constitutive activation of the MAPK pathway as well as the phosphatidylinositol 3-kinase (PI3K) pathway.[5–7]

PHOSPHATIDYLINOSITOL 3-KINASE PATHWAY

Stimulation of the PI3K pathway has been found to occur in 30% to 60% of melanomas through functional loss of the tumor suppression protein PTEN, which is associated with *BRAF V600E* mutations.[9] Also implicated in this line is the activation or amplification of serine/threonine protein kinase AKT3 in 40% to 60% of melanomas.[10–12] This pathway follows the RTK-RAS-PI3K-(PTEN)-AKT3 signal cascade to the mitochondrial antiapoptotic protein BCL2 and cellular growth regulator mTOR (mammalian target of rapamycin). Upstream of RAS, amplifications or activating mutations in the gene encoding the RTK for stem cell factor, KIT, can also activate this pathway.[2,6,12] This pathway has also been implicated in the development of melanoma brain metastases (MBM).[13]

CURRENT REGIMENS FOR *BRAF*-MUTATED ADVANCED MELANOMA

Understanding of the MAPK pathway has led to identification of therapeutic targets with development of highly specific BRAF and MEK inhibitors. BRAF inhibitors selectively target the mutated BRAF kinase, thus decreasing signal transduction through the MAPK pathway. Vemurafenib was the first approved BRAF inhibitor in 2011 on the basis of the BRIM-3 (*BRAF Inhibition in Melanoma-3*) trial.[14] This phase 3 trial conducted in 675 patients with previously untreated advanced or unresectable BRAF *V600* mutant melanoma demonstrated superior response with vemurafenib versus dacarbazine for the treatment of *BRAF*-mutant melanoma, with an overall response rate (ORR) of 48% versus 5% with dacarbazine. In the final report of this trial conducted at a median follow-up period of 13.4 months for patients on the vemurafenib arm and 9.2 months for those on the dacarbazine arm, overall survival (OS) was significantly superior for vemurafenib.[15] The median OS was 13.6 months for vemurafenib-treated patients versus 9.7 months on the dacarbazine arm (hazard ratio [HR] 0.81, 95% confidence interval [CI] 0.67–0.98, $P = .03$). The landmark analyses on vemurafenib demonstrated OS at 3 and 4 years to be 21% and 17%, respectively. It should be noted that 84 of 338 patients on dacarbazine crossed over to vemurafenib during the conduction of this study. The OS remained significant in favor of vemurafenib regardless of censoring results at crossover. In a previous report on this trial, the median progression-free survival (PFS) also significantly favored the vemurafenib arm (6.9 months vs 1.6 months, HR 0.38, 95% CI 0.32–0.46, $P<.0001$).[16] Efficacy results for other approved BRAF inhibitors, including dabrafenib and encorafenib, are very similar.[17]

Although BRAF-inhibition produces dramatic tumor response in most patients, these responses are limited by rapid development of treatment resistance at a median time of 5 to 7 months.[18] The addition of an MEK inhibitor, a downstream component of the MAPK pathway, delays the onset of resistance. Combination BRAF/MEK inhibition has also demonstrated improved treatment response, PFS, and OS compared with BRAF-inhibitor monotherapy. The current standard of care is thus to use combination targeted therapy rather than single-agent BRAF or MEK inhibitor therapy for eligible patients whose tumor harbors a mutation in *BRAF V600*. The 3 approved combination therapies are dabrafenib/trametinib, vemurafenib/cobimetinib, and encorafenib/binimetinib on the basis of several large phase 3 trials affirming superiority of the combination.[19–22]

The evolution from single-agent BRAF inhibitor therapy to combination BRAF plus MEK inhibitor therapy was rapid and with remarkably consistent results, at least for the comparator arm in this trial. In the COMBI-d study, 423 untreated patients with unresectable stage IIIC or metastatic melanoma harboring a mutation in BRAF *V600E/K* were randomized to receive combination dabrafenib (150 mg orally twice daily) plus trametinib (2 mg orally daily) versus dabrafenib alone at the same dose and schedule. Several updates with mature follow-up to the results of this trial have been published since the original report in 2014.[19,23,24] The confirmed response rate per Response Evaluation Criteria in Solid Tumors (RECIST) was 68% for the combination and 55% for dabrafenib alone, with corresponding complete response rates of 18% and 15%, respectively, for the 2 groups. The median PFS was 11.0 months versus 8.8 months, respectively (HR 0.67, 95% CI, 0.53–0.84, $P = .004$). At the time of an updated data cutoff in February 2016, the 3-year PFS and OS for dabrafenib plus trametinib were 22% and 44%, respectively, with corresponding values for the monotherapy dabrafenib arm of 12% and 32%, respectively. With this median follow-up time of $\geq$36 months for patients who were alive, 19% remained on therapy with the combination versus 3% on the monotherapy arm, without any new signals of toxicity concern, suggesting that chronic administration of these agents was safe. In a larger phase 3 trial (COMBI-v), the same doublet of dabrafenib and trametinib was compared with vemurafenib alone with remarkably similar results of efficacy.[20] The response rates were 64% versus 51%, with median PFS of 11.4 months versus 7.3 months (HR 0.56, 95% CI, 0.46–0.69, $P<.001$), all favoring the combination arm. Similarly, the 1-year OS was 72% for the combination versus 65% for vemurafenib alone (HR 0.69, 95% CI, 0.53–0.89, $P = .005$).

Given the finite time to progression that is commonly observed with targeted therapy, a pooled analysis examining the long-term efficacy of dabrafenib plus trametinib within the COMBI-d and COMBI-v trials was recently published.[25] This study reported data on 563 patients treated with this combination. The median PFS and OS were 11.1 months and 25.9 months, respectively. The PFS at 4 years was 21% and 19% at 5 years. The corresponding landmark analyses for OS were 37% and 34%, respectively. This excellent efficacy in one-third of patients treated initially with targeted therapy appears to contradict the prior notion that durable responses can only be seen with immunotherapy. Factors associated with a favorable prognosis and improved PFS and OS included older age, female sex, BRAF V600E status, normal lactate dehydrogenase, and fewer than 3 sites of visceral metastatic disease. In those patients who achieved a complete objective response to therapy (19%), the 5-year OS was an impressive 71%. An important consideration in this analysis was the fact that 88% (51/59) patients who were progression free at 5 years continued on the original therapy, either dabrafenib, trametinib, or both drugs. Conversely, in the limited available data on progression (n = 15) in responding patients who had discontinued therapy before progression, the median time to progression was only 3.7 months. Thus, the question of elective discontinuation of therapy based on depth of response remains unclear. Patients on targeted therapy should continue treatment as long as tolerable in the face of ongoing benefit of response.

The combination of vemurafenib with the MEK inhibitor cobimetinib gained regulatory approval in the United States for advanced melanoma based on the coBRIM trial, a randomized comparison of this combination to vemurafenib plus placebo in BRAF V600-mutant melanoma.[21,26] The primary endpoint of PFS was superior in the combination (12.3 months) versus the monotherapy arm (7.2 months) (HR 0.58, 95% CI 0.46–0.72, $P<.001$). Similarly, median OS was also longer at 22.3 months versus 17.4 months (HR 0.70, 95% CI, 0.55–0.90). The COLUMBUS trial similarly confirmed the superiority of yet another combination inhibiting the MAPK pathway compared with BRAF inhibition alone. In this 3-arm study, encorafenib (BRAF inhibitor) plus binimetinib (MEK inhibitor) was compared with encorafenib alone or vemurafenib alone.[27] The combination improved median PFS to 14.9 months versus 7.3 months for vemurafenib alone (HR 0.54, 95% CI, 0.41–0.71, $P<.001$). Similarly, median OS in patients treated with encorafenib and binimetinib was 33.6 months compared with 16.9 months in those who received vemurafenib (HR 0.61, 95% CI, 0.47–0.79, $P<.001$). The combination was also superior to encorafenib alone for both these comparisons.

Although the PFS and OS using encorafenib and binimetinib are numerically higher than that achieved with the other 2 combinations, it should be noted that these regimens have not been compared directly with one another, nor is that likely to occur. However, the consistency of results across the single-agent arms in these trials is remarkable. Thus, decisions on choosing a specific combination are typically made based on the predicted toxicity profile and physician-patient preference. The current National Comprehensive Cancer Network (NCCN) guidelines recommend BRAF/MEK inhibitor combination therapy with 1 of the 3 approved first-line regimens for the treatment of unresectable or distant metastatic disease in *BRAF V600* mutated melanoma.[28] There are currently no data available to guide selection of targeted therapy versus immune checkpoint inhibition as the initial therapy for unresectable or metastatic *BRAF V600* mutant melanoma; however, the NCCN guidelines suggest factoring in the rate of disease progression. Targeted therapy tends to elicit a rapid clinical response and may be more appropriate initial therapy in the setting of symptomatic disease. Vemurafenib and dabrafenib are also approved for monotherapy and only recommended in situations whereby combination therapy is contraindicated or not tolerated, and immune checkpoint inhibitor therapy is not a preferred option (eg, active auto-immune disease, organ transplant recipient, ongoing immunosuppressive therapy). There is also little definitive clinical trial data to guide selection of second-line treatment; however, all 3 combination BRAF/MEK inhibitor combinations remain reasonable options after failure of front-line immunotherapy (category 2A recommendation by NCCN).

ADJUVANT AND NEOADJUVANT THERAPY OF *BRAF*-MUTANT MELANOMA

Until recently, adjuvant systemic therapy for surgically resected cutaneous melanoma was limited to interferon or ipilimumab, both agents with substantial toxicity. The risk of relapse is predominantly linked to the depth and ulceration of the primary tumor as well as the presence of in-transit and/or nodal metastases. Before the results of the second Multicenter Selective Lymphadenectomy Trial -II, patients with positive sentinel nodes routinely underwent completion nodal dissection (CLND).[29] The lack of improvement of melanoma-specific survival with immediate CLND has markedly reduced the number of patients with sentinel node metastasis undergoing this procedure. This paradigm change in the surgical management of melanoma is important to recognize in the context of delivery of postoperative systemic therapy because all published trials of adjuvant treatment in melanoma mandated a CLND before treatment. The assumption of similar benefit of adjuvant therapy for sentinel node metastasis without CLND is thus presumed in the modern era of immunotherapy and targeted therapy.

The COMBI-AD trial was a double-blind, placebo-controlled randomized phase 3 trial aimed to assess the relapse-free survival (RFS) of combination dabrafenib and trametinib versus matched placebo administered for 12 months in resected stage III (per American Joint Committee on Cancer [AJCC], 7th edition) cutaneous melanoma harboring *BRAF V600E/K* mutations.[30,31] Patients with stage IIIA disease were required to have lymph node metastasis greater than 1 mm. Among 870 randomized patients, most (81%) had stage IIIB or IIIC disease. At mature follow-up exceeding 40 months, the median RFS had not been reached for the dabrafenib plus trametinib arm compared with 16.9 months in the placebo arm (HR 0.49, 95% CI, 0.40–0.59). The corresponding 4-year RFS rates were 54% and 38%, respectively. In the initial report at the first interim analysis for OS, the 3-year estimate for OS was 83% for the combination therapy versus 77% for placebo (HR 0.57, 95% CI, 0.42–0.79, $P = .0006$). This difference however did not cross the prespecified conservative interim boundary of statistical significance at $P = .00019$. In the follow-up report, the number of events needed for the subsequent prespecified OS interim analysis had not been reached. Using a Weibull cure-rate model, the estimated cure rate (lack of relapse) was 54% for the treatment arm versus 37% for the placebo arm. In addition, a post hoc analysis for RFS across disease stage defined by AJCC, 8th edition indicated benefit across all subgroups (stages IIIA–D) for combination therapy. This combination of dabrafenib and trametinib was approved by the Food and Drug Administration for the adjuvant therapy of completely resected stage III melanoma in 2018. Combination BRAF/MEK inhibition has not been directly compared with approved anti-PD1 agents (nivolumab or pembrolizumab)[32,33] as adjuvant therapy, and any one of these options are reasonable choices following complete resection of node-positive *BRAF V600* mutant cutaneous melanoma.

With the availability of effective systemic therapy in melanoma, there has been growing interest in neoadjuvant therapy for macroscopic nodal metastatic melanoma or disease that is considered unresectable at clinical presentation. This approach has several theoretic advantages, including control of micrometastatic disease, improved regional control, "debulking" an unresectable or borderline resectable tumor mass toward making surgery feasible, and possibly sparing a patient from unnecessary surgery in the face of progressive disease on upfront systemic therapy. In addition, this approach is suited for systematic tissue study to identify biomarkers of response and resistance as well as understanding pathologic response at the time of surgery. Given the high response rates to MAPK-targeted therapy, these agents are ideal choices for investigation in the neoadjuvant setting, although prospective data to date have been scant. In a single-institution randomized phase 2 trial, patients with surgically resectable and locally advanced clinical stage III (at least 1 palpable node with short axis >1.5 cm, or an in-transit metastasis >1 cm) or oligometastatic stage IV melanoma were randomized 1:2 to surgery upfront followed by adjuvant therapy or 8 weeks of neoadjuvant dabrafenib plus trametinib followed by surgery and 44 additional weeks of the same combination therapy.[34] This trial was halted early when clear superiority for the investigational approach was identified. The radiographic response to neoadjuvant therapy was 85%, and 7/12 (58%) patients who underwent surgery had a pathologic complete response (pCR). The median event-free survival was 19.7 months in the neoadjuvant arm compared with only 2.9 months in the standard of care arm (HR 0.016, 95% CI 0.00012–0.14, $P<.001$). Of note, only 1 patient in the latter cohort opted for adjuvant biochemotherapy, whereas the other 6 patients were observed expectantly. In an Australian prospective cohort (NeoCombi), 35 patients with stage IIIB/C melanoma were treated with 12 weeks of neoadjuvant dabrafenib and trametinib followed by surgery and an additional 40 weeks of the same systemic treatment.[35] The RECIST response was 86%, and the pCR rate was 49%. There was no progression noted during neoadjuvant therapy, and the median RFS was 23.3 months. Surgical complications occurred in 22 patients, most commonly seroma and postoperative infections requiring intravenous antibiotics. In a retrospective report from the authors' experience at Moffitt Cancer Center, 23 *BRAF V600* mutant melanoma patients with stage IIIC/IV disease were treated with neoadjuvant MAPK-targeted therapy (BRAF inhibitor monotherapy or in combination with an MEK inhibitor) for a median of 6.6 months before surgery.[36] With mature median follow-up of 43 months (range, 10–95), the radiographic response rate was 87%, and pCR was achieved in 10 patients (44%). Among the latter group, only 1 patient experienced relapse of disease, whereas 8/13 (62%) patients with residual tumor in the surgical resection specimen had relapsed. The influence of pathologic response to neoadjuvant therapy on subsequent systemic therapy has yet to be studied. The International Neoadjuvant Melanoma Consortium has made recent recommendations in an attempt to standardize study protocols in this arena for optimization of clinical care and research priorities.[37]

TARGETED THERAPY FOR MELANOMA BRAIN METASTASES

Brain metastases from melanoma are a known devastating complication with poor outcomes.[38] The treatment of MBM has historically been based on local treatment with surgery, whole-brain radiation, and stereotactic radiosurgery. Recent advances in systemic therapy have improved the median OS to 14 to 23 months.[38–40] Chemokine receptor type 4 (CCR4) is a transmembrane receptor that is overexpressed in melanoma cells that metastasize to the brain and is predictive of MBM in murine models.[13,41] CCR4 activation leads to activation of the PI3K pathway. Melanoma cells attempt to overcome the blood-brain barrier using 2 mechanisms. They secrete serine proteases, to break down occludin and claudin-5 (transmembrane proteins), and cytoplasmic plaque protein ZO-1, to disrupt the endothelial tight junction.[42] Melanoma cells then release matrix metalloproteinase-2 (MMP-2) and heparanase, which are extracellular matrix degrading enzymes, to disrupt the basement membrane.[43] At this point, melanoma cells are free to invade the brain parenchyma. The janus kinase/signal transducer and activator of transcription (JAK/STAT) pathway has been implicated in neoangiogenesis of brain metastases.[44,45] The PI3K pathway promotes MBM via upregulation of CCR4, heparanase, as well as vascular endothelial growth factor and STAT3. The MAPK pathway has also been implicated in the development of MBM. In a study of 1048 patients by Adler and colleagues,[46] the presence of *BRAF* and *NRAS* mutations was associated with increased odds of developing metastases in the central nervous system. There is evidence that downregulation of the MAPK pathway after treatment with BRAF/MEK inhibition may lead to upregulation of the PI3K pathway, leading to resistance.[47,48] As a result, melanomas that develop treatment resistance may be predisposed to metastasize to the brain.[49,50]

The BREAK-MB study evaluated activity and safety of dabrafenib monotherapy in *BRAF V600E*- and *V600K*-mutant melanomas with brain metastases.[51] Treated were 172 patients: 89 patients had not received previous local treatment (cohort A) and 83 patients had progressed after prior local treatment (cohort B). In patients with *BRAF V600E* mutations, the intracranial response rate was 39% (29/74 patients) in cohort A versus 31% (20/65 patients) in cohort B. ORR was 38% and 31% in cohorts A and B, respectively. The median PFS was approximately 4 months, and OS was approximately 8 months. Patients with *BRAF V600K* mutations (n = 33) had worse ORR; 7% (1/15) in cohort A versus 22% (4/18) in cohort B. Similarly, vemurafenib has demonstrated intracranial efficacy in a phase 2 study by McArthur and colleagues.[52] Among 146 patients enrolled, 90 were therapy naïve for MBM (cohort 1), whereas 56 patients had received prior treatment (cohort 2). The intracranial response rate was 18% in both cohorts by independent review, which was lower than extracranial response (33% and 23%, respectively). The median intracranial PFS was 3.7 months and 4 months in cohorts 1 and 2, respectively; median OS was 8.9 months and 9.6 months, respectively.

The phase 2 COMBI-MB study assessed the activity and safety of combination dabrafenib and trametinib therapy in MBM patients with *BRAF V600* mutations.[49] They established 4 patient cohorts: cohort A (n = 76), *BRAF V600E*-mutant, asymptomatic MBM without prior local brain-directed therapy and Eastern Cooperative Oncology Group (ECOG) performance status of ≤1; cohort B (n = 16), *BRAF V600E*-mutant, asymptomatic MBM with prior local therapy and ECOG performance status of ≤1; cohort C (n = 16), *BRAF V600D/E/K/R*-mutant, asymptomatic MBM with or without prior local therapy and ECOG performance status of ≤1; cohort D (n = 17), *BRAF V600D/E/K/R*-mutant, symptomatic MBM with or without prior local therapy and ECOG performance status of ≤2. Intracranial response rates were 58%,

56%, 44%, and 59% in cohorts A through D, respectively. In cohort A, extracranial response rate was 55% with median PFS of 5.6 months and median OS of 10.8 months; median duration of intracranial response was 6.5 months, and median duration of extracranial response was 10.2 months. This study demonstrated improved activity of dabrafenib + trametinib in MBM in comparison to dabrafenib monotherapy and vemurafenib.[51,52] Response rates were better than traditional local brain-directed therapies; however, the duration of disease control is shorter than in melanoma patients without brain metastases. The safety profile of dabrafenib plus trametinib was similar as previously reported studies with manageable adverse events in patients with MBM.

In an era of expanding systemic options for MBM, a multidisciplinary evaluation is essential in order to optimize outcomes using all available modalities of therapy. Studies combining targeted therapy with immunotherapy in this setting have been planned.

NRAS MUTATIONS IN MELANOMA

As discussed previously, *NRAS* mutations resulting in constitutive activation of the MAPK pathway are seen in about one-fifth of all melanomas. Given the inherent difficulty in targeting *NRAS* directly and recognition of the downstream effects of *RAS* activation, MEK inhibition has been explored as an option to inhibit the MAPK pathway in *NRAS* mutant melanoma. Binimetinib, an inhibitor of MEK 1/2, demonstrated a modest 20% response rate in *NRAS* mutant melanoma, all partial responses.[53] In a phase 3 trial of *NRAS*-mutant stage IIIC or stage IV melanoma, either untreated or with progression on immunotherapy, 402 patients were randomized 2:1 to receive binimetinib 45 mg orally twice daily or standard dacarbazine administered intravenously.[54] The response rate to binimetinib was 15% (including 1% complete response), and the median PFS was 2.8 months, compared with 1.5 months on dacarbazine (HR 0.62, 95% CI 0.47–0.80, $P<.01$). The median OS was similar in both arms. The response rate was similar (16%) in patients previously treated with immunotherapy. Binimetinib may represent an option for patients with progressive disease after front-line immunotherapy, especially in the absence of other targetable mutations or availability of clinical trial.

ABERRATIONS IN *KIT* IN MELANOMA

Melanomas harboring mutations in *BRAF* tend to occur in nonchronically sun-damaged skin. These mutations are uncommon in other histologic subtypes of melanoma, including acral-lentiginous, mucosal, and those arising in skin with chronic sun damage. Curtin and colleagues[55] analyzed 102 primary melanomas from these sites and discovered amplifications within a narrow band on chromosome 4q12, identifying a mutation in K642E, which is known to be oncogenic; this is also found in gastrointestinal stromal tumors (GIST).[56] These specimens also had elevations in KIT protein, which is a type III transmembrane RTK, thus identifying a link between *KIT* mutations and melanoma development.[57] It is now well known that *KIT* mutations can cause melanomas in mucosal regions, acral skin, and skin with sun damage.[55,58,59] *KIT*-activating mutations have been reported in 21% of mucosal melanomas, 11% of acral melanomas, 16.7% of melanomas in chronically sun-damaged skin, and 15% of anal melanomas.[55,60] The most common *KIT* mutations in melanoma are L676P and K642E translocations.[61] Imatinib mesylate is a specific inhibitor of the *bcr-abl* tyrosine kinase and is effective for the treatment of GIST and chronic myelogenous leukemia.[59] Approximately 70% of *KIT* mutations occur in the juxtamembrane region, which is a predictor of responsiveness to imatinib.

Since the identification of *KIT* mutations in melanoma, several trials have been performed to identify patients most likely to benefit from KIT inhibition. Imatinib was the first targeted drug identified to have therapeutic activity against *KIT*-mutated melanoma given its use in other malignancies harboring *KIT* mutations. Early demonstration of clinical activity of *KIT* inhibitors was published in case reports using imatinib and dasatinib.[62] Initial studies of imatinib failed to demonstrate efficacy, likely secondary to nonselection of specific molecular subtypes of melanoma more apt to harbor the target of interest.[63–65]

In an enriched population of *CKIT* mutant and/or amplified melanoma, Carvajal and colleagues[66] reported a 16% (4/25 evaluable patients) durable response rate. The median time to progression was 12 weeks, and median OS was 46.3 weeks. The 4 patients who achieved durable responses maintained disease control for more than 1 year. Guo and colleagues[67] performed a phase 2 trial of imatinib in China. Forty-three patients were evaluated with a reported ORR of 23.3% and median PFS of 3.5 months. Overall 1-year survival rate was 51%, and disease control rate (DCR) was 53.5%. Patients who experienced a partial response (PR) had significantly longer PFS and OS compared with patients with stable disease (9 vs 1.5 months; 15 vs 9 months, respectively). Patients who progressed were allowed to escalate the imatinib dose from 400 mg daily to 800 mg daily, but of these 15 patients, only 1 patient achieved stabilization of disease, whereas the others experienced progression. Hodi and colleagues[68] performed a third phase 2 trial of imatinib with 24 evaluable target-enriched melanoma patients. The trial cohort included 8 patients with *KIT* mutations, 11 with *KIT* amplifications, and 5 with both. They reported a best ORR of 29%; responses were only seen in patients harboring *KIT* mutation and not in those with *KIT* amplifications. Median time to progression was 3.7 months, and overall DCR was 50%.

These trials suggest that durable responses may be seen in *KIT* mutant melanoma treated with imatinib. Unfortunately, most patients eventually progress. The reported median times to disease progression of approximately 3 months in these target-enriched trials are significantly lower than time to progression when imatinib is used to treat GIST (median time to progression of 18 months).[68] It is unclear why there is such a difference in response between *KIT*-mutant melanoma and GIST, despite the presence of the same mutation, suggesting that there may be other pathways involved in treatment resistance that require further elucidation.

Nilotinib is another selective *bcr-abl* tyrosine kinase inhibitor similar in structure to imatinib.[69] In a phase 2 trial of nilotinib in 42 melanoma patients with *KIT* mutations, amplifications, or both, a response rate of 16.7% and DCR of 57.1% was reported. The median duration of response was 34 weeks. Most responses were again seen in patients with *KIT* mutations (6/7) rather than *KIT* amplification (1/7).

There are several ongoing studies of other novel KIT inhibitors in melanoma. PLX3397 (Pexidartinib) is being evaluated in 2 trials; the PIANO (PLX3397 KIT in Acral aNd mucOsal Melanoma) trial will investigate its efficacy in *KIT*-mutant acral and mucosal melanoma (NCT02071940). Another phase 1/2 study of this agent is underway in Asia (NCT02975700), first to determine the recommended phase 2 dose and then to assess its efficacy in patients with unresectable or metastatic *KIT*-mutated melanoma. Another novel agent under investigation is regorafenib, which is already approved for the treatment of metastatic colorectal,[70] GIST,[71] and hepatocellular carcinoma.[72] Regorafenib is a multikinase inhibitor, and the investigators propose that this will provide better efficacy in *KIT*-mutated melanomas (NCT02501551).

SUMMARY

The understanding of the pathways involved in melanoma development is essential to identifying therapeutic targets. Understanding of the MAP kinase pathway has led to successful therapeutic targeting of the *BRAF V600* mutation, accounting for 50% of melanomas arising from skin without chronic sun damage. Results for exploiting *NRAS and CKIT* mutations as valid targets have been less successful, underscoring the need to understand dominant mechanisms of melanomagenesis and resistance to therapy, whether primary or acquired. Moving the use of effective systemic therapy to earlier stages of disease may result in higher cure rates from melanoma. Trials combining targeted therapy with immunotherapy either concurrently or sequentially are currently ongoing. Results from these and other biomarker-driven trials will help shape the future armamentarium in localized and advanced melanoma, aiming to achieve a personalized therapy based on the molecular signature of an individual tumor.

DISCLOSURE

For N.I. Khushalani: Advisory board or honoraria: Array, Bristol-Myers Squibb, EMD Serono, Regeneron Pharmaceuticals, Inc, Genentech, HUYA Bioscience, Merck, Sanofi, and Immunocore. Research grants (to Institution) from Bristol-Myers Squibb, Celgene, HUYA Bioscience, Merck, Novartis, GlaxoSmithKline, Regeneron, and Amgen. Data safety monitoring committee: AstraZeneca. Common stock ownership of Bellicum Pharmaceuticals, Mazor Robotics, Amarin, and Transenetrix.

This article is the sole work of the authors and no writing assistance was received from commercial support.

REFERENCES

1. Goldinger SM, Murer C, Stieger P, et al. Targeted therapy in melanoma-the role of BRAF, RAS and KIT mutations. EJC Suppl 2013;11(2):92–6.
2. Nikolaou VA, Stratigos AJ, Flaherty KT, et al. Melanoma: new insights and new therapies. J Invest Dermatol 2012;132(3 Pt 2):854–63.
3. Sullivan RJ, Flaherty KT. Resistance to BRAF-targeted therapy in melanoma. Eur J Cancer 2013;49(6):1297–304.
4. Shtivelman E, Davies MQ, Hwu P, et al. Pathways and therapeutic targets in melanoma. Oncotarget 2014;5(7):1701–52.
5. Davies H, Bignell GR, Cox C, et al. Mutations of the BRAF gene in human cancer. Nature 2002;417(6892):949–54.
6. Tsao H, Chin L, Garraway LA, et al. Melanoma: from mutations to medicine. Genes Dev 2012;26(11):1131–55.
7. Cancer Genome Atlas Network. Genomic classification of cutaneous melanoma. Cell 2015;161(7):1681–96.
8. Munoz-Couselo E, Adelantado EZ, Ortiz C, et al. NRAS-mutant melanoma: current challenges and future prospect. Onco Targets Ther 2017;10:3941–7.
9. Dankort D, Curley DP, Cartlidge RA, et al. Braf(V600E) cooperates with Pten loss to induce metastatic melanoma. Nat Genet 2009;41(5):544–52.
10. Tsao H, Mihm MC Jr, Sheehan C. PTEN expression in normal skin, acquired melanocytic nevi, and cutaneous melanoma. J Am Acad Dermatol 2003;49(5):865–72.
11. Zhou XP, Gimm O, Hampel H, et al. Epigenetic PTEN silencing in malignant melanomas without PTEN mutation. Am J Pathol 2000;157(4):1123–8.

12. Stahl JM, Sharma A, Cheung M, et al. Deregulated Akt3 activity promotes development of malignant melanoma. Cancer Res 2004;64(19):7002–10.
13. Klein A, Sagi-Assif O, Meshel T, et al. CCR4 is a determinant of melanoma brain metastasis. Oncotarget 2017;8(19):31079–91.
14. Chapman PB, Hauschild A, Robert C, et al. Improved survival with vemurafenib in melanoma with BRAF V600E mutation. N Engl J Med 2011;364(26):2507–16.
15. Chapman PB, Robert C, Larkin J, et al. Vemurafenib in patients with BRAFV600 mutation-positive metastatic melanoma: final overall survival results of the randomized BRIM-3 study. Ann Oncol 2017;28(10):2581–7.
16. McArthur GA, Chapman PB, Robert C, et al. Safety and efficacy of vemurafenib in BRAF(V600E) and BRAF(V600K) mutation-positive melanoma (BRIM-3): extended follow-up of a phase 3, randomised, open-label study. Lancet Oncol 2014;15(3):323–32.
17. Hauschild A, Grob JJ, Demidov LV, et al. Dabrafenib in BRAF-mutated metastatic melanoma: a multicentre, open-label, phase 3 randomised controlled trial. Lancet 2012;380(9839):358–65.
18. Broman KK, Dossett LA, Sun J, et al. Update on BRAF and MEK inhibition for treatment of melanoma in metastatic, unresectable, and adjuvant settings. Expert Opin Drug Saf 2019;18(5):381–92.
19. Long GV, Flaherty KT, Stroyakovskiy D, et al. Dabrafenib plus trametinib versus dabrafenib monotherapy in patients with metastatic BRAF V600E/K-mutant melanoma: long-term survival and safety analysis of a phase 3 study. Ann Oncol 2017;28(7):1631–9.
20. Robert C, Karaszewska B, Schachter J, et al. Improved overall survival in melanoma with combined dabrafenib and trametinib. N Engl J Med 2015;372(1):30–9.
21. Ascierto PA, McArthur GA, Dreno B, et al. Cobimetinib combined with vemurafenib in advanced BRAF(V600)-mutant melanoma (coBRIM): updated efficacy results from a randomised, double-blind, phase 3 trial. Lancet Oncol 2016;17(9):1248–60.
22. Dummer R, Ascierto PA, Gogas HJ, et al. Encorafenib plus binimetinib versus vemurafenib or encorafenib in patients with BRAF-mutant melanoma (COLUMBUS): a multicentre, open-label, randomised phase 3 trial. Lancet Oncol 2018;19(5):603–15.
23. Long GV, Stroyakovskiy D, Gogas H, et al. Combined BRAF and MEK inhibition versus BRAF inhibition alone in melanoma. N Engl J Med 2014;371(20):1877–88.
24. Long GV, Stroyakovskiy D, Gogas H, et al. Dabrafenib and trametinib versus dabrafenib and placebo for Val600 BRAF-mutant melanoma: a multicentre, double-blind, phase 3 randomised controlled trial. Lancet 2015;386(9992):444–51.
25. Robert C, Grob JJ, Stroyakovskiy D, et al. Five-year outcomes with dabrafenib plus trametinib in metastatic melanoma. N Engl J Med 2019;381(7):626–36.
26. Larkin J, Ascierto PA, Dreno B, et al. Combined vemurafenib and cobimetinib in BRAF-mutated melanoma. N Engl J Med 2014;371(20):1867–76.
27. Dummer R, Ascierto PA, Gogas HJ, et al. Overall survival in patients with BRAF-mutant melanoma receiving encorafenib plus binimetinib versus vemurafenib or encorafenib (COLUMBUS): a multicentre, open-label, phase 3 trial. Lancet Oncol 2018;19(10):1315–27.
28. Coit DG, Thompson JA, Albertini MR, et al. Cutaneous Melanoma, Version 2.2019, NCCN Clinical Practice Guidelines in Oncology. J Natl Compr Canc Netw 2019;17(4):367–402.
29. Faries MB, Thompson JF, Cochran AJ, et al. Completion dissection or observation for sentinel-node metastasis in melanoma. N Engl J Med 2017;376(23):2211–22.

30. Long GV, Hauschild A, Santinami M, et al. Adjuvant dabrafenib plus trametinib in stage III BRAF-mutated melanoma. N Engl J Med 2017;377(19):1813–23.
31. Hauschild A, Dummer R, Schadendorf D, et al. Longer follow-up confirms relapse-free survival benefit with adjuvant dabrafenib plus trametinib in patients with resected BRAF V600-mutant stage III melanoma. J Clin Oncol 2018;JCO1801219. https://doi.org/10.1200/JCO.18.01219.
32. Weber J, Mandala M, Del Vecchio M, et al. Adjuvant nivolumab versus ipilimumab in resected stage III or IV melanoma. N Engl J Med 2017;377(19):1824–35.
33. Eggermont AMM, Blank CU, Mandala M, et al. Adjuvant pembrolizumab versus placebo in resected stage III melanoma. N Engl J Med 2018;378(19):1789–801.
34. Amaria RN, Prieto PA, Tetzlaff MT, et al. Neoadjuvant plus adjuvant dabrafenib and trametinib versus standard of care in patients with high-risk, surgically resectable melanoma: a single-centre, open-label, randomised, phase 2 trial. Lancet Oncol 2018;19(2):181–93.
35. Long GV, Saw RPM, Lo S, et al. Neoadjuvant dabrafenib combined with trametinib for resectable, stage IIIB-C, BRAF(V600) mutation-positive melanoma (NeoCombi): a single-arm, open-label, single-centre, phase 2 trial. Lancet Oncol 2019;20(7):961–71.
36. Eroglu Z, Eatrides J, Naqvi SMH, et al. Neoadjuvant BRAF-targeted therapy in regionally advanced and oligometastatic melanoma. Pigment Cell Melanoma Res 2019. https://doi.org/10.1111/pcmr.12813.
37. Amaria RN, Menzies AM, Burton EM, et al. Neoadjuvant systemic therapy in melanoma: recommendations of the International Neoadjuvant Melanoma Consortium. Lancet Oncol 2019;20(7):e378–89.
38. Tawbi HA, Boutros C, Kok D, et al. New era in the management of melanoma brain metastases. Am Soc Clin Oncol Educ Book 2018;38:741–50.
39. Frinton E, Tong D, Tan J, et al. Metastatic melanoma: prognostic factors and survival in patients with brain metastases. J Neurooncol 2017;135(3):507–12.
40. Sloot S, Chen YA, Zhao X, et al. Improved survival of patients with melanoma brain metastases in the era of targeted BRAF and immune checkpoint therapies. Cancer 2018;124(2):297–305.
41. Izraely S, Klein A, Sagi-Assif O, et al. Chemokine-chemokine receptor axes in melanoma brain metastasis. Immunol Lett 2010;130(1–2):107–14.
42. Fazakas C, Wilhelm I, Nagyoszi P, et al. Transmigration of melanoma cells through the blood-brain barrier: role of endothelial tight junctions and melanoma-released serine proteases. PLoS One 2011;6(6):e20758.
43. Klein A, Schwartz H, Sagi-Assif O, et al. Astrocytes facilitate melanoma brain metastasis via secretion of IL-23. J Pathol 2015;236(1):116–27.
44. Berghoff AS, Rajky O, Winkler F, et al. Invasion patterns in brain metastases of solid cancers. Neuro Oncol 2013;15(12):1664–72.
45. Xie TX, Huang FJ, Aldape KD, et al. Activation of stat3 in human melanoma promotes brain metastasis. Cancer Res 2006;66(6):3188–96.
46. Adler NR, Wolfe R, Kelly JW, et al. Tumour mutation status and sites of metastasis in patients with cutaneous melanoma. Br J Cancer 2017;117(7):1026–35.
47. Harding JJ, Catalanotti F, Munhoz RR, et al. A retrospective evaluation of vemurafenib as treatment for BRAF-mutant melanoma brain metastases. Oncologist 2015;20(7):789–97.
48. Villanueva J, Vultur A, Lee JT, et al. Acquired resistance to BRAF inhibitors mediated by a RAF kinase switch in melanoma can be overcome by cotargeting MEK and IGF-1R/PI3K. Cancer Cell 2010;18(6):683–95.

49. Davies MA, Saiag P, Robert C, et al. Dabrafenib plus trametinib in patients with BRAF(V600)-mutant melanoma brain metastases (COMBI-MB): a multicentre, multicohort, open-label, phase 2 trial. Lancet Oncol 2017;18(7):863–73.

50. Puzanov I, Amaravadi RK, McArthur GA, et al. Long-term outcome in BRAF(V600E) melanoma patients treated with vemurafenib: patterns of disease progression and clinical management of limited progression. Eur J Cancer 2015;51(11):1435–43.

51. Long GV, Trefzer U, Davies MA, et al. Dabrafenib in patients with Val600Glu or Val600Lys BRAF-mutant melanoma metastatic to the brain (BREAK-MB): a multicentre, open-label, phase 2 trial. Lancet Oncol 2012;13(11):1087–95.

52. McArthur GA, Maio M, Arance A, et al. Vemurafenib in metastatic melanoma patients with brain metastases: an open-label, single-arm, phase 2, multicentre study. Ann Oncol 2017;28(3):634–41.

53. Ascierto PA, Schadendorf D, Berking C, et al. MEK162 for patients with advanced melanoma harbouring NRAS or Val600 BRAF mutations: a non-randomised, open-label phase 2 study. Lancet Oncol 2013;14(3):249–56.

54. Dummer R, Schadendorf D, Ascierto PA, et al. Binimetinib versus dacarbazine in patients with advanced NRAS-mutant melanoma (NEMO): a multicentre, open-label, randomised, phase 3 trial. Lancet Oncol 2017;18(4):435–45.

55. Curtin JA, Busam K, Pinkel D, et al. Somatic activation of KIT in distinct subtypes of melanoma. J Clin Oncol 2006;24(26):4340–6.

56. Isozaki K, Terris B, Belghiti J, et al. Germline-activating mutation in the kinase domain of KIT gene in familial gastrointestinal stromal tumors. Am J Pathol 2000;157(5):1581–5.

57. Yarden Y, Kuang WJ, Yang-Feng T, et al. Human proto-oncogene c-kit: a new cell surface receptor tyrosine kinase for an unidentified ligand. EMBO J 1987;6(11):3341–51.

58. Patrick RJ, Fenske NA, Messina JL. Primary mucosal melanoma. J Am Acad Dermatol 2007;56(5):828–34.

59. Hodi FS, Friedlander P, Corless CL, et al. Major response to imatinib mesylate in KIT-mutated melanoma. J Clin Oncol 2008;26(12):2046–51.

60. Antonescu CR, Busam KJ, Francone TD, et al. L576P KIT mutation in anal melanomas correlates with KIT protein expression and is sensitive to specific kinase inhibition. Int J Cancer 2007;121(2):257–64.

61. Abbaspour Babaei M, Kamalidehghan B, Saleem M, et al. Receptor tyrosine kinase (c-Kit) inhibitors: a potential therapeutic target in cancer cells. Drug Des Devel Ther 2016;10:2443–59.

62. Woodman SE, Trent JC, Stemke-Hale K, et al. Activity of dasatinib against L576P KIT mutant melanoma: molecular, cellular, and clinical correlates. Mol Cancer Ther 2009;8(8):2079–85.

63. Wyman K, Atkins MB, Prieto V, et al. Multicenter phase II trial of high-dose imatinib mesylate in metastatic melanoma: significant toxicity with no clinical efficacy. Cancer 2006;106(9):2005–11.

64. Kim KB, Eton O, Davis DW, et al. Phase II trial of imatinib mesylate in patients with metastatic melanoma. Br J Cancer 2008;99(5):734–40.

65. Ugurel S, Hildenbrand R, Zimpfer A, et al. Lack of clinical efficacy of imatinib in metastatic melanoma. Br J Cancer 2005;92(8):1398–405.

66. Carvajal RD, Antonescu CR, Wolchok JD, et al. KIT as a therapeutic target in metastatic melanoma. JAMA 2011;305(22):2327–34.

67. Guo J, Si L, Kong Y, et al. Phase II, open-label, single-arm trial of imatinib mesy-late in patients with metastatic melanoma harboring c-Kit mutation or amplifica-tion. J Clin Oncol 2011;29(21):2904–9.
68. Hodi FS, Corless CL, Giobbie-Hurder A, et al. Imatinib for melanomas harboring mutationally activated or amplified KIT arising on mucosal, acral, and chronically sun-damaged skin. J Clin Oncol 2013;31(26):3182–90.
69. Guo J, Carvajal RD, Dummer R, et al. Efficacy and safety of nilotinib in patients with KIT-mutated metastatic or inoperable melanoma: final results from the global, single-arm, phase II TEAM trial. Ann Oncol 2017;28(6):1380–7.
70. Grothey A, Van Cutsem E, Sobrero A, et al. Regorafenib monotherapy for previ-ously treated metastatic colorectal cancer (CORRECT): an international, multi-centre, randomised, placebo-controlled, phase 3 trial. Lancet 2013;381(9863): 303–12.
71. Demetri GD, Reichardt P, Kang YK, et al. Efficacy and safety of regorafenib for advanced gastrointestinal stromal tumours after failure of imatinib and sunitinib (GRID): an international, multicentre, randomised, placebo-controlled, phase 3 trial. Lancet 2013;381(9863):295–302.
72. Bruix J, Qin S, Merle P, et al. Regorafenib for patients with hepatocellular carci-noma who progressed on sorafenib treatment (RESORCE): a randomised, double-blind, placebo-controlled, phase 3 trial. Lancet 2017;389(10064):56–66.

Role of Radiation in the Era of Effective Systemic Therapy for Melanoma

A. Gabriella Wernicke, MD, MSc[a], Simran Polce, BS[b],
Bhupesh Parashar, MD[c],*

KEYWORDS

- Radiation • Systemic therapy • Melanoma • Cancer • Immunotherapy

KEY POINTS

- Radiation therapy has a role in high risk resected cutaneous melanoma.
- RT has a synergistic effect with immunotherapy.
- RT with immunotherapy may induce an abscopal response.

CONVENTIONAL ROLE OF RADIATION THERAPY IN CUTANEOUS MELANOMA

As per National Comprehensive Cancer Network (NCCN) 2019, the current role of radiation therapy (RT) in cutaneous melanoma is as primary therapy in inoperable patients, either because of patient comorbidities or prohibitive surgical extent. RT is indicated as an adjuvant therapy for desmoplastic melanoma in which there is a higher risk of local regional recurrence (LRR). Risk of LRR after surgical resection is enhanced in the presence of the following pathologic features: multiple involved nodes, extracapsular extension, and positive margins. Although adjuvant RT has been shown to improve LRR, it has not been shown to improve overall survival (OS). In addition to the indications mentioned earlier, RT is indicated in recurrent and metastatic settings for palliation or enhanced local control.

THE DOSE OF RADIATION THERAPY

The following RT doses are recommended for primary and adjuvant melanoma: 64 to 70 Gy in 6 to 7 weeks in 32 to 35 fractions, 50 to 57.5 Gy in 20 to 23 fractions over 4 to 5 weeks, 35 Gy in 5 fractions over 1 week for tumors less than 3 cm^2, and 32 Gy in 4

[a] Weill Cornell Medical College, New York, NY 10021, USA; [b] Stony Brook Medical College, Stony Brook, NY 11794, USA; [c] Head and Neck Cancer Service, Zucker School of Medicine at Hofstra, Northwell Health, Center for Advanced Medicine (CFAM), 450 Lakeville Road, Suite A, Lake Success, NY 11042, USA
* Corresponding author.
E-mail address: bparashar@northwell.edu

Surg Clin N Am 100 (2020) 189–199
https://doi.org/10.1016/j.suc.2019.09.010
0039-6109/20/© 2019 Elsevier Inc. All rights reserved.

fractions over 1 week. RT doses for adjuvant RT are as follows: 60 to 66 Gy in 2 Gy/fraction over 6 to 7 weeks, 48 Gy in 20 fractions over 4 weeks, 30 Gy in 5 fractions over 2 weeks (www.NCCN.org, 2019).

EVIDENCE FOR THE ROLE OF RADIATION THERAPY IN MALIGNANT MELANOMA

There is some clinical evidence that large fractional doses of RT are better for local control of melanoma versus smaller fraction size. However, 2 randomized trials showed no difference in control rates with larger fraction size compared with a smaller fraction size.

A Dutch randomized study of 35 tumors in 14 patients treated with either 9 Gy in 3 fractions (27 Gy) or 5 Gy in 8 fractions (40 Gy). The overall response rate was 97%. Complete response was seen in 24 out of 35 (69%) and partial response was seen in 10 out of 35 (28.5%) tumors. Both regimens had acceptable and similar magnitudes of RT changes to structures. There was no difference in outcomes between the 2 groups.[1]

RTOG (Radiation Therapy Oncology Group) 83-05 was a randomized trial comparing 32 Gy in 4 fractions (hypofractionation) versus 50 Gy in 20 fractions (standard) in metastatic melanoma. There were 62 patients in the hypofractionation arm and 64 patients in standard arm. Complete response rate (24.2% and 23.4% respectively) and partial response (35.5% and 34.4% respectively) were similar in the 2 arms.[2]

To evaluate the role of adjuvant RT in patients with cutaneous melanoma, a prospective trial conducted in Australia accrued 174 patients with International Union Against Cancer (IUAC) stage I to III melanoma. The most common site was head and neck (HN). Indications of RT to the primary site included positive margins or other adverse pathologic features, such as desmoplastic histology, perineural invasion (PNI), satellitosis, and early or multiple recurrences. Nodal RT was delivered based on the following pathologic features: positive margins, extracapsular extension, PNI, lymphovascular invasion, multiple lymph nodes, and large nodes. RT dose was 30 to 36 Gy in 5 to 7 fractions over 2.5 weeks. Eleven percent of patients developed recurrence at a median of 6 months. Median disease-free survival was 25 months, and 5-year OS was 41%. The median time to develop distant metastasis was 19 months. Local recurrence (LR) if RT was delivered in less than 18 days was 4% versus 15% for RT delivered in after 18 days. Postoperative RT on a hypofractionated schedule greatly reduced LR in high-risk patients.[3]

In a retrospective study on superficial spreading or nodular melanoma of HN in 37 patients, patients received postoperative RT. Local control was 25% with RT fraction size less than 4 Gy and 71% with fractions greater than 7 Gy.[4]

Influence of Histology Subtype

Desmoplastic melanomas have a high LR rate (~50%), a high degree of neurotropism, and commonly an HN location. The role of RT has been evaluated in desmoplastic melanomas. In a retrospective review of 24 patients with desmoplastic melanoma, in which 22 lesions were located in HN, patients underwent surgical resection followed by postoperative RT. At 3 years, in-field relapse-free survival was 91%, and OS was 83%. Median thickness was 5.2 mm, and margins were less than 1 cm in 71% of patients.[5]

One hundred and twenty-eight patients with desmoplastic neurotropic melanoma were treated in the Sydney melanoma unit and Sydney cancer center between 1996 and 2007. All patients underwent excision, although 27 received adjuvant RT.

The median age at diagnosis was 65.5 years. HN melanomas were most common (51%), median Breslow thickness 4 mm, and 99% of patients had Clark level IV or V primary tumors. Patients who received adjuvant RT had thicker tumors ($P = .003$), deeper Clark level of invasion ($P<.001$), and narrower excision margins ($P<.001$). There were 8 LRs, including 6 (6%) in the surgery-only group and 2 (7%) in the adjuvant RT group. A positive margin ($P<.001$) and HN location ($P = .03$) were significant predictors of LR. The low recurrence rates after the addition of RT were lower than historical controls.[6] Compromised surgical margins were strongly correlated with higher LR rates, and the addition of RT in these cases may improve local control.

In a series of patients with desmoplastic melanoma, collected as a part of a prospectively collected database, 65 patients were evaluated. Wide excision (>2 cm in 63%, >1 cm in 100%) was performed, and no RT was given. Mean thickness was 4.2 mm, and 38% had thickness greater than 4 mm. Neurotropism was seen in 32%. With a mean follow-up of 3.7 years, and minimum 2 years, LR was seen in 4% (1 neurotropic, 1 without). Nodal metastasis was seen in 4% in tumors with no neurotropism versus 28% in patients with neurotropism ($P<.05$). LR was considerably less than historically reported, which indicates that wide excision with careful attention to margins does not require additional RT.[7]

In another retrospective analysis of desmoplastic malignant melanoma, of the 44 patients evaluated, 14 patients received postoperative RT, and 1 patient received preoperative RT. RT doses ranged from 44 to 66 Gy. Sixty-eight percent of patients had desmoplastic malignant melanoma of the HN. Forty-eight percent of patients experienced LR with a mean time of 12 months to recurrence. Clark level, primary site, and neurotropism did not predict LR; however, Clark level predicted distant metastasis. No viable tumor was found in the surgical specimen of the patient who received preoperative RT. None of 15 patients who received adjuvant irradiation had any additional recurrences (mean follow-up, 64.7 months). By contrast, 4 out of 7 patients with history of recurrence who did not receive RT had local relapse ($P = .005$). The incidence of distant metastasis did not reach statistical significance between the RT and no-RT groups. Adjuvant RT dramatically reduced LR rates, indicating that it should be added to desmoplastic malignant melanoma treatment regimens.[8]

Definitive RT may be considered for unresectable lentigo maligna (LM) or lentigo maligna melanoma (LMM). It is an excellent option for elderly patients when surgical resection is not an option. In a retrospective analysis of 150 patients with LM and LMM, RT was delivered to doses of 100 to 120 Gy at 10 to 12 Gy/fraction delivered at 3-day to 4-day intervals, and 42 to 54 Gy at 7 to 9 Gy/fraction. Recurrence rates were around 7%, and the mean time to recurrence was 45.6 months. Based on the recurrence patterns and rates in these patients, a large safety margin of 10 mm around the visible lesion is recommended.[9]

In another retrospective study in 64 patients with LM and LMM, RT dose of 100 Gy in 10 fractions over 2 weeks resulted in 0% LR in LM and 9% in LMM. All recurrences were surgically salvaged. Only a limited number of patients were identified as having hyperpigmentation and hypopigmentation around the irradiated skin. Overall clinical results were comparable with those of surgical resection.[10]

RADIATION THERAPY WITH IMMUNOTHERAPY

The 2018 Nobel Prize for physiology and medicine was given to Dr James Allison and Dr Tasuku Honjo for their seminal work on checkpoint blockade, which has significant implications in cancer pathogenesis and progression. Immune checkpoint blockage removes inhibitory signals of T-cell activation, which helps mount an effective anti-tumor response.

Regarding tumor immunology, T-cell activation is mediated by regulatory mechanisms/checkpoint signals. These regulatory mechanisms maintain the delicate balance between normal T-cell function and preventing autoimmunity. Immunologic tolerance is achieved through a central process or a peripheral process.[11] Central tolerance is achieved through clonal deletion of self-reactive clones during negative selection in the thymus, and peripheral tolerance is achieved through various other mechanisms, including T-regulatory cells (Tregs), T-cell anergy, cell-extrinsic tolerogenic signals, and peripheral clonal deletion. There is a strong selective pressure during tumor progression leading to immune tumor editing. Also, cancer development involves immune equilibrium and immune escape. The mechanism of immune escape involves upregulation of immune-suppressive ligands and cytokines as well as myeloid-derived suppressor cells. This immune-suppressive environment causes poor antigen presentation.

Radiation may reverse that and make tumor antigens more "visible" to innate and adaptive immune mechanisms.[12] RT may act through downregulation of CD47 (an antiphagocytosis signal) and release of HMBG1 (high mobility box group1).[13,14] RT also upregulates the expression of MHC-1 (major histocompatibility complex 1) on tumor cells.[15] This systemic effect may induce abscopal response to distant tumors (**Fig. 1**).

In addition, by increasing antigen presentation, RT may enhance response to CAR (chimeric antigen receptor) T-cell therapy.[16] Also, RT may improve mutation burden, increasing neoantigen levels and thereby increasing immune surveillance.[17] RT induces innate and adaptive immune response through the STING (stimulator of interferon genes) pathway. The STING pathway is important for RT-induced interferon-1 immunity.[18] Regarding the impact of RT on tumor microenvironment, RT induces transforming growth factor-beta, which promotes the suppression of cluster of differentiation (CD) 8 and CD4 T cells as well as promoting Tregs and inhibiting natural killer cells.[19,20]

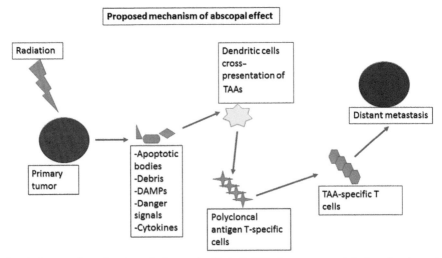

Fig. 1. Proposed mechanism of abscopal effect. DAMP, damage-associated molecular patterns; TAA, tumor-associated antigens.

PRECLINICAL AND CLINICAL EVIDENCE OF RADIATION THERAPY /IMMUNOTHERAPY SYNERGY

In a study in nude mice, 2C T-cell receptor transgenic mice were included in the study. Melanoma cell line B16 was seen to regress with ablative RT (20 Gy for 1 fraction) versus no regression in immunodeficient nude mice. This experiment provided evidence that tumor regression caused by radiation treatment is mediated by T cells. The study also showed that ablative RT induces a cytotoxic T-lymphocyte response, possibly reversing T-cell unresponsiveness, which accounts for the reduction of established tumors.[21]

In metastatic melanoma that has progressed on chemotherapy, a landmark trial published in *The New England Journal of Medicine* in 2010 showed survival benefit using ipilimumab (anti–cytotoxic T-lymphocyte-associated protein 4 [CTLA4] antibody) compared with the standard at the time, gp100 (glycoprotein 100) peptide vaccine. Patients were randomly assigned, in a 3:1:1 ratio, to receive ipilimumab plus gp100 (403 patients), ipilimumab alone (137), or gp100 alone (136). Ipilimumab was given at 3 mg/kg every 3 weeks for up to 4 treatments. Median survival was 10 months with ipilimumab versus 6.4 months with gp100. There was no detectable difference in the survival of either ipilimumab group. Grade 3/4 adverse effects happened in 10% to 15% of patients with ipilimumab and 3% with gp100. Of the 14 study drug-related deaths, 7 were associated with immune-related adverse events.[22]

In primary untreated metastatic melanoma, a 2011 article showed a survival benefit in a phase 3 study of ipilimumab (10 mg/kg) plus dacarbazine versus dacarbazine alone. Adding ipilimumab improved median survival by close to 2 months. Five-hundred and two patients were enrolled in the trial. One-year survival in the ipilimumab group was 47% versus 36% in the nonipilimumab group. Rates of complete response/partial response were 15% in the ipilimumab versus 10% in the nonipilimumab group. Grade 3/4 effects were 56% in ipilimumab plus dacarbazine group versus 27% in the dacarbazine group. There were no drug-related deaths or gastrointestinal perforations in the ipilimumab-dacarbazine group.[23]

In a 2012 phase 1 study from Oregon, 12 patients with metastatic melanoma and renal cell carcinoma received stereotactic body radiation therapy with 1, 2, or 3 RT fractions, before starting interleukin-2 (IL-2). The overall response rate was 66.6%, which was much higher than the historical response rate with IL-2 alone (20%). The investigators suggested that because the response rate of the combination was significantly higher than expected, this should be further studied. There was a significantly greater frequency of proliferating CD4+ T cells, and this could be used a predictor of response.[24]

In a study published in 2015, 418 patients with untreated metastatic malignant melanoma without BRAF (member of RAS kinase family) mutation were randomized to receive nivolumab (3 mg/kg, every 2 weeks) and dacarbazine-matched placebo every 3 weeks, or dacarbazine (1000 mg/m^2 every 3 weeks) and nivolumab-matched placebo every 2 weeks. Anti-BRAF and anti-MEK targeted agents are used for 40% of patients with these mutations. In patients without BRAF mutation, dacarbazine is the standard. At 1 year, the OS was 72.9% in the nivolumab group, compared with 42.1% in the dacarbazine group. The median progression-free survival (PFS) was 5.1 months in the nivolumab group versus 2.2 months in the dacarbazine group. The objective response rate (ORR) was 40.0% in the nivolumab group versus 13.9% in the dacarbazine group. The survival benefit with nivolumab versus dacarbazine was observed across prespecified subgroups, including subgroups defined programmed death-ligand 1 (PD-L1) status.

Grade 3 or 4 adverse events occurred in 11.7% of the patients treated with nivolumab and 17.6% of those treated with dacarbazine. There were significant improvements within OS and PFS in the nivolumab group.[25]

In a phase I study in 22 patients with malignant melanoma, a single index lesion was irradiated with 8 Gy for 2 or 3 fractions or 6 Gy for 2 or 3 fractions, followed by ipilimumab every 3 weeks. ORR was 18%. These effects were reproduced in a mouse model. In the mouse experiment, combination treatment with ipilimumab, programmed cell death protein 1 (PD1) inhibitor, and RT showed improved survival compared with ipilimumab alone.[26]

In a clinical trial in metastatic melanoma, the primary objective was to assess the safety and efficacy of combining ipilimumab with RT in patients with stage IV melanoma. Twenty-two patients with stage IV melanoma were treated with palliative RT and ipilimumab for 4 cycles. RT to 1 to 2 disease sites was initiated within 5 days after starting ipilimumab. Tumor imaging studies were obtained at baseline, 2 to 4 weeks following cycle 4 of ipilimumab, and every 3 months until progression. RT doses were variable, and 3 patients with CR had RT fractions of more than 4 Gy. ORR of ipilimumab plus RT was 27%. The study suggests that there is still a patient subset that can benefit from combined RT immunotherapy treatment, including PD1 inhibitors.[27]

In a European study in 127 consecutively treated patients with malignant melanoma in 4 centers in Germany and Switzerland, patients received either ipilimumab (82) or ipilimumab plus a local therapy (45). RT dosing was variable. Median OS in the ipilimumab plus RT group versus ipilimumab-alone groups was 93 weeks and 42 weeks, respectively ($P = .003$). There was no increase in adverse immune-related events in the combined therapy group versus the ipilimumab-only group.[28]

In a recently published study from Yale, patients with metastatic melanoma were treated with CTLA4, PD-1, or PD-L1 antibodies and local therapy to areas of disease progression in 1 to 3 sites. Four-hundred and twenty-eight patients received treatment with immune checkpoint inhibitors (ICIs) from 2007 to 2018. Seventy-seven had complete responses, whereas 69 died within 6 months of starting ICI; of the remaining 282 patients, 52 (18%) were treated with local therapy. Local therapy was associated with 3-year PFS of 31% and 5-year disease specific survival of 60%. Stratified by patterns of failure, patients with progression in established tumors had 3-year PFS of 70%, whereas those with new metastases had 3-year PFS of 6% ($P = .001$). Five-year disease specific survival after local therapy was 93% versus 31%, respectively ($P = .046$). The investigators concluded that "This experience suggests there may be an increased role for local therapy in patients being treated with immunotherapy."[29]

In a National Cancer Database (NCDB) study evaluating the role of local RT in melanoma in patients that have received ICI, multivariable Cox regression analysis was used to evaluate factors associated with OS. Subset analyses compared patients receiving RT to bone metastases versus soft tissue metastases. Of 1675 patients identified, 1387 received ICI alone, and 288 received ICI plus RT. The median OS was 15.4 versus 19.4 months in the ICI plus RT and ICI-alone groups, respectively ($P = .02$). On multivariable analysis, RT was not associated with worse OS. The poor OS in the RT group was confined to the patients who received RT to bone metastases (not soft tissue metastases). In patients irradiated to soft tissue, in whom RT was at least 30 days before ICI, OS was improved versus RT within 30 days or 30 days after ICI, median OS was 26.1 months versus 16.0 months ($P = .009$) versus 15.4 months ($P = .004$), respectively. The timing and site of RT are important variables in the effectiveness of RT plus immunotherapy regimens.[30]

In a melanoma brain metastasis study from France, clinical data from 262 patients with melanoma brain metastasis were collected via MelBase, a French multicentric

Table 1
Recent studies combining RT with ICI in patients with metastatic melanoma

Author, Year	Site of Melanoma	Design	Results	Comments
Minniti et al,[32] 2019	Melanoma brain metastasis	SRS + ipi vs SRS + nivo, 80 pts, 45 SRS + ipi and 35 SRS + nivo	Median f/u 15 mo PFS, 6 mo; 69% vs 12 mo; 42% with nivo vs 48% and 17% with ipi	Multifraction SRS (9 Gy × 3) better than single-fraction SRS. A subset developed radionecrosis
Galli et al,[33] 2019	Melanoma brain metastasis	Retrospective; 36 patients with ICI and 25 controls with no ICI treated between 2012 and 2016. 23 of 36 received anti-CTLA4 and 13 of 36 received anti-PD1	Median OS from the beginning of RT was 7 mo after first-line treatment and 4 mo in second-line treatment	No abscopal effect was seen. No synergism seen between ICI and RT
Stera et al,[34] 2019	Melanoma brain metastasis	Retrospective; 48 patients included in the study, 250 lesions. Patients received SRS plus ICI or SRS plus targeted treatment	Median 8.3-mo follow-up, the addition of ICI or systemic treatment directly before or concomitant resulted in 6-mo and 1-y survival of 75% and 50%	ICI or systemic treatment directly before or concomitant to SRS were both associated with improved OS
Rauschenberg et al,[35] 2019	Melanoma brain metastasis	Retrospective; 208 pts treated with SRS or WBRT with either ICI or TT	One-year OS 69%, 65%, 33%, and 18% ($P<0.01$) for SRS with ICI, SRS with TT, WBRT with ICI, and WBRT with TT, respectively	SRS plus ICI achieved the highest OS. A BRAF mutation is the favorable prognostic factor for OS
Amaral et al,[36] 2019	Melanoma brain metastasis	Retrospective; 163 pts, prognostic factors of OS analyzed	ICI, the median OS 13 mo, 7 mo for patients receiving TT or CT. Median OS with surgery/SRS in combination with ICI, TT, and CT was 25, 14, and 11 mo, respectively	ICI improved OS when combined with SRS

(continued on next page)

Table 1
(continued)

Author, Year	Site of Melanoma	Design	Results	Comments
Murphy et al,[37] 2019	Melanoma brain metastasis	Retrospective; 26 pts received ICI and SRS; 90 lesions treated using pembro, nivo, and ipi, sequentially, or concurrently with SRS	Median f/u 18.9 mo. Median OS was 26.1 mo. Three local failures, no significant difference between the 2 groups	Patients had a significantly longer period of intracranial PFS than those treated with nonconcurrent therapy, 19 mo vs 3.4 mo ($P<.0001$)
Schmidberger et al,[38] 2018	Melanoma brain metastasis	Retrospective; 41 pts, 15 were treated with SRS, 7 with SRS and WBRT, 19 with WBRT alone	Patients treated with ICI after RT had a censored median survival of 11 mo, compared with 3 mo for the patients who received ICI before radiotherapy. Patients who received ICI before RT had similar survival to historical controls, who had not received ICI	Long-term survivors observed after radiotherapy for brain metastases followed by ICI

Abbreviations: CT, chemotherapy; f/u, follow-up; ipi, ipilimumab; nivo, nivolumab; pembro, pembrolizumab; pts, patients; SRS, stereotactic radiosurgery; TT, targeted therapy; WBRT, whole-brain RT.

biobank prospectively enrolling unresectable stage III or IV melanoma. Two groups, patients receiving combined RT (cRT group) or not receiving cRT (no-cRT group) were identified. Ninety-three (35%) received cRT. With a median follow-up of 6.9 months, the median OS was 16.8 months and 6.9 months in the cRT and no-cRT groups, respectively. After propensity matching, cRT was associated with longer OS (hazard ratio, 0.6; 95% confidence interval, 0.4–0.8; P = .007). Median OS was 15.3 months and 6.2 months in the cRT and no-cRT groups, respectively. Systemic treatment coupled with RT results in better OS. Further prospective testing is necessary to determine the exact timing required to maximize synergistic effects.[31]

Table 1 shows a set of recently completed studies combining RT with ICI in patients with metastatic melanoma.

Multiple additional studies are published that show the benefit of ICI with SRS in patients with melanoma metastasis.[39–44]

SUMMARY

As shown earlier, RT plus ICI is a promising option for patients with melanoma, primary as well as metastatic, although the optimal dose and fractionation still need to be worked out. Also, additional prospective studies are needed to study toxicity with RT and newer ICI combinations.

CONFLICTS OF INTEREST

None.

REFERENCES

1. Overgaard J, von der Maase H, Overgaard M. A randomized study comparing two high-dose per fraction radiation schedules in recurrent or metastatic malignant melanoma. Int J Radiat Oncol Biol Phys 1985;11(10):1837–9.
2. Sause WT, Cooper JS, Rush S, et al. Fraction size in external beam radiation therapy in the treatment of melanoma. Int J Radiat Oncol Biol Phys 1991;20(3):429–32.
3. Stevens G, Thompson JF, Firth I, et al. Locally advanced melanoma: results of postoperative hypofractionated radiation therapy. Cancer 2000;88(1):88–94.
4. Harwood AR, Dancuart F, Fitzpatrick PJ, et al. Radiotherapy in nonlentiginous melanoma of the head and neck. Cancer 1981;48(12):2599–605.
5. Foote MC, Burmeister B, Burmeister E, et al. Desmoplastic melanoma: the role of radiotherapy in improving local control. ANZ J Surg 2008;78(4):273–6.
6. Chen JY, Hruby G, Scolyer RA, et al. Desmoplastic neurotropic melanoma: a clinicopathologic analysis of 128 cases. Cancer 2008;113(10):2770–8.
7. Arora A, Lowe L, Su L, et al. Wide excision without radiation for desmoplastic melanoma. Cancer 2005;104(7):1462–7.
8. Vongtama R, Safa A, Gallardo D, et al. Efficacy of radiation therapy in the local control of desmoplastic malignant melanoma. Head Neck 2003;25(6):423–8.
9. Farshad A, Burg G, Panizzon R, et al. A retrospective study of 150 patients with lentigo maligna and lentigo maligna melanoma and the efficacy of radiotherapy using Grenz or soft X-rays. Br J Dermatol 2002;146(6):1042–6.
10. Schmid-Wendtner MH, Brunner B, Konz B, et al. Fractionated radiotherapy of lentigo maligna and lentigo maligna melanoma in 64 patients. J Am Acad Dermatol 2000;43(3):477–82.

11. Wei SC, Duffy CR, Allison JP. Fundamental mechanisms of immune checkpoint blockade therapy. Cancer Discov 2018;8(9):1069–86.
12. Jiang W, Chan CK, Weissman IL, et al. Immune priming of the tumor microenvironment by radiation. Trends Cancer 2016;2(11):638–45.
13. Vermeer DW, Spanos WC, Vermeer PD, et al. Radiation-induced loss of cell surface CD47 enhances immune-mediated clearance of human papillomavirus-positive cancer. Int J Cancer 2013;133(1):120–9.
14. Yoshimoto Y, Oike T, Okonogi N, et al. Carbon-ion beams induce production of an immune mediator protein, high mobility group box 1, at levels comparable with X-ray irradiation. J Radiat Res 2015;56(3):509–14.
15. Reits EA, Hodge JW, Herberts CA, et al. Radiation modulates the peptide repertoire, enhances MHC class I expression, and induces successful antitumor immunotherapy. J Exp Med 2006;203(5):1259–71.
16. Flynn JP, O'Hara MH, Gandhi SJ. Preclinical rationale for combining radiation therapy and immunotherapy beyond checkpoint inhibitors (i.e., CART). Transl Lung Cancer Res 2017;6(2):159–68.
17. Germano G, Lamba S, Rospo G, et al. Inactivation of DNA repair triggers neoantigen generation and impairs tumour growth. Nature 2017;552(7683):116–20.
18. Deng L, Liang H, Xu M, et al. STING-dependent cytosolic DNA sensing promotes radiation-induced type i interferon-dependent antitumor immunity in immunogenic tumors. Immunity 2014;41(5):843–52.
19. Klopp AH, Spaeth EL, Dembinski JL, et al. Tumor irradiation increases the recruitment of circulating mesenchymal stem cells into the tumor microenvironment. Cancer Res 2007;67(24):11687–95.
20. Wrzesinski SH, Wan YY, Flavell RA. Transforming growth factor-beta and the immune response: implications for anticancer therapy. Clin Cancer Res 2007;13(18 Pt 1):5262–70 [Review].
21. Lee Y, Auh SL, Wang Y, et al. Therapeutic effects of ablative radiation on local tumor require CD8+ T cells: changing strategies for cancer treatment. Blood 2009; 114(3):589–95.
22. Hodi FS, O'Day SJ, McDermott DF, et al. Improved survival with ipilimumab in patients with metastatic melanoma. N Engl J Med 2010;363(8):711–23 [Erratum appears in N Engl J Med. 2010;363(13):1290].
23. Robert C, Thomas L, Bondarenko I, et al. Ipilimumab plus dacarbazine for previously untreated metastatic melanoma. N Engl J Med 2011;364(26):2517–26.
24. Seung SK, Curti BD, Crittenden M, et al. Phase 1 study of stereotactic body radiotherapy and interleukin-2–tumor and immunological responses. Sci Transl Med 2012;4(137):137ra74.
25. Robert C, Long GV, Brady B, et al. Nivolumab in previously untreated melanoma without BRAF mutation. N Engl J Med 2015;372(4):320–30.
26. Twyman-Saint Victor C, Rech AJ, Maity A, et al. Radiation and dual checkpoint blockade activate non-redundant immune mechanisms in cancer. Nature 2015; 520(7547):373–7.
27. Hiniker SM, Reddy SA, Maecker HT, et al. A prospective clinical trial combining radiation therapy with systemic immunotherapy in metastatic melanoma. Int J Radiat Oncol Biol Phys 2016;96(3):578–88.
28. Theurich S, Rothschild SI, Hoffmann M, et al. Local tumor treatment in combination with systemic ipilimumab immunotherapy prolongs overall survival in patients with advanced malignant melanoma. Cancer Immunol Res 2016;4(9): 744–54.

29. Klemen ND, Wang M, Feingold PL, et al. Patterns of failure after immunotherapy with checkpoint inhibitors predict durable progression-free survival after local therapy for metastatic melanoma. J Immunother Cancer 2019;7(1):196.
30. Gabani P, Robinson CG, Ansstas G, et al. Use of extracranial radiation therapy in metastatic melanoma patients receiving immunotherapy. Radiother Oncol 2018; 127(2):310–7.
31. Tétu P, Allayous C, Oriano B, et al. Impact of radiotherapy administered simultaneously with systemic treatment in patients with melanoma brain metastases within MelBase, a French multicentric prospective cohort. Eur J Cancer 2019; 112:38–46.
32. Minniti G, Anzellini D, Reverberi C, et al. Stereotactic radiosurgery combined with nivolumab or Ipilimumab for patients with melanoma brain metastases: evaluation of brain control and toxicity. J Immunother Cancer 2019;7(1):102.
33. Galli G, Cavalieri S, Di Guardo L, et al. Combination of immunotherapy and brain radiotherapy in metastatic melanoma: a retrospective analysis. Oncol Res Treat 2019;42(4):186–94.
34. Stera S, Balermpas P, Blanck O, et al. Stereotactic radiosurgery combined with immune checkpoint inhibitors or kinase inhibitors for patients with multiple brain metastases of malignant melanoma. Melanoma Res 2019;29(2):187–95.
35. Rauschenberg R, Bruns J, Brütting J, et al. Impact of radiation, systemic therapy and treatment sequencing on survival of patients with melanoma brain metastases. Eur J Cancer 2019;110:11–20.
36. Amaral T, Tampouri I, Eigentler T, et al. Immunotherapy plus surgery/radiosurgery is associated with favorable survival in patients with melanoma brain metastasis. Immunotherapy 2019;11(4):297–309.
37. Murphy B, Walker J, Bassale S, et al. Concurrent radiosurgery and immune checkpoint inhibition: improving regional intracranial control for patients with metastatic melanoma. Am J Clin Oncol 2019;42(3):253–7.
38. Schmidberger H, Rapp M, Ebersberger A, et al. Long-term survival of patients after ipilimumab and hypofractionated brain radiotherapy for brain metastases of malignant melanoma: sequence matters. Strahlenther Onkol 2018;194(12): 1144–51.
39. Trommer-Nestler M, Marnitz S, Kocher M, et al. Robotic stereotactic radiosurgery in melanoma patients with brain metastases under simultaneous anti-PD-1 treatment. Int J Mol Sci 2018;19(9) [pii:E2653].
40. Matsunaga S, Shuto T, Yamamoto M, et al. Gamma knife radiosurgery for metastatic brain tumors from malignant melanomas: a Japanese Multi-Institutional Cooperative and Retrospective Cohort Study (JLGK1501). Stereotact Funct Neurosurg 2018;96(3):162–71.
41. Gabani P, Fischer-Valuck BW, Johanns TM, et al. Stereotactic radiosurgery and immunotherapy in melanoma brain metastases: patterns of care and treatment outcomes. Radiother Oncol 2018;128(2):266–73.
42. Diao K, Bian SX, Routman DM, et al. Stereotactic radiosurgery and ipilimumab for patients with melanoma brain metastases: clinical outcomes and toxicity. J Neurooncol 2018;139(2):421–9.
43. Rahman R, Cortes A, Niemierko A, et al. The impact of timing of immunotherapy with cranial irradiation in melanoma patients with brain metastases: intracranial progression, survival and toxicity. J Neurooncol 2018;138(2):299–306.
44. Nardin C, Mateus C, Texier M, et al. Tolerance and outcomes of stereotactic radiosurgery combined with anti-programmed cell death-1 (pembrolizumab) for melanoma brain metastases. Melanoma Res 2018;28(2):111–9.

Current Clinical Trials in the Treatment of Advanced Melanomas

Saro Sarkisian, MD, MHA[a],*, Suresh Nair, MD[a],
Rohit Sharma, MD, FACS, FRCS(Glas)[b]

KEYWORDS

- Melanoma • Advanced melanomas • Clinical trials • Immunotherapy
- Targeted therapy

KEY POINTS

- The treatment of advanced melanoma has changed significantly with the introduction of immunotherapy and targeted therapies.
- Treatment of advanced or metastatic melanoma has promising results now with significant improvement in progression-free survival and overall survival.
- Treatment can now be individualized based on the molecular characteristics of each tumor.
- The rapid progress with newer therapies makes it more exciting and challenging at the same time. It would be interesting to see the clinical applications of the latest trials to practice.

INTRODUCTION

According to the Surveillance, Epidemiology, and End Results database, cutaneous melanoma incidence has increased substantially over the past 2 decades from approximately 38,000 in 1997 to 76,000 in 2016.[1] Age older than 50 is associated with worse prognosis and incidence in men is double that in women.[1-3] Between the ages of 15 and 39, melanoma is more commonly seen in female individuals.[2] Fortunately, 85% of melanoma cases are diagnosed at an early stage, when cure can be achieved with surgery alone.

The treatment of melanoma has witnessed significant improvements during the past decade. We describe herein historical trends in the treatment of this disease, also summarizing the latest clinical trials that would be applicable in the near future.

Before the development of immunotherapy and targeted therapy, advanced melanoma historically was treated with chemotherapeutic agents, primarily dacarbazine

[a] Department of Hematology/Oncology, Lehigh Valley Cancer Institute, 1240 South Cedar Crest Boulevard, Allentown, PA 18103, USA; [b] Department of Surgery, Marshfield Medical Center, 1000 North Oak Avenue, Marshfield, WI 54449, USA
* Corresponding author.
E-mail address: SARO.SARKISIAN@LVHN.ORG

Surg Clin N Am 100 (2020) 201–208
https://doi.org/10.1016/j.suc.2019.09.014
0039-6109/20/© 2019 The Author(s). Published by Elsevier Inc. This is an open access article under the CC BY-NC-ND license (http://creativecommons.org/licenses/by-nc-nd/4.0/).
surgical.theclinics.com

and its prodrug temozolomide. Platinum agents, vinka alkaloids, and taxanes were also used although less frequently. The outcomes in the era of chemotherapy were poor and prognosis was dismal in advanced melanoma.

Interleukin (IL)-2 is a glycoprotein T-cell growth factor that is primarily produced by Th lymphocytes and it stimulates the development of cytotoxic T lymphocyte and natural killer cells. Clinical trials investigated the use of IL-2 immunotherapy in the treatment of advanced melanoma. Across these trials, overall response was noted to be low, approximately 16% with only 6% complete response (CR) and 10% partial response (PR). Although some patients would derive benefit from IL-2, its side effects and toxicity profile make this medication useful only in patients with excellent performance status, preserved organ function, and in institutions with expertise in administering and managing its side effects.

With the low response rates observed with chemotherapeutic agents and dismal prognosis in advanced melanoma, it was paramount to have a better understanding of disease biology to develop newer treatment modalities. The understanding of the mitogen-activated protein kinase (MAPK) pathway was a revolutionary step toward this aim. The identification of driver mutations in this pathway, including BRAF and NRAS, has accelerated the development of targeted therapies either as monotherapies, or in combination. These targeted therapies were associated with significant improvement in progression-free survival and overall survival. Along with targeted therapy, immunotherapy is a novel way of stimulating the immune system, specifically T-cell activation and regulation. We summarize here the pivotal trials that were practice changing in managing advanced metastatic melanoma.

IMMUNOTHERAPY

Ipilimumab (MDX-010) is a human immunoglobulin (Ig)G1 monoclonal antibody shown to inhibit CTLA-4.[4] Early-phase studies have shown its activity in advanced, refractory melanoma. Ipilimumab was evaluated in 2 phase 3 trials. The first study (MDX010–020/CA184–020), which involved 676 HLA-A*0201–positive patients with advanced melanoma, compared ipilimumab 3 mg/kg every 3 weeks for 4 doses either singly or in combination with gp100 vaccine with a gp100-only control arm.[5] Ipilimumab administration resulted in objective responses in 11% of patients and improved progression-free and overall survival compared with gp100 alone. Of note, ipilimumab monotherapy was superior to ipilimumab/gp100 combination. A follow-up study (CA184–024) compared a higher dose of ipilimumab (10 mg/kg) in combination with dacarbazine with dacarbazine monotherapy in previously untreated melanoma. This study failed to confirm the benefit of higher dose of ipilimumab.[6] Hence, ipilimumab received regulatory approval in 2011 for the treatment of advanced melanoma at the lower dose: 3 mg/kg administered every 3 weeks for 4 doses. Survival data were strikingly similar to patterns observed in prior phase 2 studies, with survival curves plateauing after 2 years at 23.5% to 28.5% of treated patients. Ipilimumab administration resulted in an unusual spectrum of toxicities, including diarrhea, rash, hepatitis, and hypophysitis (termed immune-related adverse events, or irAEs) in up to a third of patients.

Pembrolizumab and nivolumab are humanized IgG4 monoclonal antibodies that target the PD-1 receptor found on activated T cells, B cells, and myeloid cells. Nivolumab was compared with chemotherapy in a pair of phase 3 studies involving both previously untreated (CheckMate 066) and ipilimumab/BRAF inhibitor–refractory (CheckMate 037) patients.[7,8] In both studies, nivolumab produced durable responses in 32% to 34% of patients and improved survival over chemotherapy. Compared with ipilimumab, the incidence of irAEs was much lower with nivolumab. These results led to regulatory Nivolumab approval in both indications (untreated and ipilimumab refractory melanoma) in 2014.

Pembrolizumab was evaluated in a large phase 1 study (KEYNOTE-001) of 1260 patients that evaluated 3 doses (10 mg/kg every 2 weeks, 10 mg/kg every 3 weeks, and 2 mg/kg every 3 weeks) in separate melanoma and non–small-cell lung cancer substudies.[9] Both ipilimumab-naïve and ipilimumab-treated patients were enrolled in the melanoma substudy. Objective responses were seen in 38% of patients across all 3 dosing schedules and were similar in both ipilimumab-naïve and ipilimumab-treated patients. Similar to nivolumab, most responders experienced durable remissions.

Pembrolizumab was subsequently compared with ipilimumab in untreated patients (KEYNOTE-006) in which patients were randomly assigned to receive either ipilimumab or pembrolizumab at 1 of 2 doses: 10 mg/kg every 2 weeks and pembrolizumab 10 mg/kg every 3 weeks.[10] Response rates were greater with pembrolizumab than ipilimumab, with greater 1-year survival rates. Rates of treatment-related adverse events requiring discontinuation of study drug were much lower with pembrolizumab than ipilimumab. This trial proved the superiority of pembrolizumab over ipilimumab. The US Food and Drug Administration (FDA) granted pembrolizumab accelerated approval for second-line treatment of melanoma in 2014, and updated this to include a first-line indication in 2015.

Studies have confirmed that PD-1 blockade was more effective than CTLA-4 blockade. It was hypothesized that combination blockage of PD-1/CTLA-4 would have synergistic effects. CheckMate 067 was a randomized, phase 3 study that demonstrated the superiority of ipilimumab/nivolumab combination to ipilimumab monotherapy.[11] The combination arm results in more profound responses (58%) than either ipilimumab (19%) or nivolumab (44%) alone and improvement in progression-free survival. However, there was more toxicity, including diarrhea, rash, fatigue, and pruritus that led to discontinuation of the combination drugs in 30% of patients. The durable response led to this combination to be FDA approved in 2015. In an updated analysis of the same trial published by the *New England Journal of Medicine* in 2017, the combination of ipilimumab/nivolumab resulted in significantly improved overall survival.[12]

TARGETED THERAPY

Clinical observations including the different behavior pattern of lesions in chronic sun-exposed versus nonexposed areas led to further speculation of differences at the molecular level. Whole genome sequencing data, including The Cancer Genome Atlas, identified patterns of mutations in oncogenic drivers that were different in patients with and without chronic sun exposure.[13,14] A deeper understanding of the MAPK pathway led to the identification of actionable mutations in melanoma, which led to phase III studies confirming the efficacy of drugs that would target these mutations.

Vemurafenib and dabrafenib were both studied in advanced BRAF V600E-mutated melanomas. BRIM-3 was a phase III trial evaluating vemurafenib versus dacarbazine (1000 mg/m^2 intravenously every 3 weeks) in the treatment of advanced BRAF V600E-mutated melanoma.[15] Similarly, BREAK-3 was another phase III trial evaluating dabrafenib in advanced BRAF V600E-mutated melanomas versus dacarbazine.[16] Responses for both V600 inhibitor agents were relatively similar. Single-agent BRAF inhibitors resulted in rapid and profound (approximately 50% objective responses) reductions in tumor burden that lasted 6 to 7 months. Adverse events common to both agents included rash, fatigue, and arthralgia. Clinically significant photosensitivity was more common with vemurafenib and clinically significant pyrexia was more common with dabrafenib.[16] Class-specific adverse events included the development of cutaneous squamous-cell carcinomas and keratoacanthomas secondary to paradoxic activation of MAPK pathway signaling. These trials led to regulatory approval of vemurafenib and dabrafenib in 2011 and 2013, respectively, in the treatment of advanced melanomas with BRAF V600E mutations.

Despite profound responses to BRAF inhibitors, however, these responses are short lived and temporary. Mechanisms of acquired resistance are diverse and include reactivation of MAPK pathway–dependent signaling (RAS activation or increased RAF expression), and development of MAPK pathway–independent signaling (COT overexpression; increased PI3K or AKT signaling) that permits bypass of inhibited BRAF signaling within the MAPK pathway.[17,18] These led investigators to look for other mechanisms to overcome this resistance. One way is to combine BRAF inhibition with MEK inhibition.

Three phase 3 studies confirmed the superiority of combination BRAF and MEK inhibition over BRAF inhibition alone. COMBI-d[15,19] dabrafenib/trametinib versus dabrafenib/placebo, COMBI-v[16] dabrafenib/trametinib versus vemurafenib, and coBRIM[20] vemurafenib/cobimetinib versus vemurafenib/placebo. Expectedly, compared with BRAF inhibitor monotherapy, combination BRAF and MEK inhibition produced greater responses and improved progression-free and overall survival along with lower rates of cutaneous squamous-cell carcinomas than combination therapy, reflecting the more profound degree of MAPK pathway inhibition achieved with combination BRAF and MEK inhibition. Based on these results, FDA approval was granted for both dabrafenib/trametinib and vemurafenib/cobimetinib combinations in 2015. Although the dabrafenib/trametinib combination was only approved in 2015, trametinib had independently gained FDA approval in 2013 for the treatment of *BRAF* V600E/ K–mutated melanoma on the basis of the phase 3 METRIC study.

The latest reported trial in advanced BRAF V600–mutant melanoma was COLUMBUS, which is a randomized, open-label phase III trial that compared the addition of encorafenib (BRAF inhibitor) to binimetinib versus encorafenib or vemurafenib monotherapy.[21] The combination of encorafenib and binimetinib resulted in improvement in progression-free survival and a toxicity profile comparable with either monotherapy.

CURRENT CLINICAL TRIALS IN MELANOMA

Melanoma Checkpoint and Gut Microbiome Alteration with Microbiome Intervention is a phase Ib trial sponsored by the Parker Institute for Cancer Research. It focuses on the effect of gut microbiome and activity of checkpoint inhibition in stage 4 melanoma. This study is designed to evaluate the safety and tolerability of treatment with oral microbiome study intervention (SER-401) or matching placebo in combination with anti-programmed cell death 1 (anti-PD-1) therapy (nivolumab) in participants with unresectable or metastatic melanoma. It also intends to assess clinical outcomes, the impact of microbiome study intervention administration on the microbiome profile, and its association with clinical and immunologic outcomes. Before initiating microbiome study intervention and nivolumab, participants will undergo an antibiotic or placebo treatment lead-in to prime the gut microbiome for engraftment of the oral microbiome study intervention. Intervention groups will be assessed for safety, changes in the microbiome, changes in the percentage of tumoral CD8 T cells, and antitumor activity. Participants must have measurable disease that can be biopsied and consent to baseline and on-treatment biopsies, as well as stool and blood biomarker collection throughout the study. This study is still active and participants are still being recruited.[22]

The Prospective Randomized and Phase 2 Trial for Metastatic Melanoma Using Adoptive Cell Therapy with Tumor Infiltrating Lymphocytes Plus IL-2 Either Alone or Following the Administration of Pembrolizumab is currently being conducted at the National Institutes of Health, Bethesda, MD. This trial extracts young tumor infiltrating lymphocytes (TILs) from stage 4 melanoma tumors, grows them in the laboratory and then returns the TIL with high-dose IL-2. First step is a tumor biopsy and leukapheresis, and then hospital admission for a week for conditioning chemotherapy. Pembrolizumab is administered the day after chemotherapy. It also tests the safety and efficacy of pembrolizumab addition to cell therapy. The cells are infused day −4, with up to 12 doses of high-dose IL-2 every 8 hours. Pembrolizumab is repeated every 3 weeks for up to 4 doses and patients are reassessed. Another cycle of 4 doses of pembrolizumab can be repeated. The researchers in this trial hypothesize that the addition of pembrolizumab to cell therapy would make it more effective. The safety of this approach is being addressed as well.[23]

Genetically Modified T-Cells Followed by Aldesleukin in Treating Patients with Stage III-IV Melanoma is being conducted at MD Anderson Cancer Center in Houston. This pilot phase I trial studies the side effects and best dose of genetically modified T cells followed by aldesleukin in treating patients with stage III-IV melanoma. Genes that may help the T-cells recognize melanoma cells are inserted into the T-cells in the laboratory. Adding these genes to the T cells may help them kill more tumor cells when they are put back in the body. Aldesleukin (high-dose IL-2) may enhance this effect by stimulating white blood cells to kill more melanoma cells.[24]

Talimogene Laherparepvec (TVEC) and Pembrolizumab combination in patients with Stage III-IV Melanoma (S1607) is sponsored by the National Cancer Institute (NCI) and Southwest Oncology Group (SWOG). Similar to "Coley's Toxin," first described in the nineteenth century, TVEC is an FDA-approved injectable oncolytic virus, a herpes simplex virus type 1, specifically designed for replication within tumors. It can induce antitumor immune response, both local and distant. TVEC has previously been shown to have an excellent response rate for in-transit metastases in melanoma. In this trial, the primary objective is to evaluate the durable response rate of treatment with Talimogene Laherparepvec (TVEC) in combination with pembrolizumab following progression on prior anti-PD-1 or anti-PD-L1 therapy.[25]

A Study of NKTR-214 Combined with Nivolumab versus Nivolumab Alone in Participants with Previously Untreated Inoperable or Metastatic Melanoma is sponsored by Nektar Therapeutics and Bristol Myers Squibb. Bempegaldesleukin (NKTR-214; Nektar Therapeutics, San Francisco, CA) is an investigational CD122-preferential IL-2 pathway agonist. NKTR-214 is a first-in-class, CD122-preferential IL-2 pathway agonist that provides sustained activation of the IL-2 pathway via IL-2R beta chain–biased signaling, selectively stimulating CD8+ T cells over regulatory T cells (Tregs), which require binding to the IL-2R alpha chain. NKTR-214 has proven safe and effective in increasing CD8+ T cells in the circulation and in tumor tissue in patients with a variety of cancers, including melanoma, renal, lung, bladder, and breast cancers. Interestingly, NKTR-214 significantly decreased T regulatory levels in tumors, but not in the periphery. This phase 3 trial randomizes patients to nivolumab alone or the combination in advanced melanoma. NKTR 214 with nivolumab has a breakthrough designation from the FDA based on 12-month follow-up on the first-line melanoma cohort in the phase 1 PIVOT 02 trial, presented at ASCO 2019.[26] At a median time of follow-up of 12.7 months, confirmed objective response rate (ORR) was 53% (20 of 38) in efficacy-evaluable patients, with 34% (13 of 38) of patients achieving confirmed complete responses. 42% (16 of 38) of patients achieved a maximum reduction of 100% in target lesions. DCR, also known as disease control rate (CR + PR + stable disease [SD]) was 74%.

Eighty percent (16 of 20) of patients had sustained responses. Among the 35 patients with known pretreatment PD-L1 status, ORR in PD-L1–negative patients was 6 (43%) of 14 and in PD-L1–positive patients was 13 (62%) of 21. One of 3 patients with unknown PD-L1 baseline status experienced a CR.

The most common (>30%) treatment-related AEs were grade 1 to 2 fatigue (65.9%), pyrexia (61.0%), rash (56.1%), pruritus (48.8%), nausea (41.5%), influenza like illness (39.0%), arthralgia (36.6%), chills (34.1%), and myalgia (31.7%).

An Exploratory Study of Pembrolizumab Plus Entinostat (HDAC inhibitor) in Non-Inflamed Stage III/IV Melanoma is being conducted at the University of North Carolina Lineberger Cancer Center. The first goal of this study is to understand whether entinostat can make a melanoma tumor more visible to the immune system. Participants will have a mandatory tumor biopsy 3 weeks after starting entinostat therapy. Tumor tissue collected before and after participating in this study will be compared to see if there are more immune cells in the tumor after receiving entinostat. The second goal of the study is to see if giving a combination of entinostat and pembrolizumab can shrink melanoma tumors of patients who did not have immune cells In tumors before treatment. Studies will evaluate response and side effects of the treatment.[27]

CD40 Agonistic Antibody APX005M in Combination with Nivolumab is a phase I trial sponsored by Apexigen and Bristol Myers Squibb. Subjects will receive intravenous APX005M in combination with nivolumab until disease progression or unacceptable toxicity. The cell-surface molecule CD40, a member of the tumor necrosis factor receptor superfamily, broadly regulates immune activation and mediates tumor apoptosis. CD40 is expressed by antigen-presenting cells (APCs). The engagement of its natural ligand on T cells activates APCs, including dendritic cells and B cells. CD40 agnostic antibodies have been shown to substitute for T-cell helpers provided by CD4+ lymphocytes in murine models of T-cell–mediated immunity. In tumor-bearing hosts, CD40 agonists trigger effective immune responses against tumor-associated antigens. In contrast, CD40 is also expressed on many tumor cells and its ligand in this setting mediates a direct cytotoxic effect. Ligand binding of CD40 on tumor cells results in apoptosis in vitro and impaired tumor growth in vivo. These observations have prompted efforts to use agonistic CD40 antibodies for the treatment of cancer patients and initial clinical results have been promising. Encouraging data of antiPD1 with CD40 agonists were presented at the American Association for Cancer Research (AACR) Meeting in April 2019 in advanced melanoma and pancreatic cancer.[28] Phase 1b dose-escalation portion of the clinical trial presented at AACR included patients with metastatic melanoma who had progressed when previously treated with anti-PD-1 therapy. Progression was documented by 2 consecutive tumor assessments at least 4 weeks apart. Patients were treated with 3 dose levels of APX005M (0.03, 0.1, and 0.3 mg/kg) combined with a fixed dose of nivolumab (360 mg) every 3 weeks. In the phase 1b portion of this clinical trial, APX005M was well tolerated and no dose-limiting toxicities were observed. The recommended phase 2 dose (RP2D) for APX005M is 0.3 mg/kg. Of the 5 subjects with metastatic melanoma, 1 had a confirmed PR, 2 had prolonged SD (>8 months), and 2 had progressive disease (PD) as the best overall response. The phase 2 dose-expansion portion of this clinical trial followed a Simon 2-stage design and included 2 parallel cohorts of patients treated with the RP2D of APX005M with nivolumab. In the phase 2 portion of this clinical trial, the first stage of the cohort enrolled10 subjects, in addition to the 2 subjects who carried over from the phase 1 portion. Of these 12 subjects, 2 had confirmed PR, 3 had SD, and 7 had PD as best overall response.

Pembrolizumab in Treating Patients with Stage III-IV High-Risk Melanoma Before and After Surgery (S1801) is an NCI Cooperative group trial sponsored by SWOG.

This randomized phase II trial studies how pembrolizumab works before and after surgery in treating patients with stage III-IV high-risk melanoma. The higher load of tumor neoantigens with a neoadjuvant approach may theoretically lead to a more vigorous immune response. Patients receive pembrolizumab intravenously (IV) over 30 minutes on day 1 every 3 weeks for 3 cycles, then undergo surgery within 3 weeks. Within 84 days, patients receive pembrolizumab IV over 30 minutes every 3 weeks for 15 cycles in the absence of disease progression or unacceptable toxicity. This trial is actively recruiting patients and the estimated study completion date would be in September 2022.[29]

SUMMARY

Since 2011, the treatment of advanced melanoma has seen radical improvements. A condition which would have been considered to be futile in the past decade has promising results with the introduction of immunotherapy and targeted therapies. We might witness a time when advanced melanomas would not be as life limiting as they are now for patients.

DISCLOSURE

Nothing to disclose.

REFERENCES

1. Siegel RL, Miller KD, Jemal A. Cancer statistics, 2016. CA Cancer J Clin 2016; 66:7–30.
2. Guy GP, Thomas CC, Thompson T, et al. Vital signs: melanoma incidence and mortality trends and projections - United States, 1982-2030. MMWR Morb Mortal Wkly Rep 2015;64:591–6.
3. Tarhini AA, Agarwala SS. Interleukin-2 for the treatment of melanoma. Curr Opin Investig Drugs 2005;6(12):1234–9.
4. Wolchok JD, Hodi FS, Weber JS, et al. Development of ipilimumab: a novel immunotherapeutic approach for the treatment of advanced melanoma. Ann N Y Acad Sci 2013;1291:1–13.
5. Hodi FS, O'Day SJ, McDermott DF, et al. Improved survival with ipilimumab in patients with metastatic melanoma. N Engl J Med 2010;363:711–23.
6. Robert C, Thomas L, Bondarenko I, et al. Ipilimumab plus dacarbazine for previously untreated metastatic melanoma. N Engl J Med 2011;364:2517–26.
7. Weber JS, D' Angelo SP, Minor D, et al. Nivolumab versus chemotherapy in patients with advanced melanoma who progressed receptors after anti-CTLA-4 treatment (CheckMate 037): a randomised, controlled, open-label, phase 3 trial. Lancet Oncol 2015;16:375–84.
8. Robert C, Long GV, Brady B, et al. Nivolumab in previously untreated melanoma without BRAF mutation. N Engl J Med 2015;372:320–30.
9. Hamid O, Robert C, Daud A, et al. Safety and tumor responses with lambrolizumab (anti-PD-1) in melanoma. N Engl J Med 2013;369:134–44.
10. Robert C, Schachter J, Long GV, et al. Pembrolizumab versus ipilimumab in advanced melanoma. N Engl J Med 2015;372:2521–32.
11. Larkin J, Chiarion-Sileni V, Gonzalez R, et al. Combined nivolumab and ipilimumab or monotherapy in untreated melanoma. N Engl J Med 2015;373:23–34.

12. Walchok JD, Charion-Sileni V, Gonzalez R, et al. Overall survival with combined nivolumab and ipilimumab in advanced melanoma. N Engl J Med 2017;377: 1345–56.
13. Curtin JA, Fridlyand J, Kageshita T, et al. Distinct sets of genetic alterations in melanoma. N Engl J Med 2005;353:2135–47.
14. Cancer Genome Atlas Network. Genomic classification of cutaneous melanoma. Cell 2015;161:1681–96.
15. Long GV, Stroyakovskiy D, Gogas H, et al. Combined BRAF and MEK inhibition versus BRAF inhibition alone in melanoma. N Engl J Med 2014;371:1877–88.
16. Hauschild A, Grob J-J, Demidov LV, et al. Dabrafenib in BRAF-mutated metastatic melanoma: a multicentre, open-label, phase 3 randomised controlled trial. Lancet 2012;380:358–65.
17. Johannessen CM, Boehm JS, Kim SY, et al. COT drives resistance to RAF inhibition through MAP kinase pathway reactivation. Nature 2010;468:968–72.
18. Van Allen EM, Wagle N, Sucker A, et al. The genetic landscape of clinical resistance to RAF inhibition in metastatic melanoma. Cancer Discov 2014;4:94–109.
19. Robert C, Karaszewska B, Schachter J, et al. Improved overall survival in melanoma with combined dabrafenib and trametinib. N Engl J Med 2015;372:30–9.
20. Larkin J, Ascierto PA, Dréno B, et al. Combined vemurafenib and cobimetinib in BRAF-mutated melanoma. N Engl J Med 2014;371:1867–76.
21. Dummer R, Ascierto PA, Gogas HJ, et al. Encorafenib plus binimetinib versus vemurafenib or encorafenib in patient with BRAF mutant melanoma (COLUMBUS): a multi-center, open label, randomized phase 3 trial. Lancet Oncol 2018;19(5): 603–15.
22. US National Library of Medicine. Melanoma Checkpoint and Gut Microbiome Alteration with Microbiome Intervention (MCGRAW). ClinicalTrials.gov Identifier: NCT03817125.
23. US National Library of Medicine. A Prospective Randomized and Phase 2 Trial for Metastatic Melanoma Using Adoptive Cell Therapy With Tumor Infiltrating Lymphocytes Plus IL-2 Either Alone or Following the Administration of Pembrolizumab. ClinicalTrials.gov indentifier: NCT02621021.
24. US National Library of Medicine. Genetically Modified T-Cells Followed by Aldesleukin in Treating Patients With Stage III-IV Melanoma. ClinicalTrials.gov identifier: NCT01955460.
25. US National Library of Medicine. Talimogene Laherparepved and Pembrolizumab in Treating Patients With Stage III-IV Melanoma. ClinicalTrials.gov identifier: NCT02965716.
26. Siefker-Radtke AO, Fishman MN, Balar AV, et al. NKTR-214 + Nivolumab in first-line advanced/metastatic urothelial carcinoma (mUC): updated results from PIVOT-02. J Clin Oncol 2019;37(7):388.
27. An Exploratory Study of Pembrolizumab Plus Entinostat in Non-Inflamed Stage III/ IV Melanoma. ClinicalTrials.gov identifier: NCT03765229.
28. Abstract CT089: Phase Ib/II of CD40 agonistic antibody APX005M in combination with Nivolumab (nivo) in subjects with metastatic melanoma (M) or non-small cell lung cancer (NSCLC). AACR 2019 publication. DOI:10.1158/1538-7445.AM2019-CT089.
29. US National Library of Medicine. Pembrolizumab in treating patients with stage III-IV high-risk melanoma before and after surgery. ClinicalTrials.gov identifier: NCT03698019.

Printed and bound by CPI Group (UK) Ltd, Croydon, CR0 4YY

08/06/2025

01896870-0004